An Holistic Guide to Massage

An Holistic Guide to Massage

From beginner to advanced level and beyond

Tina Parsons

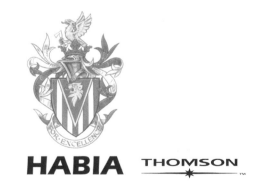

HABIA   THOMSON

Australia • Canada • Mexico • Singapore • Spain • United Kingdom • United States

THOMSON

An Holistic Guide to Massage:
From beginner to advanced level and beyond

Copyright © Tina Parsons 2004

The Thomson logo is a trademark used herein under licence.

For more information, contact Thomson Learning, High Holborn House, 50–51 Bedford Row, London, WC1R 4LR or visit us on the World Wide Web at: http://www.thomsonlearning.co.uk

British Library Cataloguing in Publication Data
A catalogue record for this book is available from the British Library

ISBN 1-86152-919-8

Typeset by 𝐓 Tek-Art, Croydon, Surrey

Printed and bound in Croatia by Zrinski d.d.

Contents

Foreword

This is an impressive book.

Tina Parsons is an impressive person. I don't know how she manages to find the time and energy to write such an amazing book, run her successful business and advise industry on a range of beauty and holistic subjects. Yet she does and with such aplomb.

I could go on about Tina's immense skills and knowledge but really we'll just let the book do the talking.

Alan Goldsbro
Chief Executive Officer
Hair And Beauty Industry Authority

Introduction

From beginner to advanced and beyond

Massage seems on the surface to need no introduction. We all know what it is and we can all do it! However, the realms of massage are very deep and far reaching, finding a base in every culture and every land since the first people roamed the earth many thousands of years ago. As a result, we now find ourselves in a time where the focus of massage is firmly rooted in the many experiences of the past, the growth of the present and the development of the future. All of this amounts to a great deal of theoretical and practical study if one is to call themselves a practitioner of massage!

This book has been written in a quest to make sense of the past by exploring the history of massage, make the most of the present through guided tuition and prepare for the future through experiential learning.

Learning is not about being told but about understanding, and one of the best teaching tools is experience. This book aims to facilitate practical and theoretical understanding of massage through guided experiential learning. It does not replace traditional teaching but attempts to complement it by means of an explorative professional and personal journey.

The book has been divided into five parts:

1   Massage overview
2   Massage skills
3   Massage preparation
4   Massage treatment
5   Massage progression.

Each part has been subdivided into chapters for ease of study and to provide further detailed information. Within the text, words in bold and italics alert the reader to important points or terms which are then explained. They are included in the glossary where appropriate.

In addition, there is the inclusion of easy to follow guides in the form of **system sorter, treatment tracker, holistic harmony** and **suggested order of work**.

- **System sorter** is a quick and easy guide to the way in which the systems of the body depend on one another for their well-being. The links between the individual systems are highlighted, encouraging a more holistic viewpoint.

- **Treatment tracker** includes a quick and easy guide to the way in which massage can be adapted to treat the different parts of the body as well as progressed to form additional treatments including mechanical, advanced, sports, remedial, Indian head, aromatherapy and reflexology massage.
- **Holistic harmony** includes information about the needs of the body in relation to massage and is subdivided into ten different categories including **pre-treatment procedures, additions, post-treatment procedures, self-help, nutrition, ageing, rest, exercise, awareness** and **special care**.
- **Suggested order of work** provides a step-by-step guide to massage of the back, hands and arms, buttocks, legs and feet, abdomen and upper body.

Fascinating facts are included throughout the text, highlighting special areas of interest.

Tip and **remember** boxes help you to recall and understand the main points concerned with system and treatment linking.

Angel advice aims to provide a source of inspiration with a thought or a deed that continues the concept of effective teaching and learning by building awareness, seeking development and initiating change.

Theory **tasks** and practical **activities** accompany each chapter helping to reinforce learning through research and experience.

Knowledge review provides the opportunity to test your knowledge with a set of short answer questions at the end of each chapter.

Website

There is an interactive website for students and lecturers to use and it provides answers to the **Knowledge review** questions.

Acknowledgements

I have once again appreciated the opportunity that Thomson Learning have given me to write this book, and would like to dedicate it to the Burghley Academy – may it remain the source of knowledge and inspiration for many years to come.

Tina Parsons
2003

Part 1
Massage overview

1 The art and science of massage

2 The historical origins of massage

3 The development of massage

4 The marketplace for massage

Learning objectives

After reading this part you should be able to:

- Recognise the differences between the art and science of massage.

- Identify the important factors relating to the history of massage.

- Understand the historical links between the Eastern and Western cultures associated with the development of massage.

- Be aware of the ways in which massage can be integrated into a variety of complementary therapies.

- Appreciate the flexibility in the use of massage as a treatment for stress and stress-related problems.

The word **massage** conjures up a myriad of images, impressions, thoughts and feelings depending on our own individual experiences of and attitudes to life. The chapters included in Part one aim to address the questions as well as dispel the myths that relate to the practice of massage as both an intuitive and personal skill and an acquired and professional treatment including:

- What is massage?
- Where does massage originate from?
- How is massage performed?
- Who is massage for?

The art and science of massage

What is massage?

Massage is a primary form of communication. It incorporates the sense of *touch*, the most powerful of all our senses and a natural means of survival. Of all the special senses including those of sight, smell, hearing and taste, the sense of touch provides us with the most immediate and effective external and internal communication system.

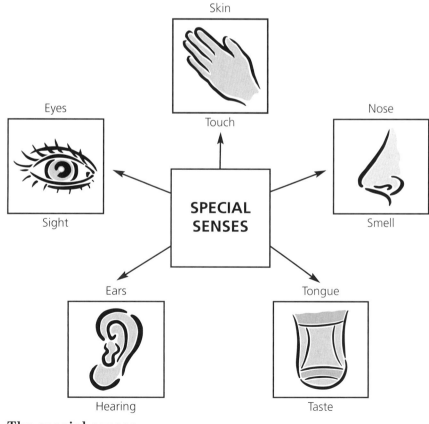

The special senses

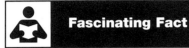

Fascinating Fact

Research has shown that humans and indeed animals that are deprived of touch experience stunted physical and emotional development.

Tip

The French words **masseur** (male) and **masseuse** (female) refer to practitioners of massage. They are commonly used words that cross the boundaries of many languages.

Touch links us with the world around us and touch also forms the connection between the body and mind.

Touch is vital to the survival of all living things:

- Touch ensures that procreation continues as a sperm meets an egg.
- Touch links us with our mothers during foetal development, continuing long after birth.
- Touch links us with the people around us enabling us to communicate both physical and emotional feelings.
- Touch enables us to develop an awareness of our surroundings.
- Touch activates physical and emotional responses.

Massage describes the many adaptations of touch that occur naturally e.g. we instinctively adjust our use of touch to stroke a crying baby, to knead an aching back, to rub our hands together to keep warm etc.

To fully appreciate the meaning of massage we can start by analysing the origins of the word, which is a derivative of the Latin *massa,* meaning 'lump' or body of matter, and *aticum,* a suffix that was added to expressive nouns and which means an act, process or function. Similarities appear in the Arabic and Greek languages with *mass* (Arabic) meaning to 'touch or feel' and *massein* (Greek) meaning to 'knead'.

The literal interpretation of the word massage can therefore be described as 'the process of touching (feeling and kneading) a body of matter'.

The French and German words for massage also share similarities in their origin:

- *Masser* (French)
- *Massieren* (German)

Massage is both an art and a science. It is an intuitive skill that forms an inherent part of each and every person and the art of massage is firmly rooted in the sense of touch. Touch offers us a way of conveying feelings and can be adapted to meet varying needs and situations, e.g. we may use touch to convey differing levels of care, both for ourselves and for others. It is not something that we always need to consciously think about – in fact it is more usually something that we just do; both intuitively and instinctively in response to a 'gut feeling'. As such, touch is the most primitive form of communication and one of the special senses that is least likely to deteriorate with age, although we can sometimes 'lose touch' or even become 'out of touch'. Touch makes us feel wanted, loved and cared for. It soothes and calms but can also stimulate and excite. Touch boosts our self-esteem and levels of self-confidence and contributes to our general feelings of well-being. In fact touch has the ability to activate every emotion imaginable and the skills associated with the giving and receiving of massage at this level are inborn. They form part of the basic

Tip

Tactile refers to the sense of touch.

Fascinating Fact

Like humans, animals use the art of touch to soothe and stimulate, as with the licking of a wound, scratching of an itch etc.

needs of a human being – that of giving and receiving love through tactile methods.

Tactile awareness is also something we are born with and continue to make use of throughout life. Intuition and experience help us develop greater tactile awareness as we learn to pick up on the various responses activated by touch both in ourselves and other people.

Massage as an art is one of the easiest skills known to man and indeed woman! It requires less practice than many other tasks we perform on a daily basis throughout our lives, as we do not seem to have to learn how to respond through touch. It is therefore an instinctive action born out of our need to survive. The different manipulations seem to come from within, forming a method of massage that is as unique and individual as our own handwriting. It is a creative skill that is enhanced through practice and experience and is controlled through the mental activity in the right hemisphere of the brain, which is associated with all aspects of creative and intuitive thinking including the natural talent we may have for any of the arts.

In the modern world, different cultures view this skill with varying degrees of confidence. This is clearly demonstrated in the way in which we communicate with other people through the sense of touch. It is a fact that a lack of personal contact results in loss of self-esteem and as such people often turn to the petting of animals in order to fulfil such needs. Research has found that those cultures who advocate more personal contact in the form of kissing as a means of greeting etc. rely less heavily on their pets as a source of comfort.

Task

Think about the many different ways we use the art of massage in our everyday lives. Make a list of at least TEN occasions when you have used touch to communicate a feeling either for yourself or for someone else, e.g. pressed your forehead in a moment of frustration or confusion or stroked a loved one to convey comfort in times of distress etc.

The study of touch has led to the development of the *science of massage,* and of certain learned skills that make up a professional treatment. The study of anatomy and physiology (structure and function) of the body as a whole provides the knowledge that underpins the treatment, forming a sound basis on which to offer massage as a professional treatment. The quality of the massage treatment then depends to a large extent on the knowledge of the physical, emotional and even spiritual condition of the person receiving the treatment.

The science of massage is therefore associated with learned skills that act as an aid to enhance the giving and receiving of massage as a professional treatment. The activity of learning by instruction requires us to make use of the left hemisphere of the brain, which controls logical and analytical thought.

Task

Have a treatment with a qualified massage practitioner and analyse the effects and benefits of the use of touch in a more structured and knowledgeable way. Make a list of the differences between applying massage to yourself and experiencing a professional massage treatment.

So what is massage?

Tip

Holistic comes from *holism* which refers to nature as a unity, made up of a whole which equals more than the just the sum of its parts.

The answer is that massage is the integration of art and science providing a means of treating the body and mind of the receiver with the body and mind of the giver. For this reason it is also classified as being an **holistic** treatment, meaning that the effects of the massage affect the *whole*.

The best massage practitioner must therefore be one who is able to use their body and hands naturally and creatively whilst concentrating on their knowledge of the person they are treating and the needs of the area on which they are working.

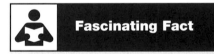

Fascinating Fact

Using your hands for massage is an instinctive, intuitive skill or *art* requiring right brain activity. The different reasons for using your hands for massage is a learned skill or *science* requiring left brain activity.

Task

Think about the ways in which the art and science of massage benefit the person giving a massage treatment as well as the person receiving the treatment.

Knowledge review

1 List the five special senses

2 From which language does the word massage originate?

3 What are the French words given to a male and female massage practitioner?

4 What does the word tactile refer to?

5 The art of massage is associated with activity from which side of the brain?

6 What can touch do to levels of self-esteem and confidence?

7 Which side of the brain is responsible for the logic associated with the science of massage?

8 Is the art of massage associated with an intuitive skill or a learned skill?

9 Is the science of massage associated with an intuitive skill or a learned skill?

10 What does holistic refer to?

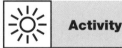

Activity

Link the art and science of massage by applying some structured self-massage. Gently rub some cream into your hands, nails and cuticles every morning and evening for a week. Use your thumbs in a circular motion to apply more pressure to specific areas. Notice how the skin responds as the texture, tone and colour improves and the circulation is stimulated. Feel how the tension eases out of the muscles and you gain greater ease of movement in the many of the individual joints. You may even find yourself taking a deep breath in and out as you start to relax into the massage. Notice how the whole of your body feels as a result of the hand massage. You may be aware of the fact that you need to visit the loo, are thirsty or even start to feel sleepy. Think about these effects and benefits but also learn to 'go with the flow' and just enjoy the experience.

The historical origins of massage

2

Where does massage originate from?

The inborn instinctive skill that is the art of massage has to be as old as humanity itself. The human race has evolved by means of reproduction and development due in part to the sensual and loving skills associated with the art of touch, and as we have already discovered, touch is the prerequisite of massage. The earliest traces of primary source evidence have been uncovered in wall drawings and cave paintings showing the giving and receiving of massage as both a sensual and caring activity.

The science or knowledge and experience of massage spans the centuries, regions and peoples of the world, yet there is no one time in history or culture that is able to claim the ownership of this inherent skill.

Instead we are able track the study of massage from as early as 3000BC to today with both written evidence and inherited practical skills that have been passed from generation to generation, each identifying the origins of massage as a means to improve health and well-being.

One of the oldest known books with reference to massage comes from China and is called the *Con Fou of the Tao-Tse* (pronounced

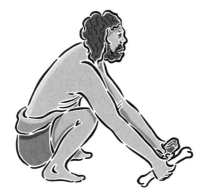

Caveperson

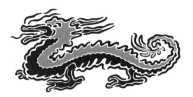

Chinese dragon

Cun Fooh of Dow Zee). It contains lists of medicinal plants, exercises and a system of massage techniques incorporating pressure points located on the body. These techniques form the basis of the modern day practices of **acupressure** and **acupuncture**, which contribute to the effectiveness of the system of health and healing known as traditional Chinese medicine.

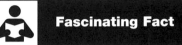

Over the centuries and various Dynasties there is evidence that the massage techniques were known as *moshou* (hand rubbing), *anmo* (press-rub), and *tuina* (push-hold).

The techniques spread from China to Japan through the teachings of Buddhism. Whilst studying in China, Japanese monks witnessed the healing methods associated with traditional Chinese medicine and both adopted and adapted the massage techniques introducing new combinations of pressure points.

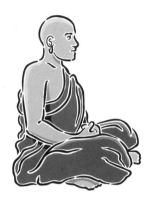

Buddhist monk

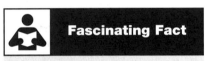

Shiatsu is a word derived from 'shi' meaning finger and 'atsu' meaning pressure.

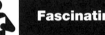

There is evidence that the Chinese *anmo* massage therapy was combined with the Korean method called *amma* by the Japanese, thus forming their own system which they also referred to as *amma*.

The Japanese went on to develop **Shiatsu**, concentrating the application of pressure on specific points or **tsubo**. This means of massage is often referred to as acupuncture without needles. Variations of this original form of massage are still very much in evidence today.

Another important historical source is the Hindu book *AyurVeda* which contains ancient medical text. Written somewhere between 1700–1800BC it describes the use of massage together with exercise as part of the daily cleansing ritual and for the treatment of various conditions.

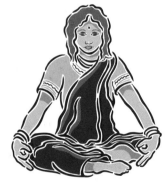

Indian

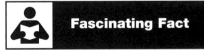

Ayurveda is a Sanskrit (ancient language of Hindu) term and is a combination of two words: 'ayu' meaning life and 'veda' meaning knowledge. It embodies a way of life that is still in existence today with many people from the East and West following its aims for a happy, healthy and inspired life.

The use of sensual massage is recorded in the *Karma Sutra* and Tantric massage to aid sexual performance and pleasure was also commonly practised together with breathing techniques and yoga.

Native Americans also passed down the practical skills associated with massage from generation to generation. The Cherokee, Penias and Navaho were amongst the many tribes who made use of massage for therapeutic purposes e.g. in the preparation of warriors venturing into war, for childbirth and the care of infants. Most often performed by healers of varying kinds, massage was also combined with the use of crushed plants, infusions of roots and warm stones to aid the effects and benefits.

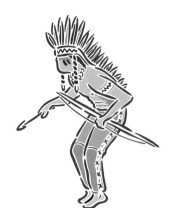

Native American

The South Pacific islanders made use of massage in and out of water. *Lomilomi* is an ancient Hawaiian massage that was used specifically for healing and is still in existence today.

In the Philippines traditional therapeutic massage, or 'hilot' as it was known, incorporated the use of a variety of techniques including those similar to Chinese acupressure.

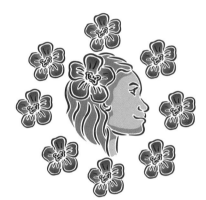

Hawaiian

 Fascinating Fact

The term 'hilot' was also used to describe a person who as part of the native healing art attended births, used techniques to set bones and applied 'fire pressure' and water massage.

The people of ancient Egypt made use of massage for cosmetic purposes as well as for therapeutic effects. Much has been written about Cleopatra bathing in milk and being massaged by handmaidens with mixtures of fats, oils, herbs and resins to maintain and enhance her beauty.

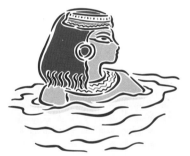

Egyptian

Over the centuries, the theory and practice of massage evolved in Europe where an holistic approach to health and well-being was also being developed.

The Greeks placed great emphasis on physical fitness in the pursuit of health and well-being. They developed many rituals that involved bathing, exercise, massage and dance for both men and women. Massage was used extensively for the preparation of gladiators and soldiers as well as post-activity to aid recovery. In addition, massage with oils and herbs was used by physicians to treat diseases and disorders.

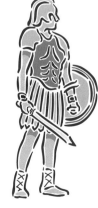

Gladiator

 Fascinating Fact

One physician of ancient Greek times was Herodicus. He advocated the use of olive oil as a muscular massage for the athletes who competed in the original Olympic Games!

Fascinating Fact

The term *anatripsis* means friction.

Fascinating Fact

Doctors today take the Hippocratic Oath which upholds the virtues instilled by Hippocrates all those years ago!

Fascinating Fact

Much has been written in history of the Roman emperor Julius Caesar. He too enjoyed the benefits of massage. It has been well documented that he experienced daily 'pinching' to ease his neuralgia (stabbing pains along a nerve/nerves)!

Fascinating Fact

Modern day spas are reminiscent of these types of baths and are often decorated in styles that date back to these times.

Hippocrates, who was alive from 460–359BC, was a pupil of the physician Herodicus. He continued the study and practice of medicinal massage which included friction and rubbing or shampooing type movements which were termed 'anatripsis'. He also noted that greater benefit could be obtained from applying massage to the body in an upward direction and that hard rubbing was 'binding', moderate rubbing caused parts to 'grow' and much rubbing caused parts to 'waste'.

Hippocrates is often referred to as the father of medicine because much of medicine was founded on his work. Evidence of this is seen in the works of the Greek physician and philosopher Galen who was alive between AD129–210.

Galen's work continued to advocate the use of massage for health and well-being. In his teens he became a *therapeutes* or attendant of the healing god Asclepius who is credited with being the founder of the world's first gymnasium. Galen went on to work with the Roman emperor Marcus Aurelius and his son who extolled the virtues of therapeutic massage.

The Romans were also famed for their development of gymnasiums incorporating hot and cold water baths, steam rooms, massage and exercise areas which they used for both health and social relaxation. Private and public baths were built and this trend continued in the countries conquered by the Romans. Examples of Roman baths can still be found today e.g. the Roman Aqua Sulis in the British city of Bath.

Although massage continued to develop in places such as China, Japan and India with acupressure, shiatsu and ayurveda, the practice of massage in Western parts started to diminish with the decline of the Roman Empire in AD500 until the Renaissance. For nearly a thousand years during the Dark and Middle Ages, the Christian era focused on the salvation of the soul. They were times of strict religious practices, with little value placed on the therapies associated with gymnasiums and baths which were thought to contribute to the abuse of sex. Anything that was seen as glorifying the human body was renounced and such practices were banned. During these times massage was associated with Satan's power and anyone who practiced such 'magic' came under great pressure from the establishment often resulting in death.

After the fall of Constantinople in 1453, the Roman baths were adopted by the Muslim Ottoman conquerors. The Islam baths or *Hamaam* as they became, once again incorporated areas for massage, relaxation and refreshment together with areas for bathing as ritual bathing and cleanliness also formed an intrinsic part of the Islamic cultures.

Just as the Roman baths followed the Roman legions, so the Islam baths followed the Ottoman and examples can still be found in Syria, Granada and Moorish Spain.

The Renaissance period was seen as a time of rebirth and a resurgence in the practice of medicinal and therapeutic massage followed.

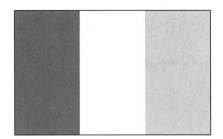

French flag

The French barber-surgeon Ambrose Pare who lived from 1517–1590 once again established the use of massage for medical purposes.

Pare went on to become the personal physician to four of France's royals and was reputed to have restored to health Mary Queen of Scots by 'the use of massage alone'. He used massage to aid the healing process and raised awareness in the value of massage categorising it into gentle, medium and vigorous. This concept was carried through medical circles of the time and further developments continued throughout the years that followed both in the West with the development of medicine and in the East with the development of traditional Chinese medicine, Ayurvedic medicine etc.

The massage we recognise today started to emerge in the eighteenth century. Often referred to as *Swedish massage*, the massage of today comes in the main from the work of Per Henrik Ling (1776–1839). Ling was a physiologist and fencing master who had completed some of his study in China. As a result he developed the Ling System of passive and active exercises, which was known as 'The Swedish Movement Cure'. It incorporated remedial exercises and massage techniques including movements he termed as 'effleurage' or stroking, 'petrissage' or pressing and 'tapotement' or striking. In 1813 the Swedish government established the Royal Swedish Central Institute of Gymnastics of which Ling was president.

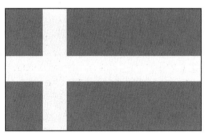

Swedish flag

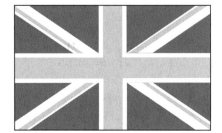

Union Jack – the British flag

Advances in the practice of massage were also being made in England. An English physician, Dr Mathias Roth, studied directly with Per Ling, bringing his 'cure' over to Britain. Dr Roth felt that massage worked on the principles associated with the law of similars – 'like cures like'. Shortly before this, the anatomical surgeon John Grosvenor (1742–1823) was amongst the first surgeons to apply massage to stiff joints and injured limbs.

Fascinating Fact

Homeopathy is based on the principles associated with the law of similars. Remedies are given in minute doses that can produce in the patient the symptoms of the disease to be cured.
Allopathy is the opposite principal on which most of Western medicine is based incorporating remedies that have an opposite effect upon the body to that caused by the disease.

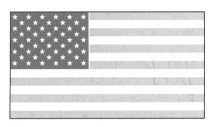

American flag

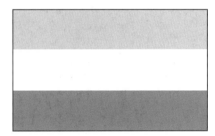

Dutch flag

Two brothers, Dr George H. Taylor and Dr Charles F. Taylor, introduced Swedish massage techniques to America in 1856. Dr Charles Taylor studied with Dr Roth in England and Dr George Taylor travelled to Sweden to further his studies. As a result they set up a practice in New York and went on to invent a mechanical massage device in 1864.

Further developments have also been recorded through the work of a Dutch physician, Dr Johann Mezgner (1839–1909). Dr Mezgner developed massage through his knowledge of anatomy and physiology, linking the effects and benefits for rehabilitation and the treatment of many diseases and disorders. He went on to develop further the techniques associated with effleurage, petrissage, tapotement, vibrations and friction which still make up the core of all massage treatments taught today.

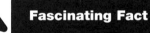

Fascinating Fact

It is unclear why French terms were commonly used to describe the forms of massage although it is thought to be due to the fact that French was the primary language associated with international scientific practices of the time.

Tip

In 1943 the Chartered Society of Massage and Medical Gymnastics was changed to the Chartered Society of Physiotherapy and in 1964 its members became state registered.

The medical professions in these countries began to encourage nurses to train as masseuses under the guidance of doctors and although massage had clear associations with the medical profession, it also began to become synonymous, due in part to poor training, with prostitution and the emergence of massage parlours. As a result, a small group of women in Britain founded the 'Society of Trained Masseuse' in 1894 in an attempt to raise the standards of massage and to establish it as a reputable profession with a strict code of practice.

The First World War saw the demand for medicinal massage increase with techniques being adapted for the treatment of mind and body e.g. shell shock, nerve damage etc. The Society of Trained Masseuse was awarded a Royal Charter in recognition of their contribution to the war effort and became the Chartered Society of Massage and Medical Gymnastics.

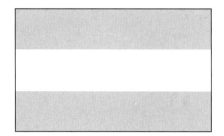

Austrian flag

Also around this time, the practice of massage was being explored within the science of psychoanalysis. Sigmund Freud (1856–1939) used massage to calm and reassure his patients before going on to develop psychoanalytic techniques. This was further developed by one of Freud's original students, an Austrian physician Wilhelm Reich, who began exploring the muscular state of his patients, concluding that 'muscular tension blocked the expression of self'. The resulting theory that emerged demonstrated that the application of massage could help to 'unblock' psychological tension in much the same way as it could unblock physical tension.

 Fascinating Fact

Reich's theories were shared by many of the Eastern cultures that had long believed that 'blocked energy' in the form of physical and psychological tension was associated with illness.

At this time, research was also being undertaken by physicians in the practice of reflexology and aromatherapy. Growing knowledge of the nervous system and its role in pain relief confirmed the effects of manual pressure and zone therapy, which gradually developed into the reflexology of today, was introduced. The use of essential oils in the perfumery industry was found to have an effect on physical and psychological aspects of the body. As a result essential oils were introduced as an effective massage medium, developing into the aromatherapy treatment we see today. However, despite this research and development massage therapy began to change in the years that followed. Whilst the Eastern countries maintained their beliefs and continued to develop their ancient systems of health and healing, Western medicine made many of its advances through scientific development and technology. The introduction of electrotherapy and drugs started to replace manual massage as a treatment for diseases and disorders. Manual massage began to be viewed as a means to merely pamper rather than heal or cure. Massage ceased to be a part of the medical training and struggled to maintain credibility as a recognised therapy.

It was not until the 1960s that massage began to regain its place as a therapeutic skill that contributed to a person's health and well-being. Awarding bodies such as City and Guilds and the International Health and Beauty Council set up courses in massage as part of Beauty Therapy training in Britain, helping to re-establish public awareness. World travel began to change public opinion as alternatives to the medical advances of the West were found in the Eastern approaches to medicine and healing. Disillusionment with some of the more impersonal medical practices associated with the taking of drugs to mask symptoms rather than heal an illness forced many people to seek such alternatives. In addition, the hippy culture of the sixties and seventies and the spread of 'flower power' encouraged people to 'get back in touch' with themselves as many people went in search of the meaning of life through massage and alternative methods of healing.

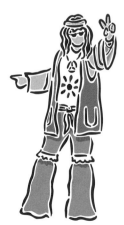

Hippy

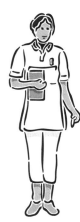

Beauty therapist

However, medical acceptance of the re-emergence of therapeutic massage was poor, with many doctors refusing to acknowledge the very real contribution that massage could make to a person's health and well-being. The earlier removal of massage from a medic's training meant that the doctors of the mid twentieth century had little or no knowledge of the effects and benefits of massage and believed that it had no rightful place within medicine. This view is still held by some, although the contributions made by the health and beauty industry since the 1960s have gone a long way to change both medical and public perception and opinion. Beauty therapists have continued to develop massage, integrating a more holistic approach as public awareness and demand has increased.

So where does massage originate from?

What has developed from the latter part of the twentieth century and is being taken forward into the twenty-first century is an amalgamation of Eastern arts and Western science. Massage has gone full circle, emerging as a treatment that is once again accepted as being *complementary* to medical practices. It is now a balanced therapy that embodies both ancient and modern day thinking, incorporating both art and science.

Tip

Alternative refers to treatment that is used *instead* of traditional Western medicine, whilst **complementary** refers to those treatments that are used to *enhance* medicinal practices. Massage is seen as being complementary.

Knowledge review

1　Where were the earliest traces of primary sources of evidence depicting the giving and receiving of massage found?

2　In which country was found the oldest reference to massage in the written form?

3　Which religious practice contributed to the spread of massage?

4　From which country did shiatsu originate?

5　What is the name of the ancient Hindu medical text that explained the use of massage in India?·

6　What was the Greek physician Herodicus reputed to have done to the competitors of the original Olympic games?

7　Which Greek physician is said to have developed a form of medicinal massage he named *anatripsis*?

8　What can we find in Britain today that provides evidence of the Romans' ritual bathing habits?

9　Who founded the original Swedish massage?

10　Which British surgeon used massage for the treatment of stiff joints and injured limbs in the late nineteenth and early twentieth centuries?

11　Give an example of what massage was used for during the First World War.

12　What was the Chartered Society of Physiotherapists originally known as?

13　Which other area of science explored the use of massage for the care of its patients?

14　What replaced massage in the advancement of medical practices in the early twentieth century?

15　Nowadays is massage seen as being an alternative or a complement to medicine?

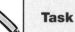

Task

Make yourself a 'time line' depicting the origins of massage through the ages. Start at 3000BC and end with the present day. Make use of the Internet for further information, adding to your time line as you discover additional references to massage through the ages. There appear to be many discrepancies in the more ancient history, but notice how the evidence gets clearer the nearer you get to the present day.

3

The development of massage

How is massage performed?

In some respects there is no answer to this question. The *art* of massage, being an intuitive, instinctive skill, needs no explanation – it just happens. No one teaches us to do it although we can learn from experience how to do it better and to greater effect. However, as a direct result of the study of the *science* of massage, various forms and structures of massage have developed i.e. methods of working that follow specific rules and guidelines.

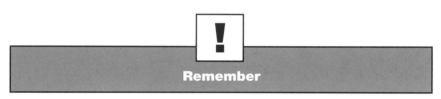

!

Remember

The *art* of massage is an intuitive skill and the *science* of massage a learned skill.

Hence massage has been used as a stand-alone treatment or in combination with other forms of treatment.

History shows us that massage was used to complement many forms of medical practices throughout the ages as well as providing a means of pleasure, relaxation, social interaction and beautification. This evidence leads us to believe that a person's physical and emotional well-being was seen as being contributory to their state of health. This view continued to be developed within Eastern cultures that used forms of traditional medicine and is still in practice today.

However, the removal of massage from the medical practices of the West in the early/mid twentieth century led to the development of two separate paths in the quest for health and well-being. As a direct result of this, massage became associated with the development of the hair and beauty industry. As such, it was used extensively in the treatment of the hair and scalp and as an accompaniment to most forms of beauty treatments including manicure, pedicure and facials. Even treatments such as wax depilation and electrical body and facial treatments incorporate an element of manual massage with the application of products.

History started to repeat itself in the West as research and development found that exercise and massage worked hand in hand. Reminiscent of the ancient Greeks and Romans, massage was once again being used both pre- and post-exercise through the introduction of public gyms, e.g. the YMCA reintroduced exercise and massage as a leisure activity in much the same way as it was used thousands of years ago.

Disillusionment in modern Western medical practices saw the introduction of alternative therapies from all over the world as well as the re-emergence of ancient massage practices.

Massage treatments began to make a re-entry into medical practices, albeit in a small way, with the referral of patients by doctors to massage therapies included within treatments such as physiotherapy, chiropractic and osteopathy etc. for the treatment of unexplained back pain.

In more recent years the development of massage has had much to do with the research being conducted into the effect of touch on human development – both physical and psychological. Medical institutes of the Western world currently undertake many forms of detailed research including:

- The application of simple massage techniques by parents to discover if it can assist in the care of brain injured children at home.
- The application of head massage to discover the effects on concentration levels in children suffering with attention deficit disorders.
- The application of massage as a means to discover the psychological effects in people suffering with post-traumatic stress syndrome.
- The application of massage in the treatment of depression to discover the effects on self-confidence and levels of self-esteem.

Research continues to develop in areas of terminal illness, for example the application of body massage as a complementary treatment of cancers and HIV, to discover its effects on boosting the immune functions of the body, as well as in many of the physical and psychological diseases and disorders that are associated with stress and affect an increasing amount of people in the world today. In addition, it has long been recognised within the hair and beauty industry that massage is one of the best forms of anti-ageing treatment.

As the demand for greater access to massage therapies has grown over recent years, so has the demand for training. Government initiatives and the introduction of the standardisation of qualifications e.g. National Vocational Qualifications (NVQs) have provided greater access to massage and massage-related training. Awarding bodies have formalised various approaches to massage incorporating separate qualifications for specific massage treatments e.g. Swedish massage, aromatherapy, Indian head massage, reflexology, sports massage etc. In addition, individual massage specialists have undertaken their own research and through personal experience have adopted and adapted ancient techniques and/or developed their own new methods of massage. These developments have almost taken us full circle: today there is an increased awareness of the benefits of combining medical practices with the application of therapeutic massage for the health and well-being of the whole person – body, mind and spirit.

Examples of the many styles of massage are highlighted in the A–Z of massage therapies that follows.

An A–Z of massage therapies

- ACUPRESSURE – probably the oldest recorded form of massage, developed in China and involves the use of pressure on points throughout the body to stimulate the flow of energy through the energy channels and/or meridians. Similar to Japanese shiatsu which developed later although pressure is generally applied with the thumbs or fingers only.

- AMATSU – a massage treatment taking its origins from the Japanese traditional healing systems incorporating manual physical testing and manipulations to restore balance and health.

- AROMATHERAPY – combines ancient and modern massage techniques together with essential oils from plants, fruits, flowers, bark, roots or resin to bring about physiological and psychological well-being. Essential oils are added to a base/carrier oil to create a unique blend suited to each person's individual needs.

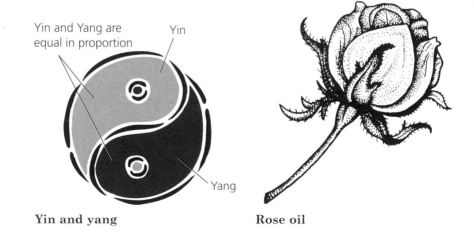

Yin and Yang are equal in proportion

Yin

Yang

Yin and yang   **Rose oil**

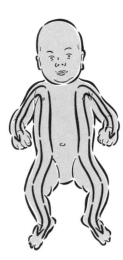

Baby massage

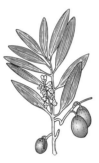

Bach flower remedy – olive

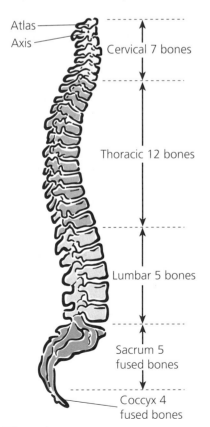

The spine

Atlas
Axis
Cervical 7 bones
Thoracic 12 bones
Lumbar 5 bones
Sacrum 5 fused bones
Coccyx 4 fused bones

- AYURVEDIC MASSAGE – traditional Indian techniques for balancing the body and mind. Ayurveda is a Sanskrit term that can be translated as 'knowledge of life' and Ayurvedic massage is seen as being an essential part of this paradigm.

- BABY/INFANT MASSAGE – the intuitive use of touch combined with the adaptation of massage techniques to soothe and nurture a child through the stresses of infancy. Can be used by those involved in professional childcare as well as by parents.

- BACH FLOWER MASSAGE – manipulation of the skin with a combination of massage movements and the thirty-eight different Bach Flower essences to aid inner conditions associated with psychic imbalance e.g. fear, anxiety, obsessions etc.

- BIODYNAMIC MASSAGE – concerned with the integration of mind and body, biodynamic massage involves a broad range of manual techniques that work on both physical and psychological levels, helping to dissolve the blockages of accumulated tension and bringing the body back into balance to improve health and well-being.

- BOWEN TECHNIQUE – a non-invasive hands-on therapy that incorporates gentle rolling movements over the skin and underlying muscles to relieve built up stress and tension followed by a period of rest between moves allowing the body to reset itself in an attempt to bring about an increased sense of physical well-being.

- CHAVUTTI THIRUMAL MASSAGE – born of the ancient Indian fighting system known as Kalarippayattu – a part of Ayurvedic medicine. Chavutti thirumal means 'massage by foot pressure' and is applied using one foot at a time whilst holding onto a support rope which runs at head level across the treatment room.

- CHIROPRACTIC – from the Greek words *chier* meaning 'hand' and *praktikos* meaning 'done by', chiropractic is a manual therapy incorporating examination and manipulative techniques that work on the skeletal/muscular systems by focusing on the spine and its effects on the nervous system. This therapy aims to improve bone structural problems resulting from injury and wear and tear as well as improve body functions through the links associated with body structure and function.

- DAOYIN TAO – Chinese face, neck and shoulder massage. A combination of ancient Chinese and modern Western massage techniques.

- DEEP LYMPHATIC THERAPY – deep tissue massage performed systematically on each part of the body followed by the use of heat e.g. steam, helping to liquefy and drain excessive fluid reducing oedema (swelling) and aiding lymphatic drainage and flow.

- DEEP TISSUE MASSAGE – a means of working manually with the layers of the body (skin, fat, muscles) to relax, lengthen and release using the knuckles, fists, forearms and/or elbows to penetrate deeply into the tissue.

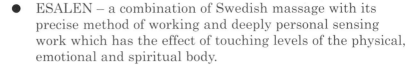

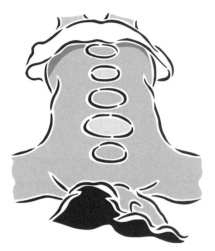

Hot and cold stones

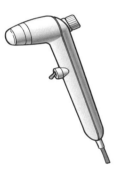

Mechanical massage – audio sonic vibrator

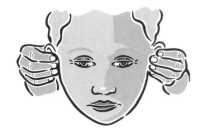

Ear massage

- ESALEN – a combination of Swedish massage with its precise method of working and deeply personal sensing work which has the effect of touching levels of the physical, emotional and spiritual body.

- HELLERWORK – developed by Joseph Heller in the 1970s, Hellerwork is a combination of movement education and/or re-education to realign the body and deep tissue massage to release the rigid physical, mental and emotional patterns that contribute to misalignment. Hellerwork is a derivative of ROLFING.

- HYDROTHERAPY – incorporating the use of water and massage and sometimes referred to as 'water healing'. Pressurised water can be used to apply a water massage and/or manual massage can be applied in water. Often used for rehabilitation after injury due to the supportive nature of water.

- INDIAN HEAD MASSAGE – traditionally practised by the people of India and passed from mother to daughter and from father to son through the generations. It involves the manual application of massage movements to relieve the physical, psychological and spiritual effects of stress bringing about a sense of inner peace and tranquillity.

- LASTONE THERAPY – developed in the early 1990s by a massage therapist, it involves the use of water-heated volcanic black basalt stones and cold white marble stones. Used over the body in various combinations to stimulate circulation, reduce inflammation and/or swelling as well as relieve muscular problems and pain.

- LOMILOMI – an ancient healing art practised by Hawaiians incorporating massage performed with fingers, palms of the hand and/or elbows using a lubricant e.g. kukui nut, macadamia nut and coconut oils. May also include a style of treatment known as 'walking the body' or 'A'e' in which the practitioner walks on the person receiving the massage.

- MANUAL LYMPHATIC DRAINAGE (MLD) – light, rhythmical massage movements following the lymphatic vessels of the body in an attempt to aid drainage of toxins from the system.

- MASSAGE AS PART OF A BEAUTY TREATMENT – variations of traditional Swedish massage are applied as part of a beauty treatment i.e. massage movements are used for the application of cleansers during facials, wax depilation and epilation. A more comprehensive massage accompanies the application of nourishing products such as hand creams in manicures, foot lotions in pedicure and moisturisers in facials.

- MASSAGE AS PART OF AN HOLISTIC TREATMENT – variations of Eastern and Western massage are applied as part of an holistic treatment i.e. ear and/or face massage following Thermal Auricular therapy, massage for stress management etc.

- MECHANICAL MASSAGE – the use of electrotherapy to imitate the effects of manual massage e.g. gyratory and vibratory, vacuum suction, audio sonic.

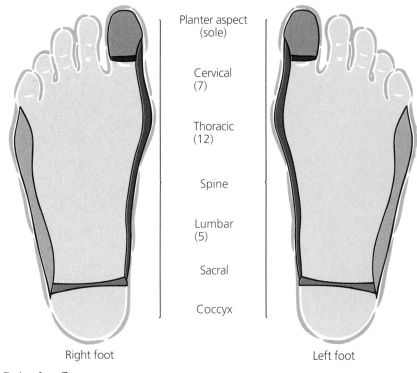

| | Planter aspect (sole) |
| Cervical (7) |
| Thoracic (12) |
| Spine |
| Lumbar (5) |
| Sacral |
| Coccyx |

Right foot   Left foot

Spinal reflexes

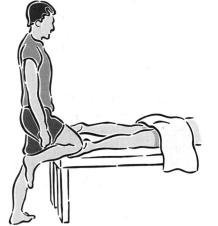

No hands massage

- METAMORPHIC TECHNIQUE – a form of manipulation therapy, similar to that of reflexology, that has the effect of stimulating energy. The spinal reflexes are worked on the feet, hands and head relating to stages in a person's life from conception onwards to bring about an emotional, behavioural and/or physical transformation.

- NEUROMUSCULAR THERAPY – nerve pressure and pain is reduced through the application of thumb/finger pressures applied to irritated/congested areas of muscles. It is also known as trigger point therapy or myotherapy.

- NO HANDS MASSAGE – the use of body parts other than the hands to perform massage e.g. forearms, elbows, knees, feet in an attempt to conserve healthy hands and wrists of the practitioner by minimising repetitive strain and/or to apply a deeper, firmer massage when required.

- ON-SITE MASSAGE – massage in the workplace or other public place e.g. shopping centre, beach, aeroplane etc. Massage is applied through clothing without the use of a product and a special portable massage chair is often used. On-site massage provides accessible massage for the relief of everyday stress-related symptoms.

- OSTEOPATHY – a manipulative therapy which works on the whole body through the skeleton, muscles, ligaments and tendons to relieve pain and improve and maintain general mobility. This in turn benefits the functions of the body as a whole as the belief is that the body functions as a complete system. Cranial osteopathy is a technique

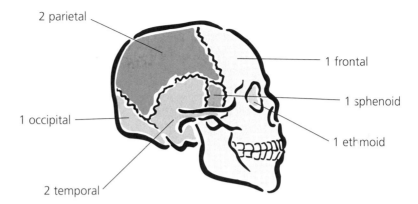

2 parietal

1 frontal

1 sphenoid

1 occipital

1 ethmoid

2 temporal

Bones of the cranium

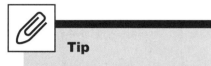

whereby the bones of the skull are manipulated using finely tuned palpatory skills.

● PHYSIOTHERAPY – the application of massage and the use of exercise to re-establish the use of the skeletal/muscular systems in cases of illness, injury and/or surgery.

● POLARITY THERAPY – developed by Randolph Stone as a science of balancing opposite energies within the body to promote mental, physical and emotional well-being. Massage is applied to specific body points using one or more of three levels of touch: very light classified as neutral, stimulating classified as positive and deep classified as negative.

● REFLEXOLOGY – incorporates the application of finger/thumb pressure techniques to points on the feet, hands or ears to stimulate the body's own healing mechanisms. These parts are viewed as being microcosms or miniature representations of a larger system, the whole body, based on the belief that by stimulating the part one can stimulate the whole.

● REIKI – Reiki comes from the Japanese words '*Rei*' meaning 'universal' and '*Ki*' meaning 'energy'. It

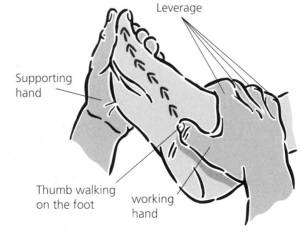

Leverage

Supporting hand

Thumb walking on the foot

working hand

Reflexology

incorporates a technique that works on balancing energy flow to aid healing. There are three stages to Reiki: Reiki 1 – which teaches the practitioner to use the energy on themselves, their friends, families and pets as well as plants and food. Reiki 2 – takes the principles a stage further with the use of ancient symbols that activate the use of energy to greater benefit and may be used on clients. Finally, Reiki Master – allows the teaching of Reiki to be passed from a Master to a layperson.

- REMEDIAL MASSAGE – the treatment of specific injuries, RSI (repetitive strain injury) and work-related problems through deep and superficial massage to bring about pain relief and correction of the body's muscles and soft tissue.

- ROLFING – developed in the 1930s by Dr Ida Rolf, Rolfing is a method of realigning the body's structure through manipulation. Using the fingertips, hands and knuckles, it has the overall effect of realigning the body with the forces of gravity, enabling the body to heal itself more efficiently and effectively. HELLERWORK is a derivative of rolfing and works on the same basic principles.

- SELF MASSAGE – a means of applying massage techniques to oneself to aid in the relief of muscular tension and associated pain to bring about a greater sense of well-being.

- SHIATSU – meaning 'finger pressure' incorporating relaxed pressure at various points or 'tsubo' on the body with the use of the fingers, palms, thumbs as well as an easy leaning of the forearms, elbows, feet or knees or simple rotation of a limb. Known as acupuncture without needles, it originated in Japan as an holistic treatment for the mind, body and spirit.

- SPORTS MASSAGE – a combination of Swedish massage and deep tissue massage applied either pre-activity to aid performance and/or post-activity to aid recovery. Pre-sports massage is usually applied vigorously with speed and post-sports massage is usually applied rhythmically and slowly.

- SWEDISH MASSAGE – traditional form of massage incorporating effleurage or stroking, petrissage or kneading and tapotement or striking movements to aid health and well-being.

- SYNCHRONISED MASSAGE – traditionally a form of Ayurvedic massage combining special strokes and rhythms with the application of medicated oils. May also refer to the performance of any style of massage by two practitioners. Both sides of the body are massaged in sync helping to create greater relaxation with a more balanced application of treatment.

- THAI YOGA MASSAGE – a massage therapy combining acupressure, gentle stretching and applied yoga from the traditional Thai massage or 'nuad Thai'. It is based on the belief in a life force or prana that circulates the body within an energy line system called ten sen. The treatment aims to rebalance the energy system to bring about increased health and well-being.

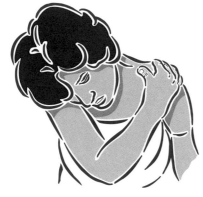

Self-massage

Tapping the hands

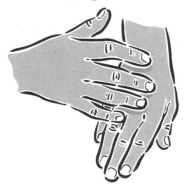

Tapotement

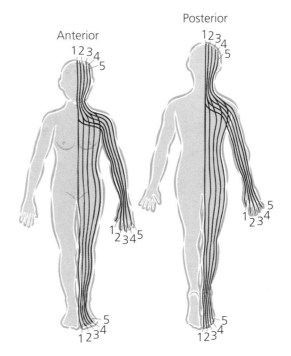

Zone therapy

- TUI NA MASSAGE – meaning 'push-hold' Tui Na massage takes its origins from traditional Chinese medicine and specialises in injury repair and body maintenance by adjusting energy flow.
- ZONE THERAPY – the application of pressure at a point within a zone or pathway to stimulate the flow of energy in the whole zone. Extreme pressure may be used as a means of blocking extreme pain.

Tip

A good way of researching a treatment is to book an appointment with a local practitioner. Alternatively, try to attend health and beauty exhibitions and complementary health fairs where practitioners and trainers are available to discuss their therapies in more detail. In addition, the Internet provides a wealth of information.

Task

Choose five of the therapies listed in the A–Z. Using whatever resources are available to you, complete further research on each one. Include in your research the following:

- Historical origins of the treatment
- Effects and benefits
- Application of the treatment

Make a resources file in which you can place this information. Add to it as you continue to develop your knowledge.

So how is massage done?

Touch is the stimulus and adaptations in the use of touch bring about varied levels of stimulation.

Massage incorporates the application of varied pressure and speed to bring about a reaction. As we have seen, massage can be applied with the hands or other body parts e.g. forearms, elbows, knees, feet etc. and/or electrical machines, stones etc. The sensory functions of the skin pick up the stimulus through the sensory nerves present in the dermis (layer of skin).

The sensory nerves convert the stimulus into electrical impulses or messages that pass along a network of nerves through the body to the brain. The brain in turn interprets the messages and decides upon a course of action – hopefully to lie back and enjoy! The brain formulates messages of its own as electrical impulses that are passed along a corresponding network of nerves, which in turn activate a reaction, for example stimulating blood flow to the area being massaged.

A reaction may therefore be experienced by both the giver and receiver of massage, confirming its role as a vital method of communication. In this way massage has also been used to great effect in the treatment of animals and many veterinary practices, zoos and trusts all over the world advocate the use of massage in animal welfare.

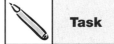

Task

Think of the different ways in which you may have instinctively used the art of massage in the care of a family pet. Think also about the effect this has had on you, your relationship with the animal and your life generally.

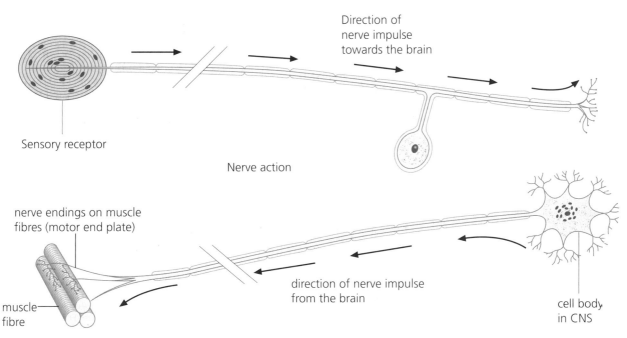

Nerve action

Knowledge review

1   What is the difference between the *art* and *science* of massage?

2   With which industry did massage develop in the West during the twentieth century?

3   What were introduced in the West as a means of combining exercise and massage and were reminiscent of the ancient Greeks and Romans?

4   In recent years, what type of research has the development of massage been associated with?

5   What has long been recognised by the hair and beauty industry as being one of the benefits of massage?

6   Which massage therapy incorporates the use of essential oils as a primary part of its application?

7   How many flower essences make up the Bach Flower Remedies?

8   What does palpation mean?

9   What is the name given to the Hawaiian traditional massage therapy?

10   Which electrical machines are associated with mechanical massage therapy?

11   Which massage therapy incorporates the application of massage without the need for the client to remove their clothes?

12   Which three parts of the body are commonly used for the application of reflexology?

13   When is sports massage applied vigorously and quickly – pre- or post-sport?

14   Which type of massage therapy commonly incorporates the application of massage by two practitioners simultaneously?

15   How do sensory nerves contribute to the effects of massage on the body?

 Activity

Use your increasing knowledge as a base to determine the direction in which you would like your study of massage to take you. You will soon realise that the acquisition of new massage skills is endless – there is always something new to learn, and who knows you may even go on to develop a new method of your own someday!

The marketplace for massage

4

Who is massage for?

The answer to this question has got to be everyone!

Tip

Massage is potentially suitable for everyone. However there are a few exceptions when massage would not be appropriate. These are known as **contraindications** and include occasions when cross-infection may occur or when the application of massage may worsen an existing condition e.g. bruising, varicose veins etc. This will be covered in greater detail in later chapters.

In fact we can make that statement even broader and say that massage is suitable for every living thing! As we saw in the previous chapter, massage is known to be of benefit to animals and there is no reason why the basic principles cannot be applied in much the same way to the care of plants. Think about the way in which the branches of a tree sway in the wind or the way a flower opens its petals in response to the sun's rays. It could be said that these responses are a direct result of the vibrations created by air and light, which perform their own unique form of 'massage' on the surface of the plant or flower!

Task

Make a list of as many different ways in which you think massage occurs naturally e.g. the sea massaging the land etc.

However, although the theory of massage may be loosely applied to all living things, the main focus of this book is in the application of massage for humans and there are many occasions when the reactions experienced during massage are of benefit, and none more so than in the treatment of stress.

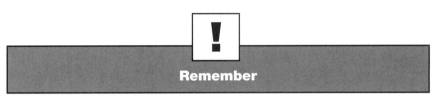

Remember

You can adapt the theories, principles and practice of massage for the care of any living thing.

Stress or the 'pressure associated with any factor which can adversely affect the functioning of the body as a whole' has the potential to disturb and seriously disrupt natural homeostasis and well-being.

Tip

Homeostasis refers to the natural balance and stability of the body, mind and spirit needed to maintain optimum health.

Tip

Stress may be described as something that is actually happening to us and/or something that we imagine may happen and is associated with high demands, high constraints and low support.

Stress is a fact of life and has been since the beginning of time. Throughout the ages our ancestors faced the stresses associated with survival in much the same way as we do today. The basic stressors or causes of stress may have changed but the body's reactions to stress have stayed much the same. The special sense organs pick up stressors through touch, sight, hearing, smell and taste.

System sorter

STRESS AND THE SPECIAL SENSES

Sight

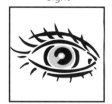

Sight is a sophisticated sense, providing the body with an early warning system alerting it to a possible stressor through vision, e.g. we can avoid potential dangers when we see them.

Touch

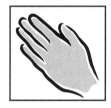

Touch provides physical communication alerting the body to any potential physical stressor, e.g. we quickly move away from something that is too hot, too cold, too sharp etc.

SPECIAL SENSES

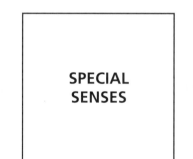

Hearing

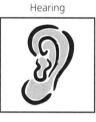

Hearing enables us to sense the distance and direction of a possible stressor and provides a means to determine the associated danger through the interpretation of sound, e.g. strong emotions are communicated through sound.

Taste enables us to detect a possible stressor once it has entered the body through the mouth alerting us to the need to eliminate it before additional harm is caused, e.g. spitting out foul-tasting food.

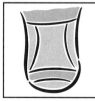

Taste

Olfaction refers to our sense of smell and the means by which the body is able to detect a possible stressor, e.g. air that may be harmful.

Olfaction

The combination of these senses provides the body with a means of avoiding stress in the first instance and is a skill that can be further enhanced through experience of the stressors associated with our everyday lives, i.e. we may learn to avoid certain known stressors.

The initial encounter with a stressor at this level is known as the *alarm phase*. In response to touch, sight, hearing, smell and taste, the body initiates the release of the hormone **adrenalin** into the bloodstream. This is sometimes referred to as an 'adrenalin rush' and is responsible for the following physiological responses:

- Increased blood flow to the brain to improve mental activity.
- Increased blood flow to the muscles to improve muscle strength and endurance.
- Increased levels of breathing to improve oxygen intake.
- Conversion of glycogen (carbohydrate) in the liver for additional energy production.
- Reduced blood flow to the digestive and urinary organs, slowing down digestion and the release of waste from the body.
- Increased sweating to reduce body temperature.
- Dilation of the pupil to increase vision.

As a result, the body experiences an increase in mental alertness, energy and strength which stem from the body's natural ability to defend itself in order to maintain homeostasis or essential balance and harmony.

However, as a result of this change in function, the body may also experience physical reactions in the form of:

- Racing heart and rapid breathing
- Trembling
- A rush of energy
- 'Butterflies' in the tummy
- Clammy hands.

In this way, the body is built to cope well when faced with short, sharp bursts of stress. Once the stressor has passed, the body returns to normal and is able to counteract any adverse effects in a short period of time.

Fascinating Fact

Adrenalin is also known as the fight or flight hormone as it prepares the body for increased physical and mental exertion either to meet the stressor head on (fight) or run away from the stressor (flight)!

Task

Think about the reactions you may expect to experience in the event of being told you are to be tested on the theory content of this book. You will experience all of the aforementioned reactions but as soon as you realise that you can use the book to find the answers, your body will very quickly go back to normal.

Often in life we find ourselves subject to excessive and/or prolonged periods of stress and this in turn initiates another set of responses and reactions within the body that is known as the *resistance phase*. This involves another hormone known as **cortisol.** Along with adrenalin, cortisol is also released into the bloodstream during the alarm phase, but is slower acting and longer lasting. It helps to regulate the body's resistance to stress by maintaining the responses experienced during the alarm phase. As a result the organs and body systems involved with combating stress come under increasing pressure and gradually start to weaken. The body craves a period of rest after a period of increased activity. If this is not available then the body starts to experience further reactions in the form of:

- Loss of concentration
- Muscle fatigue
- Indigestion
- Loss of energy.

Added to which, over a period of time, the body may become more susceptible to conditions that are **acute** in nature i.e. they are sudden, often severe and usually short in duration. These include:

- Headaches
- Eye strain
- Aches and pains in joints and muscles
- Digestive problems e.g. diarrhoea or constipation
- Urinary problems e.g. cystitis
- Common cold and/or associated symptoms e.g. sore throat, cough etc.
- Anxiety
- Allergies.

Task

Now imagine that the test is on the whole of the book and it is necessary for you to pass it in order to gain your qualification. However, this time you cannot use the book to get the answers and you have only a limited period of time in which to prepare. Think about the possible responses and reactions as your body tries to maintain resistance in order to achieve the goal. Think also about the additional forces that may contribute to this phase, making it easier to cope, e.g. lots of support or harder to cope, e.g. lots of constraints.

In turn, long-term stressors have the affect of increasing the release of the stress-related hormones adrenalin and cortisol and finally lead to what is known as the *exhaustion phase*, commonly referred to as 'burn out'. This results in a further weakening of the organs and body systems responsible for coping with stressful situations, reducing the natural defences and leaving the body vulnerable and at risk. Existing conditions worsen as the body is unable to counteract the effects of stress and a degeneration of the body starts to occur resulting in conditions that are more **chronic** in nature i.e. long lasting, increasingly severe and seriously debilitating, including:

● Migraine
● High blood pressure
● Repetitive strain injury (RSI)
● Irritable bowel syndrome (IBS)
● Depression
● Skin disorders e.g. eczema.

Task

Make a list of TEN possible situations in which a person may face the alarm, resistance and exhaustion phases associated with varying stress levels e.g. the death of a loved one, the birth of a baby etc.

Statistics show that 70% of modern day diseases are the result of long-term stress. This relates to times in our lives when the demands and constraints are high and the support is low.

Massage is a means of counteracting the everyday stressors that affect our society, helping to boost physical and psychological immunity in the form of:

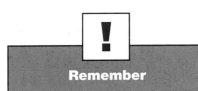

● A 'one-off' massage treatment offers a short-term solution to an annoying stressor e.g. the effects of a busy day studying are aided by relieving the physical symptoms i.e. aching muscles, tired eyes etc. preparing the body for rest.

● Regular massage treatment offers more long-term stress relief. Regular treatments encourage greater self-awareness as well as providing time out in which to rejuvenate and regenerate both body and mind.

Massage offers an essential ingredient in the prevention of stress as well as a natural complement to the treatment of stress-related conditions. The market for massage is potentially enormous, as can be seen in the A–Z of massage practices that follows.

An A–Z of massage practices

Tip

Many people experiencing high levels of stress turn to alcohol, drugs and food as a means of short-term relief. As stress levels intensify, the need for relief increases often resulting in a form of dependency.

- ADDICTION CENTRES – massage is being used with high levels of success in cases of high alcohol and drug dependency. It can be used to balance and maintain a drug/alcohol free state in recovering addicts as well as help in the various stages of becoming drug/alcohol free. Massage may also be used to aid in the treatment of eating disorders.

- AIRPORTS AND AEROPLANES – massage is being offered in many major airports as well as part of the in-flight entertainment. It acts as a pleasurable way of passing the time involved with travel as well as a means to reassure and relax nervous passengers who view flying as a major stressor.

- BEACH – massage is becoming a popular easy access treatment with on-site massage being offered in beach locations across the world. The warm, relaxed and beautiful locations help to enhance the therapeutic value of the treatment.

- BEAUTY SALONS – massage has always played an important role in beauty and is used as a stand-alone treatment of the whole body or as an integral part of a treatment of the hands, feet, face, ears and scalp in manicures, pedicures, facials, Indian head massage etc., helping to combat the general adaptation syndrome associated with varying stress levels.

- CARE HOMES – massage is being used with great success as part of the treatment given to those people who find themselves in care. Whether it is children because of behavioural problems or the elderly because of personal circumstances massage provides a means to combat the stressors associated with either situation.

- CLINICS – massage therapists often operate out of private clinics offering a specific form of massage and/or bringing together a number of like-minded professionals each specialising in massage related treatments.

- COMPLEMENTARY – massage is often used as an additional service in establishments that offer complementary therapies such as homeopathy, iridology, kinesiology, crystal therapy etc.

- CRUISE LINERS – many cruise liners have on-board spas and health/beauty salons. Being on holiday provides people with the time to relax and enjoy the benefits that can be gained from massage treatments.

- GENERAL PRACTICES – massage is becoming increasingly accepted as a complementary therapy and is often incorporated in the general facilities offered as part of a programme promoting good health by nurses, midwives, counsellors etc.

- HAIR SALONS – hair salons have always made use of massage in shampooing and conditioning treatments.

However, hairdressers are increasingly adding to their massage skills by offering their clients additional treatments such as Indian head massage etc.

- HEALTH CLUBS, CENTRES AND HYDROS – increasing awareness amongst athletes has prompted the use of massage in a sports context both pre- and post-exercise to reduce and prevent excessive physical stress and to create greater mental alertness and focus.

- HOME – many people seeking massage would prefer to be treated in the comfort of their own home, making it a popular mobile treatment. Treatment in the home often eliminates the stress associated with entering a busy salon/clinic environment which many people find intimidating.

- HOSPICES – massage is used with increasing popularity and success in the treatment of the terminally ill and their families. It can be used as a means of helping people come to terms with stresses associated with illness and loss.

- HOSPITALS – massage is being used increasingly for medical rehabilitation, prevention and maintenance of the body as a whole.

- MATERNITY UNITS – massage is used to great effect prior to and during childbirth as well as in the care of infants immediately after birth. Massage may be performed by medical staff, e.g. midwives, but equally by partners and parents and self massage may also be used to help relieve the stresses associated with childbirth for the mother.

- MEDICAL CENTRES – nurses are once again being encouraged to train in massage in order to offer the therapy to day patients as well as part of care in the home.

- MENTAL HEALTH – massage offers a simple and effective method of communication for people of all ages providing a means of gaining trust, reassurance and security in an often frightening and confusing world.

- NURSING HOMES – massage provides very real benefits for the elderly in terms of their physical and psychological well-being with many nursing homes introducing massage as part of a care programme.

- RETREATS – massage is a popular treatment for people seeking physical, emotional and spiritual enlightenment in an attempt to 'find their true self' and eliminate the stresses of life.

- SCHOOLS – massage is being used to aid disruptive and hyperactive children and is seen as an important tool in assisting in communication problems and antisocial behaviour.

- SPAS – massage is used as a complementary treatment both in and out of water. Day spas are becoming a popular way of de-stressing and are reminiscent of the Roman baths.

- SPORTS CENTRES – massage is once again seen as providing the link between physical fitness and well-being, helping in the preparation of the body before and after exercise to combat physical and psychological stressors associated with competitive sports.

- SPORTS CLUBS – most professional sports clubs – football, rugby etc. – will make use of massage therapy as part of the preparation of their athletes for sporting activities as well as for the treatment of sports-related injuries.

- WORKPLACE – many employers are realising the benefits that massage has on the stress levels of their workforce and are introducing the provision of on-site massage for both short and long-term relief.

So who is massage for?

Potentially massage is for everyone.

- There are no age restrictions – just adaptations of pressure.
- There is no sexual discrimination – just a professional code of practice.
- There are no cultural barriers – just variations of techniques.

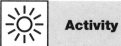

Activity

As you progress through your massage training and beyond, consider offering your services to one or other of these practices locally. Initially work experience in an environment in which you would ideally like paid work is a good way of determining your suitability as well as getting yourself known. Ultimately, we may choose to put something back into our community by offering our services free of charge in an environment where massage is not readily funded. As well as providing a worthwhile service to others it is also a valuable tool in self-development.

Knowledge review

1   Who is massage potentially for?

2   What does the term homeostasis refer to?

3   What is a stressor?

4   List the five special senses.

5   Name the three phases associated with the general adaptation syndrome.

6   What is the name given to the hormone associated with fight or flight?

7   With which phase of the general adaptation syndrome is the hormone cortisol associated?

8   Which phase of the general adaptation syndrome is commonly associated with 'burnout'?

9   What are the differences between acute and chronic conditions?

10   What do the initials RSI and IBS stand for?

11   Give two types of addictions that may be aided through massage therapy.

12   Name three beauty treatments that incorporate the use of massage.

13   Which two hairdressing treatments incorporate massage therapy?

14   Which type of massage practice is commonly visited in order to find spiritual enlightenment?

15   Give two ways in which massage is used in a sporting context.

Task

Monitor the ways in which you respond to stress. Make a list of the things that 'stress you out' and answer the following questions:

1 List the ways in which you respond to the stressors and which phase of the general adaptation syndrome is connected with each.

2 How could having one massage treatment be of help to you?

3 How could regular massage treatments help you?

Use the outcomes of this task to help you when you begin to work with clients. Your experiences will help you to empathise with others as well as provide a possible solution through the provision of massage and associated aftercare advice.

Part 2

Massage skills

Learning objectives

After reading this part you should be able to:

- Recognise the skills needed for the application of massage.

- Identify the relevant anatomy and physiology associated with the application of massage.

- Understand the links between the theory and practice of massage.

- Be aware of the different methods of applying massage.

- Appreciate the physiological and psychological factors associated with the giving and receiving of massage.

Massage as a treatment requires the use of intelligent as well as intuitive touch and as such incorporates a combination of skills that may be learned and indeed experienced. The massage of today has been founded on the intuitive experiences of our worldwide ancestors as well as the intellectual experimentation of our more modern day forefathers. The massage of the future lies with the natural integration of both aspects of this art and science and the following chapters aim to address the key learning points including:

- How does the body work?
- How are massage movements performed?
- How does the body respond to massage?

5

The theory

How does the body work?

In order to find the answers to this question we need to study the anatomy and physiology of the human body as a whole.

Tip

Anatomy refers to the *structure* of the body whilst physiology refers to the *function* of the body.

Millions and millions of individual microscopic cells provide the building blocks which make up the human body. Together **cells** build to form **tissue, glands, organs**, **body systems** and, finally, the **human organism.**

Cells

A new human organism is formed when an egg cell or **ovum** from the female fuses with a sperm cell from the male during fertilisation. Each egg cell and sperm cell contains 23 chromosomes that in turn contain the inherited characteristics from each parent. This fusion between the egg and sperm cells forms a single complete cell called a **zygote** containing the necessary 46 chromosomes needed to form a complete new person. This process is known as **meiosis.**

What follows is a process called **mitosis** or simple cell division whereby the zygote is able to reproduce itself many millions of times forming the embryo and foetus.

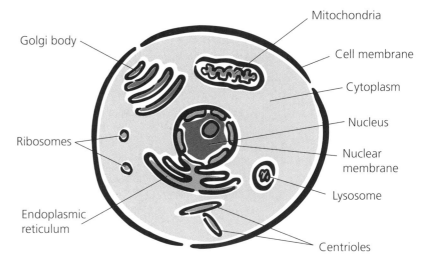

Structure of a cell

As development continues through the process of mitosis, individual cells form which all share a similar basic structure and function.

Cell structure and function

- Cell membrane – semi-permeable outer layer of a cell allowing substances to pass through.
- Nucleus – the information centre of the cell containing **DNA** (deoxyribonucleic acid) that carries the materials needed to form chromosomes.
- Cytoplasm – semi-fluid containing organelles or 'little organs' in the form of mitochondria, ribosomes, golgi body, lysosomes, endoplasmic reticulum and centrioles.
- Mitochondria – the powerhouses of the cell containing the power to create energy.
- Ribosomes – the 'protein houses' of the cell storing protein that is needed for the growth and repair of individual cells.
- Golgi body – providing the cell with a 'sorting and delivering system' for proteins to other parts of the cell.
- Lysosomes – the 'disposal units' of the cell breaking down damaged and worn out parts.
- Endoplasmic reticulum – providing the cell with a 'transportation system' for substances around the cell.
- Centrioles – the 'reproductive units' of the cell involved in the process of mitosis.

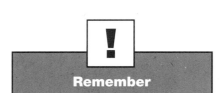

Remember

Meiosis is the process whereby a new organism is created through the fusion of an egg cell and a sperm cell. **Mitosis** is the process whereby the cells subdivide for growth and development.

As further development continues, certain cells begin to specialise in their structure and function. As a result, specialist groups of cells form which are known as tissue.

Tissue

There are four different types of tissue: **epithelial, connective, muscular** and **nervous**.

Epithelial tissue is produced from groups of cells to form the lining or coverings of many organs and vessels of the body including:

- The uppermost layers of the skin
- The linings of the heart and lungs
- The linings of the nose, windpipe, arteries and veins
- The linings of the stomach and digestive organs
- The linings of the bladder and genito-urinary organs.

Epithelial tissue contains cells that have developed to specialise in providing a *protective* function. Some of the cells develop tiny hair-like structures called **cilia** which are found in areas such as the nose and windpipe and help to prevent unwanted particles from entering the body by initiating the sneeze and cough reflexes.

Connective tissue is produced from groups of cells that specialise to form either a solid, semi-solid or a liquid including:

Solid connective tissue in the form of:

- **Bones** – **compact** or hard outer layer and **cancellous** or spongy inner layer.
- **Cartilage** – *fibro* forming disks between the bones of the spine, *elastic* forming the outer ear and *hyaline* forming the ends of bones at joints.
- **Fibrous** – **tendons** that attach muscles to bones and **ligaments** that attach bone to bone at joints.

Semi-solid connective tissue in the form of:

- **Areolar** – connecting and supporting other tissue
- **Adipose** – storing of fat
- **Elastic** – providing elasticity
- **Lymphoid** – engulfing bacteria.

Liquid connective tissue in the form of:

- **Blood** – transporting substances around the body.

Connective tissue contains cells that have developed to specialise in providing a connecting, protective and supportive function.

Muscular tissue is produced from groups of cells that specialise to create internal and external movement including:

- **Skeletal** – voluntary movement e.g. walking, chewing etc.
- **Visceral** – involuntary movement e.g. the movement of food and waste through the digestive system.

 Fascinating Fact

Peristalsis is the term given to the involuntary wave-like movement that takes place in tubular organs

- **Cardiac** – the movement of the heart to maintain the heart beat.

Nervous tissue is produced from groups of cells that specialise to respond to *sensation* e.g. changes in temperature, levels of pressure and pain etc. in the form of:

- **Neurons** – receive and respond to stimuli.
- **Neuroglia** – support and protect neurons.

Fascinating Fact

Most cells are able to reproduce themselves when damaged through mitosis e.g. simple cell division enables damaged skin to repair and heal etc. However, neurons are less able to perform this function and so need the extra protection provided by the neuroglia to prevent such damage which can if extreme lead to irreversible paralysis.

Glands

Glands are formed from epithelial tissue and contain specialist cells that produce a substance in the form of:

- **Mucus** – produced by cells that make up the linings or mucous membranes of the digestive and respiratory tracts.
- **Sweat** – produced by the sudoriferous (sweat) glands in the skin in response to changes in body temperature.
- **Sebum** – the natural oil of the skin and hair is produced by the sebaceous glands in the skin.
- **Cerumen** – earwax produced by the ceruminous glands of the ear.
- **Tears** – formed by lacrimal glands in the face.
- **Digestive juices** – produced by the stomach and pancreas in response to digestion.
- **Bile** – produced in the liver and stored in the gall bladder in response to digestion.
- **Hormones** – chemical messengers produced from the food we eat by the endocrine glands.

Tip

Most glands pass their substances into ducts (tubes) and are known as **exocrine glands**. However **endocrine glands** are the exception as they pass their substances (hormones) directly into the bloodstream.

Organs

Organs are complex structures that have developed from two or more different types of tissue including:

- Heart and lungs
- Brain
- Skin
- Liver
- Stomach
- Kidneys and bladder.

Due to their complex structure which is a combination of tissue types and specialist cells, the organs are multifunctional.

Body systems

Body systems are formed from associated organs and glands that have a common function and include the **integumentary, skeletal/muscular, respiratory, circulatory, digestive, genito-urinary, nervous and endocrine** systems.

Human organism

All body systems are interrelated and function together to form a human organism.

How does the body work?

Each body system relies on the others for its health and well-being and the term **homeostasis** refers to the harmonious interaction between systems in order to maintain a stable internal environment required for the survival and maintenance of every cell, tissue, gland, organ and system that is the human organism.

There follows an outline of each of the body systems with a set of tasks, activities and knowledge reviews. More specific anatomical and physiological information accompanies the treatment section in Part four.

System sorter

CELLS

Integumentary system

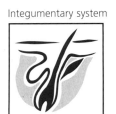

The cells of the surface of the skin, hair and nails form stratified keratinised epithelial tissue. This means that they are formed in layers, are hard and dry and contain the protein keratin contributing to the protection of the body as a whole. Skin cells are constantly being renewed and massage stimulates this process.

Skeletal/muscular systems

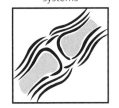

Specialised cells form the dense tissue associated with bones and the different types of muscular tissue needed for voluntary and involuntary movement of the body as a whole. Massage helps to stimulate all forms of movement making the body perform more effectively as a whole.

Respiratory system

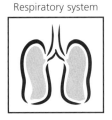

The respiratory tracts – nose, throat and windpipe – that lead into the lungs contain a lining that is ciliated. This means there is a covering of tiny hairs (cilia) which trap unwanted particles, preventing them from entering the body. Massage helps to relax the body which in turn relaxes the airways, allowing improved breathing.

Circulatory system

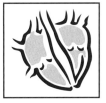

Blood cells form fluid connective tissue. They are able to move around the body within tubes (arteries and veins) transporting substances to and from all of the other cells of the body for growth, repair and maintenance. Massage stimulates blood flow, speeding up its transportation functions.

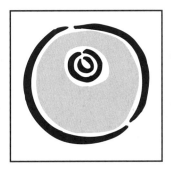

Endocrine glands are formed from epithelial tissue and contain cells which are able to secrete a hormone (chemical messenger) directly into the blood stream. The blood transports hormones to target cells which 'pick up' the associated message and act accordingly. Massage helps to stimulate blood flow and so improve the transportation of hormones.

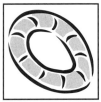

Endocrine system

Specialist cells known as neurons and neuroglia form nervous tissue which enable the body to respond to external and internal stimuli because of their function of sensitivity. Massage helps to stimulate nerve responses, making the system more efficient and effective.

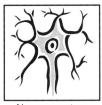

Nervous system

The lining of the bladder is formed from transitional epithelial tissue which is contractible, allowing the bladder to expand when full of urine and deflate when empty. Massage stimulates the release of toxins which are ultimately released from the body in urine.

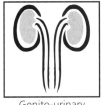

Genito-urinary system

The lining of the digestive tract is made up of goblet cells that are responsible for the secretion of mucus. This mucus helps the flow of nutrients and waste through the system. Massage can stimulate the action within the lower part of the digestive system allowing more effective and efficient removal of waste.

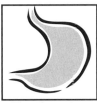

Digestive system

Integumentary system

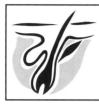

What is the integumentary system?

The integumentary system consists of the skin, hair and nails. The skin forms two main layers, the **epidermis** (top layer) and **dermis**, under which lies a layer of fatty tissue known as the **hypodermis**. Lying directly under these layers are the muscles and then bones and/or organs of the body.

The epidermis

The uppermost section of the skin is made up of five individual layers or *strata*.

- **Stratum germinativum or basal layer** – deepest layer in which cells continuously reproduce through mitosis pushing the old cells up towards the surface of skin. As the old cells make their way up to the surface they change in composition, forming the next four layers until they are finally shed as part of the natural exfoliation process called

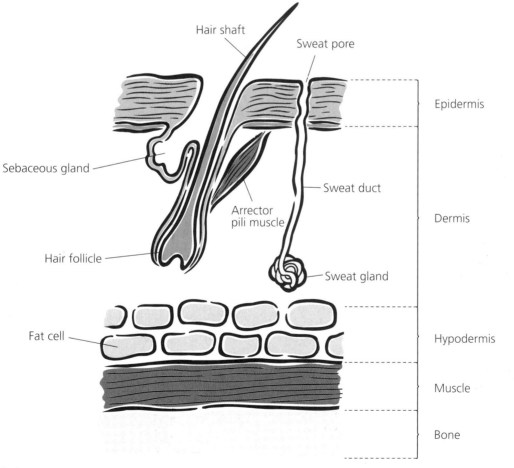

Structure of the skin

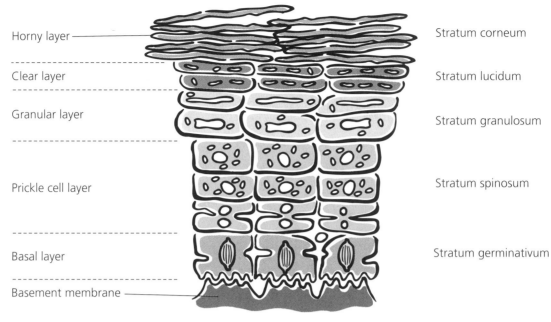

Horny layer	Stratum corneum
Clear layer	Stratum lucidum
Granular layer	Stratum granulosum
Prickle cell layer	Stratum spinosum
Basal layer	Stratum germinativum
Basement membrane	

The epidermis

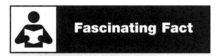

Fascinating Fact

It takes one month on average for the cells of the stratum germinativum to reach the stratum corneum.

desquamation. Specialist cells known as *melanocytes* present in this layer contribute to the colour of the skin. Melanin is the term given to the colour pigment produced by these cells. Nails also develop from cells of the stratum germinativum and form into three layers of hard, clear cells providing additional protection to the ends of the fingers and toes.

- **Stratum spinosum or prickle cell layer** – as the old cells of the stratum germinativum are pushed up to form this layer they begin to go through a process known as *keratinisation*. The cells are less able to reproduce through mitosis and as a result of keratinisation become hard and spiky.

- **Stratum granulosum or granular layer** – the cells continue to move towards the surface and as they form this layer they become granule-like in composition contributing to the protective functions of the skin.

- **Stratum lucidum or clear layer** – the cells gradually become flatter and harder as they form this layer. The melanin content is lost and the cells become clear and transparent contributing to the waterproofing function of the skin.

- **Stratum corneum or horny layer** – the cells have finally reached the surface to form the uppermost layer of skin. It takes approximately one month for the cells to develop from the stratum germinativum to eventually become the stratum corneum at which point they are constantly being shed to allow for the process to continue.

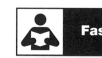

Fascinating Fact

We shed or desquamate in the region of 4 % of our total skin cells every day which is approximately 18 kg of skin in a lifetime! A large percentage of household dust is made up of these skin cells!

The dermis

The dermis lies directly below the epidermis and forms two layers – the upper *papillary* layer and the lower *reticular* layer. The papillary layer contains cells that interact with those of the stratum germinativum. The reticular layer forms the greater part of the dermis and contains the bulk of the structures associated with the functions of the skin.

- **Hair follicle and hair shaft** – hairs are produced within the hair follicle and extend up and out of the skin to form the hair shaft. There are three different types of hair: *lanugo, vellus* and *terminal*. Lanugo hair (soft and fine) is present on the body prior to birth. This is replaced with vellus hair (downy) that covers the whole of the body except for the palms of the hands and soles of the feet. Terminal hair (coarse) develops in areas requiring extra protection.

- **Sebaceous glands** – produce sebum, which is the skin's natural oil.

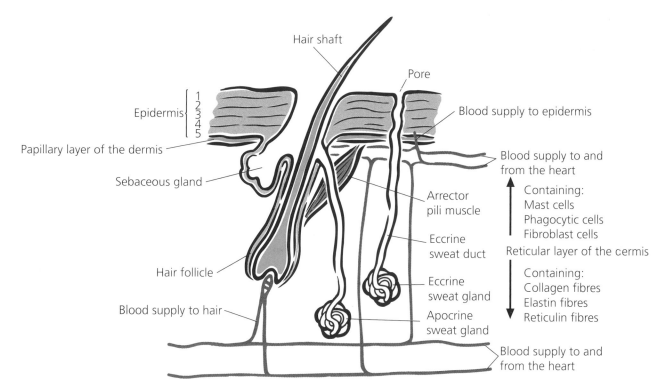

The dermis and its structures

- **Arrector pili muscle** – minute muscles which are attached to the hair follicles and epidermis and are able to contract to form 'goose bumps'.

- **Sweat glands, ducts and pores** – sweat glands are collectively known as sudoriferous glands of which there are two types; *eccrine* and *apocrine*. Eccrine sweat glands are found all over the body but are more numerous on the palms of the hands, soles of the feet and armpits whilst apocrine glands are present mainly in the underarm and pubic areas.

- **Collagen, elastin and reticulin fibres** – provide the skin with strength, elasticity and support. Strength to protect the underlying structures, elasticity to cope with fluctuations in size and support for the blood vessels and nerve endings which supply this layer. Together they contribute to the ageing process of the skin and are associated with the firmness of a youthful skin and the formation of lines and wrinkles of an ageing skin.

- **Mast, phagocytic and fibroblast cells** – provide the skin with the means to react to damage, defend against disease and produce new cells.

- **Blood supply** – provides a link between the integumentary system and the other systems of the body.

- **Nerve supply** – provides a link between the skin and the brain and vice versa.

The hypodermis

The hypodermis or subcutaneous layer as it sometimes referred to contains a loose network of cells in the form of areolar tissue. In addition a network of fat cells is also present in the form of adipose tissue providing a storage area for the excess fat in our diet.

What does the integumentary system do?

Fascinating Fact

The papillary layer of the dermis contains cells which contribute to the formation of the characteristic fingerprints.

The skin, hair and nails provide the whole body with a waterproof outer covering that is resilient and flexible, contributing to our unique personal appearance.

The integumentary system has many functions which contribute to its general well-being as well as helping to maintain its links with the other systems of the body including protection, temperature regulation, absorption, secretion, excretion, sensation and production.

Protection

The skin protects like a living suit of armour keeping vital organs safely *in* and environmental enemies *out*!

- Acid mantle – skin cells, sweat and sebum together produce the acid mantle forming a protective covering to the skin and helping to maintain a natural pH of between 4.6 and 6.

- Melanin production – melanocytes in the stratum germinativum produce melanin in response to exposure to the ultraviolet rays of the sun as part of the tanning process helping to safeguard against sunburn.

- Fat cells – in the form of adipose tissue deposited in the hypodermis they act as a 'cushion' against damage to underlying structures i.e. muscles, bones and organs.

- Touch – the skin's links with the nervous system alert the body systems to respond when it senses danger acting as an early warning system e.g. pain, pressure, excessive temperature is communicated through touch.

- Healing – the skin is able to repair and renew through the process of mitosis (simple cell division). When the skin is damaged blood rushes to the area forming a fine covering over the wound. Blood cells accumulate forming a clot that dries to form a scab. Meanwhile the scab prevents blood from leaving the body and germs from entering. New skin develops beneath the scab, which drops off once the skin is completely renewed.

- Hair and nails – vellus hair offers general protection to the whole of the body whilst terminal hair protects the more vulnerable areas i.e. hair on the head protects the skull, the eyebrows and eyelashes protect the eyes, the pubic hair protects the genitalia etc.

Temperature regulation

The skin contributes to maintaining normal body temperature of 36.8° Centigrade in the following ways:

- **Sweating** – the eccrine sweat glands produce sweat in response to a rise in body temperature. The sweat travels up the duct and exits the body through a pore. As the sweat evaporates on the surface of the skin it has a cooling effect.

Tip

The apocrine sweat glands are activated during puberty and produce a stickier form of sweat which exits the body via the hair follicle and, as it begins to break down, contributes to body odour.

- **Vasodilation and vasoconstriction** – when there is a rise in body temperature the surface blood capillaries dilate (widen) allowing the blood to flow near the skin's surface. As a result the skin reddens creating what is known as an erythema and excess heat is lost from the body. The opposite occurs when the body temperature drops. The surface blood capillaries constrict (tighten) forcing the blood away from the skin's surface to flow closer to the internal organs. As a result the skin appears pale as the blood warms the internal organs.

- **Fat cells** – in the hypodermis act as insulation helping to conserve heat and prevent heat loss.
- **Goose bumps** – created by the contraction of the arrector pili muscles in the dermis, which lifts the individual hairs trapping a layer of warm air beneath them in an attempt to conserve heat when body temperature drops.

Absorption

Cells are semi-permeable, which means that they allow a certain amount of substances to pass through them. The cells of the epidermis become hardened as they reach the surface and the formation of the acid mantle helps to ensure that enough absorption is possible to keep cells hydrated. Hair and nails are also able to absorb water and moisture helping to maintain their condition through hydration. Certain substances with a particular molecular structure are able to penetrate the skin further through diffusion. The molecules are able to pass through the epidermis and are picked up by the blood vessels circulating in the dermis. Examples of such substances include:

- Aromatherapy oils
- Hormone replacement therapy (HRT)
- Nicotine patches.

Secretion

Secretion refers to the cellular process of releasing a substance. The skin secretes sebum:

- Sebum – produced by the sebaceous glands, sebum acts as a lubricant for the skin and hair, helping to maintain condition. Sebum is secreted into the hair follicles and onto the skin via a pore where it travels the length of the hair during combing/brushing. Sebum contributes to the suppleness of the skin and the lustre of hair.

Fascinating Fact

Sebum production is controlled by hormones. As a result, puberty is a time when sebum production is increased due to the associated hormone release, often resulting in oily skin.

Excretion

Excretion refers to the elimination of waste from the body and the skin contributes to this process in three ways:

- Sweat contains water together with small amounts of waste products in the form of urea, uric acid, ammonia and lactic acid and is excreted from the sweat glands present in the skin.
- Skin cells excrete waste products associated with energy production e.g. carbon dioxide into the blood vessels circulating in the dermis. Carbon dioxide is carried to the lungs where it is breathed out.
- Skin cells also excrete waste products and water associated with energy production that are collected up by the blood and lymphatic vessels and taken to the kidneys. The waste products and water are excreted from the body in the formation of urine.

Sensation

The sensations associated with touch, pressure, pain and temperature are transmitted to the brain via an elaborate network of sensory nerves and receptors in the skin in the form of electrical impulses. The brain interprets these sensations and transmits messages to organs and glands via motor nerves in order to initiate a response. This process takes less than one tenth of a second to activate.

Fascinating Fact

A reflex action occurs when a reflex arc is produced i.e. the impulses reach the spinal cord where a quick response is made without needing to inform the brain first. This occurs in cases of inherited and learned experiences e.g. knee jerk reflex and touching a hot plate etc.

Production

The skin produces vitamin D:

- The action of sunlight converts a fatty substance called ergosterol present in the skin into vitamin D.
- Vitamin D helps the body store calcium.
- Calcium is needed for the maintenance of healthy bones.

The integumentary system as a whole therefore contributes to the well-being of its own structures i.e. the skin, hair and nails, as well as that of the whole of the body through the links it maintains with all of the body systems.

Knowledge review

1 Which part of the skin contains five individual layers or strata?

2 Which layer of skin contains the hair follicle and hair shaft?

3 What is melanin and where is it produced?

4 What does desquamation refer to?

5 What is the term given to the process of reproducing new cells in the stratum germinativum?

6 What is sebum and which glands are responsible for its production?

7 What is the difference between lanugo, vellus and terminal hair?

8 Which sweat glands contribute to the production of body odour?

9 What are the arrector pili muscles responsible for?

10 What is the name given to the tissue that contains fat cells?

11 How does the production of melanin contribute to protecting the body?

12 What happens to the surface blood capillaries when the body temperature drops?

13 What do the terms excretion and secretion refer to?

14 Which vitamin is produced in the skin?

15 Are skin cells semi-permeable, permeable or non-permeable?

Activity

Develop your knowledge of the integumentary system by noting the skin's reactions when you complete the following activities:

Rub your feet with the following:

- Hot flannel
- Brush
- Cold flannel
- Hand.

Task

Note how different the skin appears on different parts of the body and in different age groups. Make a list of the characteristics you have noted in the skin of various parts of your own body. Compare this with what you notice in the skin of your friends and family. Make a list of at least TEN factors which you think may contribute to the differences.

Skeletal/muscular systems

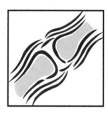

What are the skeletal/muscular systems?

Bones and muscles are active living tissue, which are capable of both growth and repair.

Bones are composed of approximately:

- 25% water;
- 30% organic substances e.g. bone-forming cells known as osteoblasts; and
- 45% inorganic materials e.g. calcium and phosphorus.

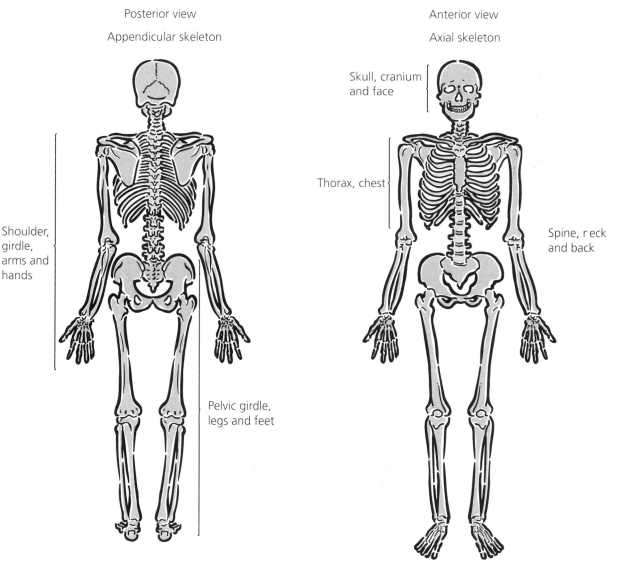

Posterior view

Appendicular skeleton

Anterior view

Axial skeleton

Skull, cranium and face

Thorax, chest

Shoulder, girdle, arms and hands

Spine, neck and back

Pelvic girdle, legs and feet

The skeleton

Muscles are composed of:

- 75% water;
- 20% organic substances e.g. muscle-forming cells known as myoblasts; and
- 5% inorganic substances e.g. mineral salts.

Bones are soft during childhood allowing for rapid growth, hardening as we age to form solid structures that can withstand a great deal. They contain a combination of **cancellous** and **compact** bone tissue depending on their size, function and shape:

- Cancellous bone tissue is spongy in texture and loose in structure forming the inner portion of most bones. It contains red bone marrow which is responsible for the formation of new blood cells as well as yellow bone marrow which provides an additional storage area for fat cells.
- Compact bone tissue is hard in texture and solid in structure providing a covering for cancellous bone tissue.

Bones are grouped together to form the core of the body or *axial* skeleton and the girdles and limbs or *appendicular* skeleton.

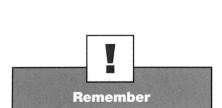

Remember

Excess fat is also stored in the cells of the hypodermis.

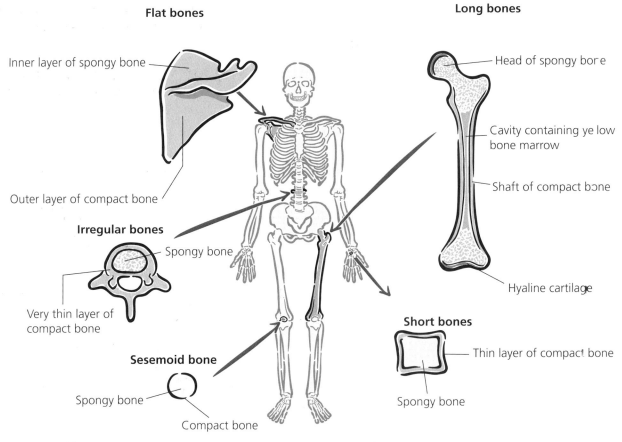

Structure of bones

Five different types of bones composed of varying amounts of spongy (cancellous) and hard (compact) bone tissue form the axial and appendicular skeleton including: long, short, irregular, flat and sesemoid bones.

Tough connective tissue forms an outer covering to most bones in the form of *periostium* and *cartilage:*

- Periostium covers the length of bones, producing new bone cells for growth and repair and linking the bones to the circulatory and nervous systems.
- Cartilage covers the ends of bones at joints, helping to prevent wear friction as bones move against one another.

Bones form three different types of joints – **fibrous, cartilaginous** and **synovial** which are classified according to the amount of movement they allow:

- Fibrous joints are fixed joints allowing no movement between bones. Examples include the joints between the bones of the skull in adults.
- Cartilaginous joints are slightly moveable joints which contain pads of cartilage between the bones allowing only a limited amount of movement. Examples include the joints between the bones of the spine.
- Synovial joints are freely moveable joints which are made up of a cavity between the bones containing a fluid allowing ease of movement. Examples include the joints of the shoulder, hip, elbow, knee etc.

Bones are linked together at synovial joints by **ligaments**. Also made from tough connective tissue, ligaments allow bones to move freely within a safe range.

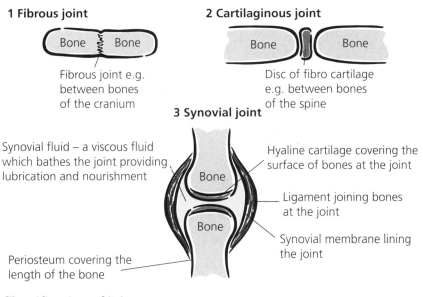

1 Fibrous joint

Bone / Bone

Fibrous joint e.g. between bones of the cranium

2 Cartilaginous joint

Bone / Bone

Disc of fibro cartilage e.g. between bones of the spine

3 Synovial joint

Synovial fluid – a viscous fluid which bathes the joint providing lubrication and nourishment

Bone

Hyaline cartilage covering the surface of bones at the joint

Ligament joining bones at the joint

Bone

Synovial membrane lining the joint

Periosteum covering the length of the bone

Classification of joints

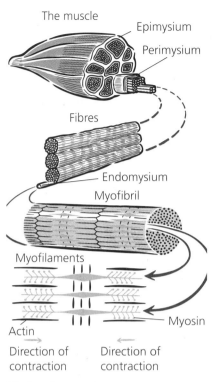

The muscle
Epimysium
Perimysium
Fibres
Endomysium
Myofibril
Myofilaments
Actin
Myosin
Direction of contraction   Direction of contraction

Skeletal muscle structure

Skeletal muscles are needed to perform such movements and are attached to bones by **tendons** e.g. Achilles tendon attaches the calf muscle to the foot at the ankle.

There are over six hundred muscles in the body made up of fibres containing thread-like structures called myofibrils extending from one end of the fibre to the other. Each myofibril is made up of a combination of thick and thin threads called myofilaments which work together in much the same way as an extending ladder to form concentric (shortening of the muscle) and eccentric (lengthening of the muscle) contractions.

Also present within the muscle fibres are **mitochondria**. These are responsible for generating the energy needed for the muscle to make a movement, which in turn moves the whole body. Mitochondria are often referred to as powerhouses as they store **glycogen, water** and **myoglobin**:

- Glycogen and water are the end products of the carbohydrates, fruit and vegetables we eat and the fluid we drink and are needed to create energy.
- Myoglobin holds the oxygen brought to the muscles by the blood and is needed to activate the energy.

Muscles form four basic shapes: spindle, flat, triangular and ring and generally attach to bones at a fixed point or origin at one end and a moveable point or insertion at the other. Muscle power needs to be forceful in order to move the corresponding bones.

What do the skeletal/muscular systems do?

There are many functions expected of the skeletal/muscular systems including **shape, support, posture, protection, movement, storage** and **production**.

- The skeleton provides a framework to which tendons attach the skeletal muscles thus forming our unique shape.
- Muscles work in groups to maintain body posture incorporating **agonist** muscles or prime movers, **antagonists** or apposing muscles, **synergists** or 'helper' muscles aiding the agonistic action and **fixator** muscles helping to 'fix' the position of the body when a specific movement takes place.

Remember

Skeletal muscles are responsible for voluntary movement, e.g. the muscles of the legs when walking whilst **visceral** muscles are responsible for the involuntary movements that carry the food through the digestive system etc. and **cardiac** muscles are associated with the movement of the heart.

Tip

Muscles contract in one of two ways depending on the type of movement generated – a *concentric* contraction incorporates the shortening of a muscle whilst an *eccentric* contraction incorporates a lengthening of the muscle.

- Muscles and bones form a barrier helping to protect the internal organs from external attack.
- For skeletal muscles to contract to produce a movement, they are stimulated by the nervous system through motor nerves. The decision to make a voluntary movement is initiated by the activity within the brain. A message is formulated in the form of an electrical impulse which reaches the muscle via a network of motor nerves leading from the brain to the spinal cord branching out to enter the muscle at a motor point. From this point, the nerves branch out with motor end plates that attach to each muscle fibre where the message is received and a movement is created.
- Bones take organic matter from the blood i.e. minerals and fat to be stored.
- Red bone marrow produces new blood cells supporting the blood circulatory system.
- Muscle movement produces heat helping to maintain body temperature.

 Fascinating Fact

A person starts to shiver when body temperature drops. This physical action incorporates the use of the muscles which in turn generates heat helping to raise body temperature!

The body relies on the integration of muscles and bones to produce movement but they cannot do so alone. Muscles and bones in turn rely on the interaction of the circulatory and nervous systems to produce the required energy and initiate the appropriate action.

- Muscles produce chemicals as part of the process of generating movement. Glycogen stored in the mitochondria and oxygen in the myoglobin of the muscle together produce ATP (adenosine triphosphate) which forms the fuel needed to create movement. As a result of this process carbon dioxide and water are produced in the muscles. This is associated with aerobic energy.

Tip

Anaerobic energy production also results in breathlessness as the body struggles to take in enough oxygen to fuel its energy needs.

- The use of ATP generates the production of another chemical called **pyruvic acid** and this is utilised by the oxygen in the muscles to create more energy.
- When the body's need for energy is high, excessive amounts of pyruvic acid are produced which in turn produces the chemical **lactic acid**. This is associated with anaerobic energy and aching muscles.

The skeletal/muscular systems rely heavily on each other for all of their actions and functions. In addition they cannot perform without input from the other systems of the body including:

- Circulatory systems transporting chemicals to and from the muscles.
- Digestive system supplying fuel for energy production in the form of glycogen from the food we eat.
- Respiratory system supplying oxygen to activate energy production from the air we breathe.
- Nervous system informing the muscles when and how to move.

Specific information relating to the position and action of bones, joints and muscles of each part of the body will accompany the massage treatment in Part 4.

Activity

Bend your elbows and feel the muscle action in your upper arms. In order for the movement to take place the brain has first of all instructed the muscles via the network of nerves. The muscles of the upper arm are attached at their origin (fixed point) to the shoulder joint and their insertion (moveable point) to the elbow joint. Feel the muscles at the front of the upper arm (biceps). They are contracting concentrically (shortening) to produce the force to lift the hand and lower arm and are the agonist muscles (prime movers). Now feel the muscles at the back of the arm (triceps). They are contracting eccentrically (lengthening) and are the antagonist muscles (apposing muscles). There is a smaller muscle in the middle of the front of the arm (brachialis) that acts as the synergist muscle, helping the action of the biceps. Place your hand in the crook of the elbow and feel the action of this muscle as you bend your elbow. In addition, other muscles are acting as fixators 'fixing' body posture as you move your arm.

Knowledge review

1   Which contain the most amount of water – muscles or bones?

2   What are the names given to spongy and hard bone tissue?

3   What is the term used that refers to the part of the skeleton forming the girdles and limbs?

4   What covers the length of bones?

5   What covers the ends of bones at joints helping to prevent friction?

6   Name the three types of joints.

7   Which type of joints are freely moveable?

8   What is the function of ligaments?

9   Which structure attaches muscles to bones?

10   What are muscles made up of?

11   What is the name given to the 'powerhouses' present in muscles that are responsible for storing glycogen, water and oxygen?

12   Name the fixed and moveable points of muscle attachment.

13   Which system contributes to the action of voluntary movement?

14   Where is red bone marrow found and what does it produce?

15   What is stored in yellow bone marrow?

Task

Using an anatomy and physiology text book research the different types of synovial joints under the following heading:

- Plane
- Pivot
- Hinge
- Ellipsoid
- Condyloid
- Saddle
- Ball and socket.

Respiratory system

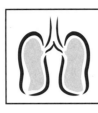

What is the respiratory system?

The respiratory system can be divided up into two main parts – the upper and lower respiratory tracts:

1 Upper respiratory tract consisting of the **nose, sinuses, pharynx** and **larynx**

2 Lower respiratory tract consisting of the **trachea, bronchi and lungs:**

Upper respiratory tract

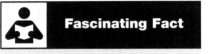

Fascinating Fact

Particles picked up in the nose initiate the sneeze reflex ensuring exit out of the body!

- Nose – providing the main point of entry for air coming into the body and the main point of exit for air leaving the body. The nostrils form two separate openings into the nasal cavity which is lined with ciliated mucous membrane forming layers of hair-like cells called cilia which filter air as it enters. Mucus is produced by goblet cells and is thick and slimy trapping any minute particles in the air as it enters the nose.

- Sinuses – air spaces in the bones of the skull which open onto the nasal cavity. These sinuses are lined with epithelial tissue containing cells that secrete mucus.

Fascinating Fact

Lacrimal glands or tear glands are situated in recesses in the frontal bone (forehead). They secrete fluid in the form of tears which leave the glands by small ducts passing over the front of the eyes under the lids where they drain into the nasal cavity through a small canal.

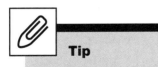

Tip

Adenoids and tonsils consist of lymphatic tissue and contribute to the immune functions of the body by filtering harmful substances from the incoming air.

- Pharynx – the back of the throat leading on from the nasal cavity. It is divided into three sections – naso, oro and laryngo. The nasopharynx contains the **Eustachian tube** linking the nasal cavity with the ears. The oropharynx provides a passageway for food and air entering the body via the mouth and the laryngopharynx provides the passageway for food to enter the oesophagus. The adenoids and tonsils are located within the naso- and oropharynx respectively.

- Larynx – leading on from the pharynx, the larynx forms the upper throat and contains the vocal cords. The larynx also contains a lid-like structure called the epiglottis which prevents food from entering the lower respiratory tract when we swallow.

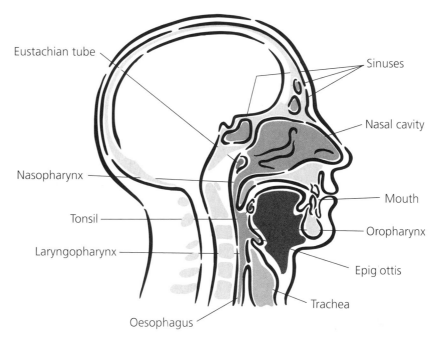

Structures of the upper respiratory tract

Lower respiratory tract

- Trachea – leading on from the larynx, the trachea is commonly known as the windpipe. It forms a semi-solid passageway for air.
- Bronchi – the trachea divides into smaller passageways forming the left and right bronchi which lead into each lung.
- Lungs – soft, spongy balloon-like structures situated on either side of the heart. Within the lungs, the bronchi subdivide to form smaller tubes called bronchioles which end in tiny sac-like structures called alveoli where the exchange of gases, e.g. oxygen and carbon dioxide, takes place.

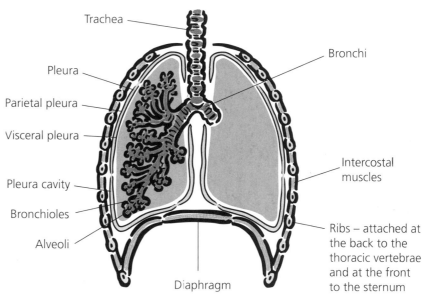

Structures of the lower respiratory tract

Tip

Filtering of the incoming air continues into the lower respiratory tract by the trachea and bronchi. Any trapped particles initiate the cough reflex.

Tip

The left lung is smaller than the right to allow room in the chest for the heart.

What does the respiratory system do?

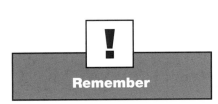

The heart is made from cardiac muscular tissue and acts like a pump. It is the centre of the blood circulatory system and is involved with the transportation of blood to and from all parts of the body.

The respiratory system is responsible for respiration involving five individual processes: **breathing, external respiration, transportation, internal respiration** and **cellular respiration**.

1 Breathing – can be defined as the movement of air in and out of the lungs by inspiration or inhalation and expiration or exhalation.
2 External respiration – the exchange of oxygen from the air with carbon dioxide in the blood takes place within the alveoli in the lungs.
3 Transportation – the pulmonary blood circulation ensures that oxygen is transported to the heart (via pulmonary veins) for distribution around the body and that carbon dioxide is transported from the heart (via pulmonary arteries) to the lungs for exit out of the body.
4 Internal respiration – oxygenated blood from the heart and lungs is received by the cells of the body where it is replaced with carbon dioxide. Deoxygenated blood is then transported back to the heart and lungs and the whole process repeated.
5 Cellular respiration – the utilisation of oxygen in the cells and the production of carbon dioxide. The individual cells use the oxygen to form energy and as a result produce carbon dioxide.

It is important to appreciate that every living cell is dependent on the act of breathing for survival, and care should be taken to ensure that the rate and depth of breathing matches the needs of the body. Although this is controlled by the nervous system, everyday factors such as stress (changing the rate of breathing) and poor posture (constricting the organs associated with breathing) can put excessive strain on the respiratory system resulting in inadequate breathing techniques. This in turn affects the performance of the cells, tissues, organs and systems of the body.

Fascinating Fact

The **solar plexus** located in the centre of the chest provides the link between the nervous and the respiratory systems through a set of nerves which stimulate the lungs in response to stress. Solar refers to the sun and plexus refers to a network of nerves i.e. the nerves radiate out like the sun's rays.

Knowledge review

1. Name the parts that make up the upper respiratory tract.

2. Name the parts that make up the lower respiratory tract.

3. What structures are present in the nose to filter incoming air?

4. What does the Eustachian tube link?

5. How many parts make up the pharynx?

6. What is the function of the epiglottis?

7. What is the trachea commonly referred to as?

8. Which is the smaller lung and why?

9. Give the technical terms for breathing in and out.

10. What does internal respiration refer to?

11. How is oxygen transported around the body?

12. What do the cells use oxygen for?

13. What is produced as a result of the cells using oxygen?

14. Which systems are linked by the solar plexus?

15. Where is the solar plexus located?

Activity

Practice breathing exercises in order to gain greater breath control. Breathe in deeply through the nose and then let as much air out of the mouth as possible. Repeat twice more before returning to normal breathing. Note how you feel as a result of deep breathing both physically and emotionally. You should feel calmer and more in control as your body has been replenished with maximum amounts of oxygen whilst at the same time been able to release maximum amounts of carbon dioxide.

Task

All forms of exercise rely on efficient breathing. In turn the body as a whole relies on some form of exercise to maintain its efficiency and effectiveness. Find out how breathing is improved through exercise and how exercise improves breathing.

Circulatory systems

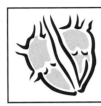

What are the circulatory systems?

The circulatory systems comprise two complementary systems, blood and lymphatic circulation, which work together providing the body with a transportation system for nutrients to be transported to the cells of the body and waste transported away.

The **heart** is the centre of the circulatory systems; **blood** and **lymph** form the transportation mediums with **vessels** forming a complex network of tubes for transportation of nutrients and waste to and from the cells.

Heart

The heart is located in the thorax between the lungs and slightly towards the left side of the body. It is a hollow, muscular organ that acts like a pump. The heart is divided into four sections or chambers separated by a muscular wall known as the septum. Valves form a connection between the chambers.

Blood

Blood is a fluid connective tissue containing **cells** that are suspended in a liquid called **plasma**. There are three main types of blood cells:

- Erythrocytes or red blood cells containing haemoglobin which carries oxygen and carbon dioxide. Erythrocytes contribute to the colour of blood.

- Leucocytes or white blood cells which defend the body against disease

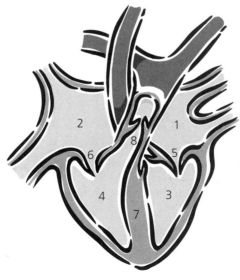

1 Left atrium
2 Right atrium
3 Left ventricle
4 Right ventricle
5 Bicuspid valve
6 Tricuspid valve
7 Septum
8 Valves

The heart

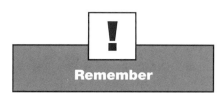

Remember

Dehydration results in blood and lymph losing much of their water content which contributes to sluggish circulation. Blood and lymph circulate much more effectively when fluid levels are high. Alcohol and caffeine are diuretics which encourage the body to lose water and should be avoided in excess because of this.

● Thrombocytes or platelets which contribute to the formation of blood clots at the site of an injury.

Plasma is made up of approximately 10% protein and 90% water in which chemical substances are dissolved or suspended.

Lymph

Lymph is a straw-coloured liquid containing lymphocytes, leucocytes and water contributing to the defence of the body.

Blood vessels

Blood is circulated around the body by a network of vessels called **arteries** and **veins:**

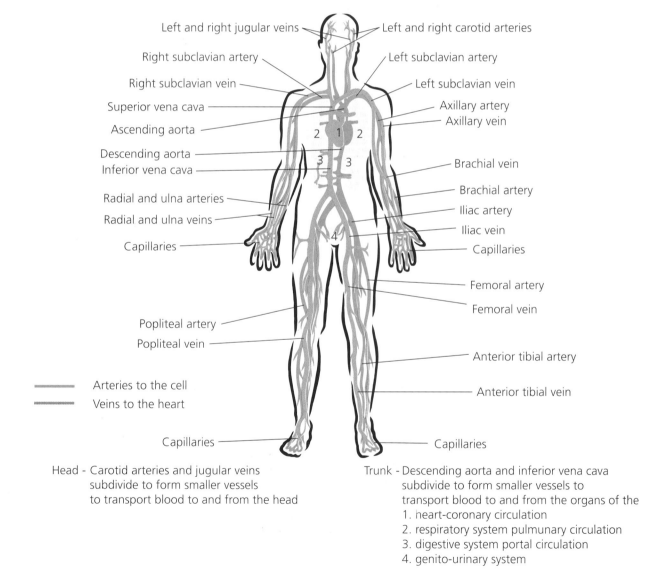

Left and right jugular veins
Right subclavian artery
Right subclavian vein
Superior vena cava
Ascending aorta
Descending aorta
Inferior vena cava
Radial and ulna arteries
Radial and ulna veins
Capillaries
Popliteal artery
Popliteal vein

Left and right carotid arteries
Left subclavian artery
Left subclavian vein
Axillary artery
Axillary vein
Brachial vein
Brachial artery
Iliac artery
Iliac vein
Capillaries
Femoral artery
Femoral vein
Anterior tibial artery
Anterior tibial vein

———— Arteries to the cell
------- Veins to the heart

Capillaries   Capillaries

Head - Carotid arteries and jugular veins subdivide to form smaller vessels to transport blood to and from the head

Trunk - Descending aorta and inferior vena cava subdivide to form smaller vessels to transport blood to and from the organs of the
1. heart-coronary circulation
2. respiratory system pulmunary circulation
3. digestive system portal circulation
4. genito-urinary system

The main arteries and veins of the body

- Arteries always carry blood *away* from the heart. They are thick-walled hollow tubes that subdivide into smaller vessels called **arterioles.**
- Veins always carry blood *towards* the heart. They are thin-walled hollow tubes that subdivide into smaller vessels called **venules**.

Capillaries form at the end of arterioles and venules and provide the link between the blood circulation and the cells.

Lymphatic vessels

Lymph is circulated around the body by a network of lymphatic vessels that start as small single cell structures called lymphatic capillaries that provide the link between the lymph circulation and the cells. Capillaries develop into larger tubes that follow the course of venules and veins through the body. These tubes pass through **nodes**, **tissue** and **ducts** before connecting with veins:

- Lymphatic nodes are situated in strategic places around the body and act as a filtering system for lymph. They contain cells responsible for defending the body against antigens by producing an antibody.

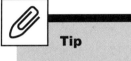

Tip

An **antigen** is an unwanted and harmful substance e.g. bacteria and an **antibody** is substance capable of counteracting their effects.

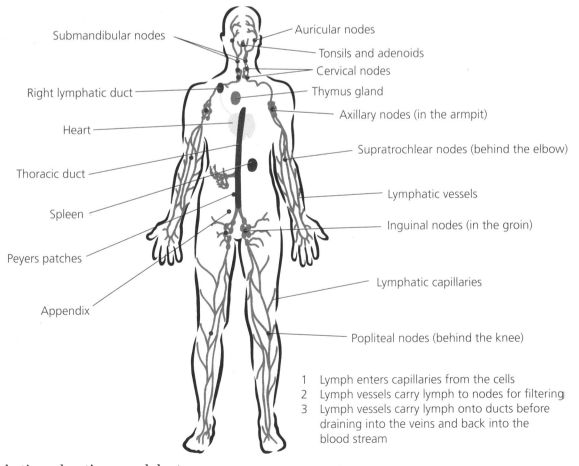

1 Lymph enters capillaries from the cells
2 Lymph vessels carry lymph to nodes for filtering
3 Lymph vessels carry lymph onto ducts before draining into the veins and back into the blood stream

Lymphatic nodes, tissue and ducts

- Lymphatic tissue collects in various parts of the body to form areas that continue to defend the body and include the spleen, thymus gland, tonsils, adenoids, lacteals and appendix.

- Lymphatic ducts collect filtered lymph before draining it into veins and include the thoracic duct and the right lymphatic duct.

Tip

The thoracic duct collects lymph from the left side of the head, neck and thorax, the left arm and both legs as well as the abdominal and pelvic areas, draining it into the left subclavian vein. The right lymphatic duct collects lymph from the right side of the head, neck and thorax as well as the right arm, draining it into the right subclavian vein.

What do the circulatory systems do?

The circulatory systems contribute to the well-being of every system, organ, gland, tissue and individual cell linking each with one another in a quest for homeostasis. The specific functions of the systems include **circulation, transportation, defence** and **regulation**:

Circulation

The blood circulation is a two-way system that:

- Transports the vital resources such as oxygen, water and food *to* every cell of the body via arteries, arterioles and capillaries.

Tip

Pulmonary circulation refers to blood flow between the heart and lungs and **systemic circulation** refers to blood flow between the heart and the cells of the body. **Portal** (blood flow between the heart and digestive system) and **coronary** (blood flow between the heart itself) circulation are both subsidiaries of systemic circulation.

- Transports unwanted substances such as carbon dioxide and waste products *away* from every cell via capillaries, venules and veins to be released out of the body.

Blood vessels

A   Main artery Aorta taking oxygenated blood *away* from the heart to the cells

B   Pulmonary artery taking deoxygenated blood *away* from heart to lungs

C   Superior and inferior vena cava (veins) bringing deoxygenated blood *to* the heart

D   Pulmonary veins bringing oxygenated blood *to* the heart

Blood circulation

The heart

1   Left atrium receives oxygenated blood from the lungs

2   Right atrium receives deoxygenated blood from the cells

3   Left ventricle sends blood to the cells

4   Right ventricle sends blood to the lungs

5   Bicuspid valve separates upper and lower chambers preventing back flow of blood

6   Tricuspid valve separates upper and lower chambers preventing back flow of blood

7   Septum separating left and right sides of the heart

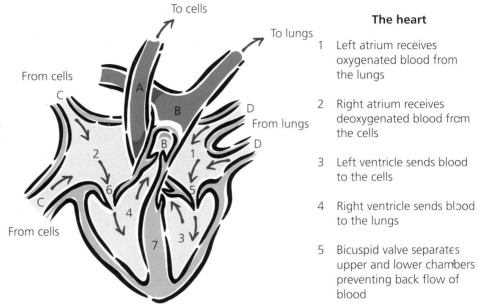

The lymphatic circulation is a one-way system that supports the blood circulation by:

● Picking up the waste from the cells that the blood is unable to collect transporting it via lymphatic vessels, nodes and ducts.
● Picking up fats from the digestive system.

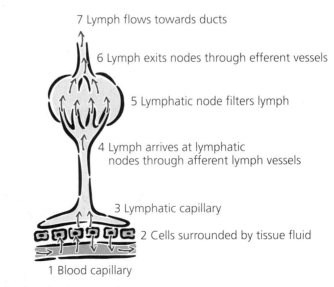

7 Lymph flows towards ducts

6 Lymph exits nodes through efferent vessels

5 Lymphatic node filters lymph

4 Lymph arrives at lymphatic nodes through afferent lymph vessels

3 Lymphatic capillary

2 Cells surrounded by tissue fluid

1 Blood capillary

Lymph circulation

Circulation of blood and lymph relies on the involuntary movement of the heart, voluntary movement by the skeletal muscles and involuntary movement of the visceral muscles:

- The pumping action of the heart determines the speed (heart beat) and force (blood pressure) by which the blood leaves the heart via arteries and arterioles.

- The blood returning to the heart via venules and veins relies on the action of skeletal and visceral muscles e.g. the muscles associated with walking, running etc. and the muscular action associated with breathing, eating etc.

- Lymph circulation is one way and also relies on the action of skeletal and visceral muscular action.

Tip

Veins, venules and lymphatic vessels contain valves which prevent back flow of blood and lymph.

Transportation

Blood and lymph are responsible for transporting substances *to* the cells including:

- Oxygen from the respiratory system
- Nutrients including water, carbohydrates, minerals, vitamins, proteins and fats from the digestive system
- Hormones from the endocrine system
- Antibodies.

Blood and lymph are responsible for transporting substances *away* from the cells including:

- Waste products including carbon dioxide and lactic acid etc.
- Excess water
- Worn out and dead cells
- Used hormones.

Defence

The circulatory systems form a part of the immune system helping to safeguard the body against disease through leucocytes (white blood cells) and lymphocytes. In addition, lymphatic tissue helps to protect specific areas of the body including:

- Adenoids and tonsils help to purify air coming into the body through the nose and mouth.

- Appendix contributes to the purification of waste in the intestines.
- Thymus gland produces a group of hormones to stimulate the production of T-lymphocytes for protection against antigens.
- Spleen acts as a reservoir storing blood which can be diverted to other parts of the body when needed.

Regulation

The circulatory systems contribute to the regulation of the following:

- Body temperature through vasoconstriction and vasodilation of surface blood vessels by either conservation or convection of body heat.
- Fluid balance through the composition of blood and lymph.
- PH through chemical systems in the blood called buffers helping to maintain a pH of approximately 7.4.
- Changes in the body e.g. growth, puberty etc. through the transportation of hormones.

It is important to appreciate the many vital tasks the circulatory systems perform in helping to maintain homeostasis.

Activity

Check the beating of your heart.

- Find the pulse in your neck by pressing the fingers of your right hand against the left side of your neck. What you are feeling is the force of the heart pumping blood into an artery during each beat of the heart.
- Count the number of beats in the space of one minute.
- Then jog on the spot for at least one minute at the end of which check your pulse once again counting the number of beats in one minute.
- Notice how your pulse rate has raised in response to the need for more oxygen as you jogged.
- Check your pulse again after a further ten minutes. Notice how it has returned to normal, as the body's need for oxygen has decreased.
- Take note of your breathing throughout this activity and determine what type of breathing you used and why.

Knowledge review

1   Name the two complementary systems that make up the circulatory systems.

2   Which organ is at the centre of the circulatory systems?

3   What are the two forms of transportation medium?

4   What is the name given to the network of tubes that transport substances to and from cells?

5   What is blood made up of?

6   What are erythrocytes, leucocytes and thrombocytes?

7   What does lymph contain?

8   Name the two main types of blood vessels.

9   What do these blood vessels subdivide to form?

10 What vessels link the circulatory systems with the cells of the body?

11 What course do lymphatic vessels follow through the body?

12 What happens to lymph in the nodes?

13 Give an example of lymphatic tissue.

14 Name the two lymphatic ducts.

15 What does systemic circulation refer to?

Task

Many people suffer with high or low blood pressure. High blood pressure places additional strain on the heart and low blood pressure places additional strain on the brain. Conduct some research trying to find the possible causes of such conditions together with the physical effects. Include the ways in which a person can try to prevent and/or avoid such conditions.

Digestive system

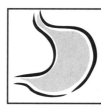

What is the digestive system?

The digestive system begins at the mouth and ends at the large intestine and it is collectively known as the **alimentary canal**.

The alimentary canal consists of the following structures:

- Mouth – comprising the hard and soft palate, lips, muscles, teeth, salivary glands and tongue. The mouth provides the starting point for the ingestion of food and fluid.

- Pharynx – linking the respiratory and digestive systems, the pharynx provides a passageway for the ingested food and fluid from the mouth and into the oesophagus as it is swallowed.

- Oesophagus – a long muscular tube (approx 25 cms in length) extending from the pharynx to the stomach. It lies behind the trachea and in front of the spine. Its muscular layers contract to move the ingested food down in the involuntary action known as **peristalsis** through a ring of muscle called the **cardiac sphincter** and into the stomach.

- Stomach – a j-shaped sac which lies under the diaphragm on the left side of the body where the next stages of the digestive process take place. It contains folds or rugae that allow it to stretch out when full and contract when empty. At the end of the stomach there is a ring of muscle called the **pyloric sphincter** which controls the entry of digested food into the small intestine.

- Small intestine – a long coiled tube (approx 6 m in length) which fills the bulk of the abdominal cavity. It is made up of three sections: the **duodenum,** the **jejunum** and the **ileum.** Absorption of nutrients from the digested food into the circulatory systems takes place within the small intestine.

- Large intestine – known also as the bowel, it is divided into five sections: the **caecum**, the **colon**, the **rectum**, the **anal canal** and the **anus**. The large intestine is responsible for moving the waste products of digestion through the system for elimination from the body.

In addition to the alimentary canal, the digestive system also relies on three **accessory organs:**

- **Liver** – the largest internal organ of the body lying below the diaphragm in the upper right section of the abdominal cavity. The liver is one of the most important links between body systems and has many functions, some of which are directly associated with the digestive system. Functions include: filtering, detoxification and deamination of blood, storage of nutrients e.g. some vitamins, glycogen and iron, production of bile to aid digestion and the production of heat to maintain body temperature.

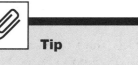

Tip

The diaphragm is a sheet of muscle separating the internal organs of the chest i.e. heart and lungs from those of the abdomen.

Tip

Deamination refers to the breaking down of amino acids and the formation of urea in the liver.

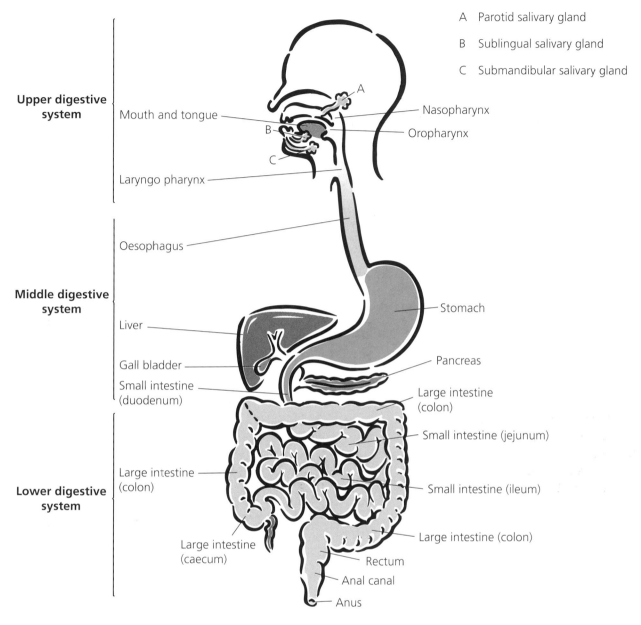

A   Parotid salivary gland

B   Sublingual salivary gland

C   Submandibular salivary gland

Upper digestive system

Mouth and tongue

Nasopharynx

Oropharynx

Laryngo pharynx

Middle digestive system

Oesophagus

Liver

Gall bladder

Small intestine (duodenum)

Stomach

Pancreas

Large intestine (colon)

Lower digestive system

Large intestine (colon)

Small intestine (jejunum)

Small intestine (ileum)

Large intestine (colon)

Large intestine (caecum)

Rectum

Anal canal

Anus

The digestive system

- **Gall bladder** – a pear-shaped sac located just above the duodenum and under the liver. It is connected to both the duodenum (first section of the small intestine) and the liver by ducts. It receives bile from the liver which it stores until needed by the duodenum to aid in the process of digestion and absorption.

- **Pancreas** – a long thin organ lying across the abdominal cavity on the left side of the body. It has an endocrine function producing hormones associated with blood sugar levels and an exocrine function producing juices associated with digestion. These digestive juices pass from the pancreas into the duodenum via a duct. The hormones pass directly into the bloodstream.

What does the digestive system do?

Together the alimentary canal and the accessory organs perform many functions which in turn have an effect on the well being of the whole of the body including: **ingestion, digestion, absorption** and **elimination**.

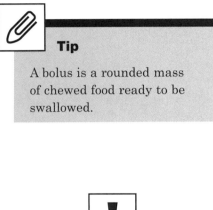

Tip

A bolus is a rounded mass of chewed food ready to be swallowed.

!

Remember

Peristaltic action refers to the involuntary action associated with visceral muscular tissue.

Fascinating Fact

The cardiac sphincter is a weak muscle allowing regurgitation of food from the stomach if necessary.

- Ingestion of food and fluid takes place in the mouth where it is checked for temperature by the sensitive skin of the lips, held within the mouth by the facial muscles, tasted by the papillae (taste buds) of the tongue, broken down by the teeth and the action of the jaw, bound together with saliva and formed into a bolus before being passed to the pharynx where swallowing takes place.

- Peristaltic action sends the bolus down the oesophagus, passing through the cardiac sphincter and into the stomach.

- Digestion also begins in the mouth and carries on in the stomach. In the mouth mastication (chewing) takes place which breaks down the food into a bolus. Chemical digestion takes place through the action of saliva in the mouth and digestive juices in the stomach breaking the food down further to form a semi-liquid known as chyme. This passes from the stomach through the pyloric sphincter and into the small intestine.

- Vital nutrients from the chyme are passed from the stomach and small intestine into the circulatory systems for transportation around the body. Small amounts of water, alcohol and some drugs are absorbed directly into the bloodstream from the stomach and the rest of the nutrients are absorbed from the three sections of the small intestine. This process is aided by the secretion of bile from the gall bladder and pancreatic juices from the pancreas.

- As the chyme reaches the latter stages of the small intestine any remaining matter forms into faeces. Peristaltic (involuntary) muscular action forces the faeces along the rectangular colon from the ileocaecal sphincter linking the small and large intestines into the caecum, ascending, transverse, descending and sigmoid colon, through the rectum and into the anal canal for elimination out of the body via the anus. Any remaining water is absorbed along the way.

The healthy functioning of the digestive system contributes to the health of the whole body. Vital nutrients in the form of food and fluid are a necessary part of the survival of every cell, tissue, gland, organ and system in order to sustain life.

Knowledge review

1 Name the main parts that make up the alimentary canal.

2 What are the three accessory organs?

3 What mixes with food in the mouth to produce a bolus?

4 Name the tube that links the pharynx with the stomach.

5 What is peristalsis?

6 What is chyme?

7 Where is the stomach located within the body?

8 Where is bile formed and stored?

9 Which is the largest internal organ of the body?

10 Give three functions of the liver.

11 What does the pancreas produce to aid digestion?

12 What happens in the small intestine?

13 What is the large intestine responsible for?

14 What happens to any water present in the large intestine?

15 Which part of the large intestine is responsible for the final elimination of faeces?

Activity

Monitor your eating habits over the next week. Try to eat three meals a day. Include a variety of foods associated with a healthy diet. Take time out to eat, chewing each mouthful well before swallowing. Make time to relax for at least half an hour immediately after eating. Avoid eating 'on the run' and fast food. Start to take note of how your digestive system responds and how your body feels as a whole. You should start to experience greater energy levels and reduced adverse effects e.g. bloating, flatulence, indigestion etc.

Task

Many people experience problems associated with their digestive system as a result of stress. Research the following disorders that may be caused/aggravated by stress:

- Irritable bowel syndrome (IBS)
- Obesity
- Stomach ulcer
- Anorexia and bulimia.

Genito-urinary system

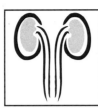

What is the genito-urinary system?

The genito-urinary system consists of the male and female **genitalia**, the **kidneys**, **bladder, ureter** tubes leading from the kidneys to the bladder and a **urethra** tube leading from the bladder to the outside of the body.

Male genitalia

The male genitalia include the **testes**, the **vas deferens**, the **prostate gland** and the **penis**.

● Testes – develop in the abdomen of a male foetus and drop into a sac of skin and muscle located behind the penis known as the scrotum just before birth. After puberty the testes produce sperm which passes along a tightly coiled tube called the epididymis extending to form the vas deferens.

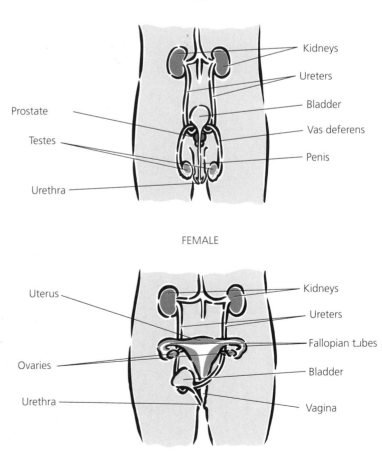

The male and female genito-urinary systems

- Vas deferens – peristaltic action forces the sperm along the vas deferens towards the penis. Each vas deferens passes by sac-like structures called **seminal vesicles** which secrete the fluid that mixes with the sperm to form semen. This fluid passes from the seminal vesicles to the vas deferens through ducts. Each vas deferens then passes through the prostate gland.
- Prostate gland – a chestnut-shaped structure which secretes a milky fluid contributing to the formation of semen. The prostate gland opens onto the urethra tube to create an exit out of the body through the penis.

Female genitalia

The female genitalia include the **ovaries**, the **fallopian tubes**, the **uterus** and the **vagina**.

- Ovaries – there are two ovaries on either side of the pelvic girdle about the size and shape of almonds, which store ova (eggs).
- Fallopian tubes – each approximately 10 cm in length opening just above the ovaries to create a passageway for released ovum to travel from the ovaries to the uterus.
- Uterus – or womb is the site for the development of an ovum which has been fertilised by a sperm or for the release of the unfertilised ovum during menstruation. The uterus opens out into the vagina at the neck of the womb or cervix which together form the route for the birth of a baby.

Accessory glands

The breasts are glands which develop in females in response to activity within the genitalia. They are present in males but are not

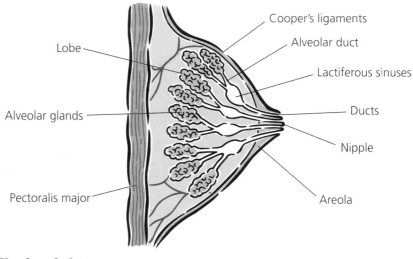

The female breast

activated into development in the same way. The female breasts are known as mammary glands and develop during puberty. Each breast consists of about twenty lobes each containing alveolar glands and ducts. Milk is produced in the glands in response to pregnancy. It is passed through the ducts to the lactiferous sinuses where it is stored before passing into further ducts and out of the nipple. The external portion of the breast forms a pigmented area of skin or areola around the nipple containing sebaceous glands that secrete sebum in order to lubricate the area.

Urinary system

The structures of the urinary system are common to both sexes and include the kidneys, ureters, bladder and urethra.

- Kidneys – there are two bean-shaped kidneys located either side of the spine at the waistline. The kidneys produce urine which is passed out of the kidneys into the ureter tubes.
- Ureter tubes – two long, thin tubes extending from each kidney to the bladder. Peristaltic (involuntary) muscular action forces urine along the ureter tubes.
- Bladder – a pear-shaped structure when empty, becoming oval in shape as it fills with urine. The bladder contains folds called rugae which extend as the bladder fills. Nerve endings in the bladder wall detect an increase in size and activate an internal sphincter muscle which relaxes as the bladder contracts, allowing a passageway through to the urethra.
- Urethra tube – a single narrow muscular tube leading from the bladder to the outside of the body. It contains an external sphincter muscle closing off the exit to prevent release of urine. In a male the urethra is longer than in a female and has dual function providing exit out of the penis for either urine or semen.

What does the genito-urinary system do?

The functions of the genito-urinary system may be divided into two categories:

1 Functions of the genitalia which include the **production of hormones** and **reproduction.**
2 Functions of the urinary system which include **filtration, re-absorption, production, excretion** and **regulation**.
   - The testes and ovaries are also known as gonads or sex glands and are responsible for producing the male and female sex hormones.
   - The onset of puberty equips a male and female to reproduce a new human being with the production of sperm and the release of ova.

- Large amounts of blood pass continuously through the kidney to be filtered of unwanted substances. Many other vital substances are also filtered out of the blood during this process.

- Reabsorption of these vital substances takes place prior to the production of urine as the kidneys regulate the amount of water and minerals needed by the body.

- The excess water, minerals and waste are finally excreted from the body.

The dual functions of the genito-urinary system contribute to many vital functions of the body. The body gives out many signs that this system is working and will alert the body when stressed e.g. the feeling associated with needing to empty the bladder, sexual tension etc.

Activity

The external sphincter muscle responsible for preventing the release of urine from the body is inactive in babies, hence the need for nappies. In later years it is important to maintain strength in this muscle in order to prevent the onset of urinary problems e.g. incontinence. To test your muscle strength try the midstream test. As you pass water first thing in the morning when your bladder is at its fullest, try to stop mid flow for a few seconds. If this is difficult to do, then try to strengthen the muscle by doing some simple exercises. Squeeze the muscle tightly, hold for a few seconds and release. You will gradually strengthen the muscle helping to prevent future problems.

Knowledge review

1 Name the male genitalia.

2 Name the female genitalia and accessory glands.

3 What do the testes produce?

4 What do the ovaries produce?

5 What does the pigmented skin around the breasts contain?

6 Where are the kidneys located within the body?

7 What is produced in the kidneys?

8 Which structures connect the kidneys and bladder?

9 What is peristalsis?

10 What is the purpose of the folds or rugae in the bladder?

11 What is the name given to the tube that leads from the bladder?

12 Is this tube is longer in males or females?

13 Which genito-urinary organs are also known as gonads?

14 What happens to the blood that passes through the kidneys?

15 What does excretion mean?

Task

The kidneys contribute to maintaining the body's fluid balance by conserving or releasing water. As such, water is needed to maintain every bodily function and we each require approximately one and a half to two litres of water per day.

- Make a list of the type of foods that have a high water content thus contributing to this daily amount.
- Why are herbal teas better for the body than tea and coffee?
- How does alcohol contribute to dehydration?
- Why is still water served at room temperature better for the body than carbonated water served chilled?

Nervous system

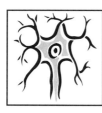

What is the nervous system?

The nervous system is the body's main communication centre and can be divided into three main parts:

1 **The central nervous system** (CNS) or control centre consisting of the brain and spinal cord.
2 **The peripheral nervous system** (PNS) consisting of nerves linking the various parts of the body with the central nervous system.
3 **The autonomic nervous system** (ANS) consisting of the sympathetic and parasympathetic systems.

The nervous system is made up of highly specialist cells known as **neurons** together with supportive cells called **neuroglia**. Neurons

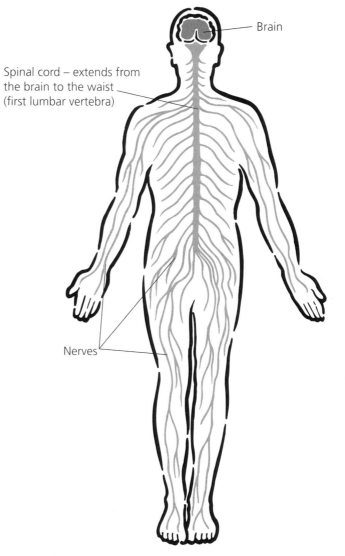

Brain

Spinal cord – extends from the brain to the waist (first lumbar vertebra)

Nerves

The nervous system

group together to form **nerves** and bundles of nerves form **white** or **grey matter**:

- White matter is found on the *inside* of the brain and the *outside* of the spinal cord and provides a link between the whole of the nervous system.
- Grey matter is found on the *outside* of the brain and *inside* of the spinal cord and is responsible for coordinating the action within the nervous system.

Branching off from the central nervous system is the peripheral nervous system which consists of twelve pairs of **cranial** nerves leading to and from the brain and thirty-one pairs of **spinal** nerves leading to and from the spinal cord.

Finally, the autonomic nervous system supplies nerves to all of the internal organs of the body that are not under our conscious control and is divided into two opposing parts, the **sympathetic** and **parasympathetic** systems. The sympathetic system is responsible for stimulating the body into activity and the parasympathetic system prepares the body for rest.

Tip

The bundles of nerves associated with white matter are more fast acting than those that make up grey matter.

What does the nervous system do?

Fascinating Fact

Reflexes are functions used to describe the automatic responses such as swallowing, vomiting, coughing, sneezing, as well as the reflexes associated with moving away from a hot plate and the knee jerk reflex etc. As such, reflexes enable the body to perform various functions without conscious effort as well as enable the body to limit the damage caused by different stimuli.

As a whole, the nervous system acts as a two-way communication network and is responsible for **sensory, integration, motor, reflex** and **regulatory** functions:

- **Sensory** or afferent nerves carry messages in the form of electrical impulses from the sensory organs i.e. skin, eyes, ears, nose and tongue *to* the spinal cord and onto the brain.
- The brain receives the impulses which are then **integrated** to form a complete message, interpreted to formulate a suitable response and stored in the form of a memory.
- **Motor** or efferent nerves then carry messages *away* from the brain via the spinal cord and peripheral nerves to the parts of the body needed to respond e.g. muscles and organs.
- A mixture of sensory and motor nerves are found in the spinal cord where there is a two-way fast tracking system enabling impulses to travel both ways without having to bypass the brain. This process forms a **reflex arc** and

Fascinating Fact

The sympathetic system is associated with stress responses and the parasympathetic system is known as the 'peace maker'.

activates very quick responses associated with **reflex actions**.

- The involuntary actions of the body including breathing, digestion etc. are **regulated** by the autonomic nervous system. The sympathetic system is responsible for stimulating the body into activity and the parasympathetic system for counteracting the effects of such stimulation by preparing the body for rest.

Task

Using your anatomy and physiology book for reference, make a chart outlining the effects that both the sympathetic and parasympathetic systems have on the following organs and their functions:

- Eyes and sight
- Heart and blood pressure
- Muscles and movement
- Lungs and breathing
- Liver and the conversion of glycogen and the secretion of bile
- Stomach and intestines and the processes of digestion and absorption
- Kidneys and bladder and the excretion of waste.

Activity

Take note of how your body responds to a stressful situation – learn to recognise the actions of the sympathetic nervous system. Take note also of how the body relaxes – learn to recognise the actions of the parasympathetic nervous system.

Knowledge review

1   What is the central nervous system made up of?

2   What does the peripheral nervous system contain that links it with the central nervous system?

3   Name the two systems that make up the autonomic nervous system.

4   Name the specialist and supportive cells that make up the nervous system.

5   Where is white and grey matter found?

6   How many pairs of cranial nerves are there?

7   How many pairs of spinal nerves are there?

8   Which part of the autonomic nervous system prepares the body for rest and which prepares the body for activity?

9   What is the function of sensory nerves?

10   What is the function of motor nerves?

11   How does the brain respond to the impulses it receives?

12   Which types of nerves are responsible for reflex actions?

13   What is a reflex arc?

14   What types of actions are associated with the autonomic nervous system?

15   Give two actions that are regulated by the sympathetic nervous system.

Task

The special senses include sight, smell, hearing, taste and touch. Make a chart highlighting the special senses and the sensory organ involved with their performance. State how they each contribute to the well-being of the whole body.

Endocrine system

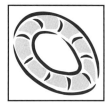

What is the endocrine system?

The endocrine system is closely linked to the nervous system. Together they act as communication centres of the body. The nervous system communicates its messages via electrical impulses and the endocrine system communicates with chemical messengers in the form of hormones. The nervous system is fast acting with immediate responses e.g. reflex actions, whilst the endocrine system is more slow acting and responsible for gradual changes within the body e.g. growth.

The endocrine system consists of a set of ductless glands which are widely spaced around the body with each one being responsible for the production of hormones.

Hormones are chemical substances formed from the components of the food we eat and are either protein-based or fat-based. Hormones have the ability to affect changes in other cells and are secreted directly into the bloodstream and transported to the various systems of the body. Target calls receive the hormones and allow the body to respond to the message and initiate the appropriate changes.

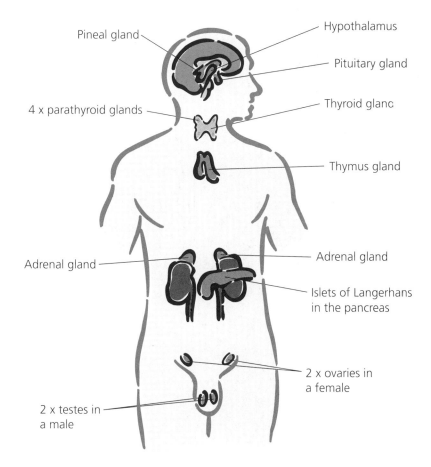

The endocrine system

Endocrine glands and their hormones

Pituitary gland

Situated at the base of the brain behind the nose and consists an anterior (front) and posterior (back) lobes.

Anterior lobe

Produces hormones that control other endocrine glands and other body systems:

- ACTH (adrenocorticotrophic hormone) – controls the cortex of the adrenal gland.
- TSH (thyroid stimulating hormone) (throtrophin) – controls the thyroid gland.
- Gonadotrophins (FSH) (follicle stimulating hormone) and LH (luteinising hormone) – control the ovaries and testes.
- GH (growth hormone) (somatotrophin) – promotes growth of the skeletal and muscular systems.
- PRL (prolactin) – promotes growth of the ovaries, testes and mammary glands and stimulates lactation (milk production) in the breasts.
- MSH (melanocyte stimulating hormone) – promotes the production of melanin (colour pigment) in the skin.

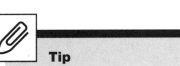

Fascinating Fact

The pituitary gland is also known as the master gland because of its controlling effect on the other glands.

Posterior lobe

Produces two hormones that have an effect on the kidneys and the reproductive organs in females.

- ADH (antidiuretic hormone) (vasopressin) – decreases urine production by the kidneys to regulate fluid balance.
- OT (oxytocin) – stimulates the uterine and mammary gland contraction in preparation for childbirth and breast feeding.

Pineal gland

Situated deep within the brain between the cerebral hemispheres. It is often referred to as the 'third eye' because of its position. Responsible for the hormone melatonin, also known as 'the chemical expression of darkness' as it is produced at night in response to fading daylight.

- **Melatonin** – regulating the daily sleep/wake cycle. monthly menstrual cycle and body rhythms i.e. the cycles of life.

Tip

The pineal gland is thought to be associated with the seasonal affective disorder (SAD). The darker winter months bring about an increased production of melatonin making a person feel tired and sad!

Thyroid gland

Situated just below the larynx and in front of the trachea in the neck. Consists of two lobes and is responsible for the secretion of three hormones in response to the production of TSH in the pituitary gland:

- **Thyroxine** and **Triiodothyronine** – regulate metabolism.
- **Calcitonin** – helps to maintain calcium and phosphorus levels by stimulating the storage of calcium and phosphorus in the bones and the release of excess in urine.

Parathyroid glands

Situated in two pairs on either side of the back of the lobes of the thyroid gland. Responsible for assisting the thyroid gland in the regulation of calcium and phosphorus levels with the production of parathormones:

- PTH (parathormone) – stimulates the reabsorption of calcium and phosphorus when levels in the body are low, from the bones and decreases the amount lost in urine.

Thymus gland

Situated behind the sternum in between the lungs. It is made of lymphatic tissue contributing to the immune functions of the body by producing a group of hormones called thymosins:

- **Thymosin** – stimulates the production of T-lymphocytes to protect the body against antigens (harmful substances).

Adrenal glands

Situated on top of each kidney. Each gland consists of an outer cortex and inner medulla:

Cortex

Produces hormones known as steroids in response to the production of ACTH in the pituitary gland:

- **Glucocorticoids** including cortisol and cortisone – stimulating metabolism, development and inflammation.
- **Mineralocorticoids** including aldosterone – regulating mineral concentration in the body.
- **Gonadocorticoids** including androgens – stimulating sexual development.

Medulla

Produces stress hormones in response to stimulation by the sympathetic nervous system to prepare the body for 'fight or flight':

- **Adrenalin and noradrenalin** – responsible for stimulating body systems needed for physical action e.g. muscular and respiratory, and shutting down those not needed e.g. digestive and urinary.

Islets of Langerhans

Situated in small clusters at irregular intervals within the pancreas. Responsible for the regulation of blood sugar levels with the production of two hormones:

- **Insulin** – reduces blood sugar levels by promoting the storage of excess sugar (glycogen) in the liver and muscles.
- **Glucagon** – increases blood sugar levels by promoting the release of sugar (glycogen) from the liver and muscles.

Ovaries

Situated within the female pelvic girdle on either side of the uterus. Responsible for the secretion of female sex hormones:

- **Oestrogen** and **progesterone** – responsible for the development of secondary sexual characteristics e.g. menarche (start of menstruation), development of breasts, widening of hips and the growth of pubic and axillary hair.

Testes

Situated in the male scrotum which hangs externally from the body under the penis. Responsible for the secretion of the male sex hormone:

- **Testosterone** – responsible for the development of secondary sexual characteristics e.g. production of sperm and semen, the change in voice, development of muscles, bones and male pattern hair growth.

What does the endocrine system do?

The functions of the endocrine system ensure that the changing needs of the body are met in terms of **homeostasis, growth** and **sexual development**.

- Homeostasis is the maintenance of a constant state e.g. body temperature, mineral balance, blood pressure, fluid balance etc.
- Growth occurs in natural phases throughout life with rapid growth in the first year of life, slow, steady growth during

childhood, rapid growth during puberty with growth ceasing at the average age of 16–17.

- Sexual development occurs in stages throughout life starting with puberty in both sexes and ending with menopause in females and andropause in males.

These functions are controlled, communicated and maintained by the links between the nervous and endocrine systems.

The nervous tissue of the hypothalamus in the brain provides the link between the nervous and endocrine systems. It forms an attachment with the pituitary gland allowing two-way communication to take place between the systems.

The hypothalamus receives information from the body through its nerve connections in the cerebrum of the brain. This stimulates the production of releasing hormones in the hypothalamus which regulate the hormone secretion of the pituitary gland. As a result the pituitary gland then produces hormones which control the other endocrine glands. The brain provides additional methods of stimulating hormone production in other endocrine glands by alerting the appropriate glands to changes in the internal and external environment, e.g. the islets of Langerhans in the pancreas are alerted to the changes in blood sugar levels and the adrenal medulla is stimulated by stressful situations.

 Activity

A female between the time of puberty and menopause goes through various stages of hormone release associated with menstruation and the monthly cycle. As a female we should be aware of the fluctuations in hormone release and the effects this has on our body. Pay particular attention to your body over the next month and note the changes that take place and the reactions from those close to you. As a male you should be also be aware of the changes this brings about in the females around you. Pay particular attention to the changes that occur in those close to you. Try to discuss these changes and create greater awareness on all levels.

Knowledge review

1   What is the difference between the endocrine and nervous systems?

2   What is a hormone?

3   What are hormones made from?

4   Which endocrine gland is referred to as the master gland?

5   What is the hormone melatonin associated with?

6   How does the antidiuretic hormone vasopressin contribute to maintaining the body's fluid balance?

7   Where are the parathyroid glands located within the body?

8   Which endocrine glands produce the stress hormones cortisol and adrenalin?

9   Which endocrine gland contributes to the immune functions of the body?

10   Where are the Islets of Langerhans located?

11   Which endocrine glands are responsible for producing male and female sex hormones?

12   Which endocrine gland is often referred to as the 'third eye'?

13   Which endocrine gland is associated with metabolism?

14   Which structure in the brain releases hormones that regulate the hormone secretion in the pituitary gland?

15   What is the meaning of homeostasis?

Task

The menopause is a time when females begin a process that leads to the cessation of menstruation. Research has found that males of a similar age group also experience changes and have named this andropause. Conduct your own research into the effects of menopause and andropause on females and males. Include in your research the possible effects that drugs, complementary treatments and positive thinking may have.

6

The practice

How are massage movements performed?

Although massage as an art is primarily an intuitive skill and as such one that comes from within us, massage as a science is more of an exacting skill requiring the acquisition of knowledge. A balanced use of such skills results in a form of massage that is performed with both intuition and intelligence.

In addition to having a working knowledge of the anatomy (structure) and physiology (function) of the human body, it is also necessary to have knowledge of the specifics pertaining to massage itself including:

- **Terms of reference** – anatomical positions of the body.
- **Classification of movement** – anatomical movements of the body.
- **Tools and Products** – manual/mechanical, use/maintenance
- **Techniques** – massage movements
- **Indications** – suitability for massage
- **Contraindications** – unsuitability for massage
- **Actions** – effects and benefits of massage
- **Contra actions** – possible after effects of massage

Angel advice

In order to perform massage to the greatest good and for the benefit of others, it is necessary to have gained this knowledge. Then and only then can you call yourself a masseuse/masseur in the true sense of the word.

Terms of reference

These are used to describe the various *anatomical positions* of the body and include:

- Median/midline – the centre line through the body
- Anterior – the front of the body
- Posterior – the back of the body
- Medial – towards the midline
- Lateral – away from the midline
- Inferior – closer to the feet
- Superior – closer to the head
- Proximal – nearer to the point of attachment of a limb to the trunk
- Distal – further from the point of attachment of a limb to the trunk
- Palmar – the palm or underside of the hand
- Plantar – the sole or underside of the foot
- Dorsal – the upper or posterior surface
- Longitudinal – running along the body from and to the head and feet.
- Transverse – running across the body.

Technical terms are also used to refer to the *anatomical position* of a client during massage treatment:

- Prone – lying horizontal with the face down
- Supine – lying horizontal with the face up.

Tip

Lateral flexion of the trunk refers to side bending away from the midline.

Classification of movement

These are used to describe the various *anatomical movements* that the body can perform and include:

- Flexion – bending at a joint e.g. bending the elbow.
- Extension – straightening a joint e.g. straightening the elbow.
- Abduction – movement away from the midline of the body e.g. moving the leg outwards.
- Adduction – movement towards the midline of the body e.g. moving the leg inwards.
- Circumduction – a circular movement of a limb and/or its parts in combination with flexion, extension, abduction and adduction e.g. circling the wrist.
- Rotation – circling of a whole limb e.g. circling the arms.
- Dorsiflexion – moving the foot to point the toes upwards e.g. standing on your heels.
- Plantarflexion – moving the foot to point the toes downwards e.g. standing on tiptoes.

- Supination – turning the forearm so that the palm faces upwards.
- Pronation – turning the forearm so that the palm faces downwards.
- Inversion – turning the foot inwards.
- Eversion – turning the foot outwards.

Tools

Massage may be performed manually, mechanically and/or by using a combination of the two.

- Manual massage primarily incorporates the use of the hands although other areas of the arms may be used including forearms and elbows. Massage using the hands is the most common form of massage.
- Mechanical massage incorporates the use of machines that simulate manual massage. They include vibratory, gyratory and vacuum suction machines.

Manual massage

Manual massage relies on the use of the hands to perform different massage techniques that each produce a variety of stimulating effects on the body, mind and spirit.

A prerequisite for performing manual massage is having a knowledge of the anatomy and physiology of the parts of the body as well as of the 'tools of the trade' i.e. the hands and arms.

The bones of the hands and arms form a part of the appendicular skeleton and consist of:

- The shoulder girdle – flat bones called scapulae form the shoulder blades and long bones called clavicles form the collarbones.
- Upper arms – long bones known as humerus bones form the length of the upper arms from shoulders to elbows.
- Lower arms or forearms – long bones known as the ulna and radius form the length of each forearm from elbow to wrist. The ulna is on the little finger side of the forearm and the radius on the thumb side.
- Wrists – eight individual short bones collectively known as the carpals form each wrist.
- Hands – five miniature long bones called metacarpals form the length of each hand from the wrist to the attachment of the fingers/thumb.
- Fingers/thumb – fourteen miniature long bones called phalanges form the fingers and thumbs of each hand. There are three phalange bones to each finger and two to each thumb.

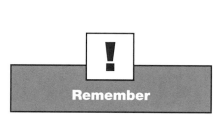

Remember

Other body parts may be used in the application of massage including the feet and/or knees as in **Chavutti Thirumal massage**, **Lomilomi** and **No hands massage**.

Angel advice

A human being is believed to be made up of more than the sum of its parts.

Fascinating Fact

The prominence of the elbow or funny bone as it is commonly referred to is known as the **olecranon process**.

☀ **Activity**

Feel each of the bones of your own hands and arms. Track the length of these bones gently feeling for the joints. Notice how the shape of the bones gives your arms and hands their own unique shape. Compare your hands and arms with those of others and notice the differences in the length and width associated with the shape of the bones.

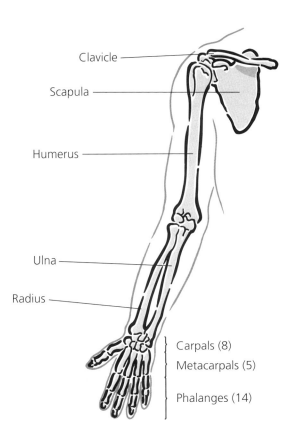

Clavicle

Scapula

Humerus

Ulna

Radius

Carpals (8)
Metacarpals (5)
Phalanges (14)

The shoulder girdle and arm

The bones of the hands and arms are attached to each other by ligaments and form synovial (freely movable) joints including:

- Shoulder – classified as a **ball and socket** joint allowing a maximum range of movement.
- Elbow – where the humerus, ulna and radius meet at the elbow the joint is classified as a **hinge** joint allowing movement of flexion (straightening) and extension (bending) of the lower arm. The joint between the ulna and radius at the elbow is a **pivot** allowing rotational movements as well. These rotational movements allow the arm to **supinate** – turn so that the palm of the hand is facing upwards, and **pronate** – turn so that the palm of the hand is facing downwards.
- Wrist – the joint between the radius and carpals is an **ellipsoid** joint allowing movements of **flexion, extension, abduction** (away from the body) and **adduction** (towards the body). **Plane** joints exist between the individual carpals offering limited **gliding** movements between the bones.
- Fingers – the fingers form **condyloid** joints where the phalange bones meet the metacarpal bones allowing movements associated with flexion, extension, abduction, adduction and limited **rotation**. **Hinge** joints exist

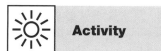

Activity

Starting at your shoulders and extending down to the fingers and thumbs, go through the range of movements in each joint. Check that your joints allow you the freedom of movement stated.

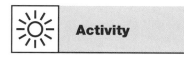

Activity

If you touch your thumb and little finger together you will see the puffy formation on the palm of the hand of the thenar and hypothenar eminences. These muscles help the hand to **grip**.

between the individual phalange bones of each finger allowing flexion and extension only.

- Thumbs – the thumbs form **saddle** joints with the carpal and metacarpal bones allowing an almost full range of movement. Hinge joints exist between the phalange bones of the thumbs themselves allowing flexion and extension only.

The skeletal muscles of the hands and arms are attached to the bones by tendons and include:

- Deltoid muscle – covers the top of the arm and shoulder from the clavicle to the upper part of the humerus. Assists in the movement at the shoulder joint, lifting the arms up, back and forwards.

- Biceps – situated at the front of the upper arm and is responsible for flexion (bending) of the arm at the elbow and supination of the forearm and hand turning the palm upwards.

- Triceps – situated at the back of the upper arm and works in opposition with the biceps to extend the arm.

- Brachialis – situated at the front of the arm below the biceps and works with the biceps to flex (bend) the arm at the elbow.

- Flexor and extensor muscles – situated in the forearm, hand and fingers and responsible for flexing and extending (bending and straightening) the wrist, hand and finger joints.

- Muscles of the **thenar eminence** form at the base of the thumb on the palm and extend down to the wrist.

- Muscles of the **hyothenar eminence** form at the base of the little finger on the palm and extend down to the wrist.

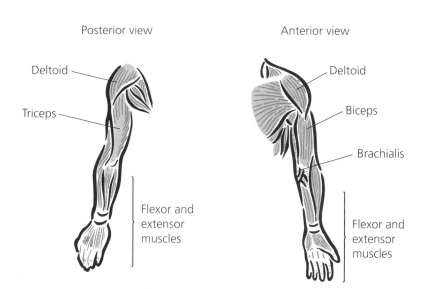

Muscles of the shoulders and arms

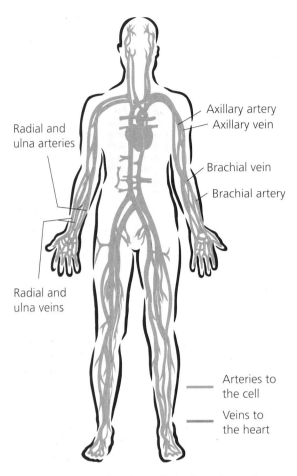

The arteries and veins of the hands and arms

Radial and ulna arteries

Radial and ulna veins

Axillary artery
Axillary vein

Brachial vein

Brachial artery

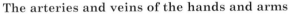

Arteries to the cell

Veins to the heart

Axillary nodes (in the armpit)

Supratrochlear nodes (behind the elbow)

Lymphatic vessels

The lymph nodes of the arm

Circulation

Oxygenated blood is carried to the cells of the hands and arms from the heart by the **axillary, brachial, radial** and **ulnar** arteries.

Carbon dioxide is transported away from the cells of the hands and arms to the heart by the **ulnar, radial, brachial** and **axillary** veins.

Lymph is carried away from the cells of the hands and arms by lymphatic vessels that follow the course of the veins, passing through the following nodes before draining into the thoracic and right lymphatic ducts:

- **Supratrochlear lymph nodes** – in the crook of the elbow draining lymph from the forearm.
- **Axillary lymph nodes** – in the armpit draining lymph from the whole of the arm.

Nerve supply

The peripheral nervous system supplies the hands and arms with a network of nerves radiating from the spinal cord called the

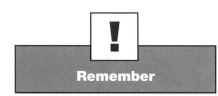

Remember

Manual massage is associated with the use of the hands and as such is a skill that relies on intuition as well as instruction.

brachial plexus. The brachial plexus contains the **radial** and **ulna** nerves that affect the triceps and biceps as well as the skin and muscles down the arm to the fingertips.

This nerve supply enables us to perform and respond to massage through the special sense of touch linking the body and mind to induce feelings of physical and psychological well-being.

Mechanical massage

The introduction of mechanical massage occurred as a direct result of medical developments in the West largely contributing to the fall in the application of manual massage by physicians. Many of the machines developed for the medical profession have been adopted and adapted for the beauty, sports and holistic industries. Their use complements that of manual massage providing the masseur/masseuse with an additional means of massage (detailed information can be found in Part 5).

- Vibratory massage machines – create a tremulous motion causing rapid movements to and fro. Examples include percussion and audio sonic vibrators. Vibratory machines may be used on the body and adapted for use on the face.
- Gyratory massage machines – create a convolution causing circular movements around a central point. Examples include hand-held and free-standing gyratory machines

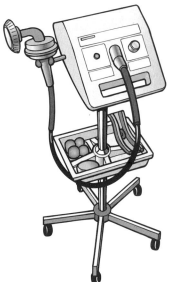

Gyratory machine

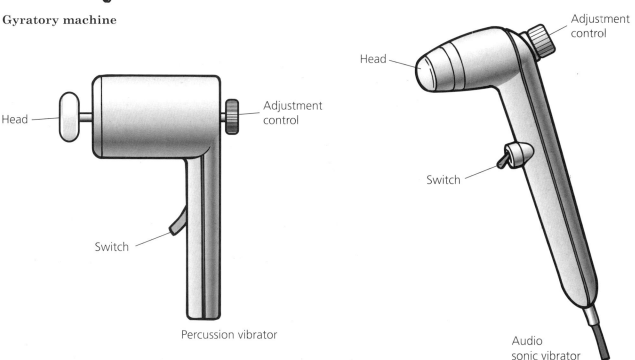

Percussion vibrator

Audio sonic vibrator

Vibratory machines – audio sonic and percussion

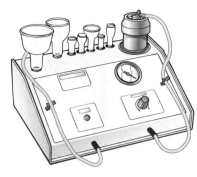

Vacuum suction machine

that are used on the body only and brush cleanse machines that are used on the face and body.

- Vacuum suction massage machines – create a vacuum causing a mild suction effect through pressure. Suction may be intermittent or continuous and can be used on the face and the body.

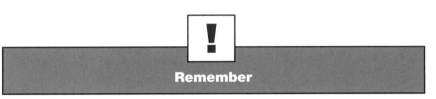

Remember

Mechanical massage is associated with the use of electrical machines and as such is a skill that relies heavily on instruction. Further training in mechanic and electric treatments plus manufacturer's guidance is needed for the application of each machine as they may vary slightly in their application and function.

Tip

Massage oils often contain traces of nuts that are known allergens (a substance that can produce an allergic reaction) e.g. peanut oil etc. Checking the ingredients will avoid unnecessary complications.

Tip

The use of massage cream often encourages desquamation (natural exfoliation) due to the fact that it is easily absorbed. Frequent application of cream will prevent this.

Products

In addition to the tools of the trade manual and mechanical massage also relies on the use of products to enhance their effectiveness including **oil, cream/emulsion, gel** and **powder**:

- Oil – most commonly used massage medium as it provides 'slip' making it easier to perform massage and more comfortable to receive massage.
- Cream/emulsion – a mixture of oil and water. They tend to be more easily absorbed by the skin making the choice of creams and emulsions suitable for smaller, specific areas e.g. hands/feet/face.
- Gel – a jelly-like substance that has a more matt effect on the skin than oils and creams/emulsions making them a good choice for normal and combination skin types.
- Powder – encourages deeper application of massage as it prevents excessive slip. Powder is also useful for greasy skin as it absorbs excess sebum and does not leave the residue commonly associated with oils and creams. It may be necessary to use powder on excessively hairy skin, as it is generally more comfortable.

Fascinating Fact

Swedish massage was traditionally performed using powder as the choice of massage medium. It is not so commonly used in the present day due to the complications associated with excessive inhalation.

Use of products and tools

When using any of the products for massage it is important to discuss their preferences with the person receiving the massage as well as offer advice as to the suitability of each product for the area being treated. Further information relating to the choice and use of products and tools will accompany the **preparation** and **consultation** sections in Part 3 and the **treatment** section in Part 4.

When using any of the tools for massage it is important to be aware that they cannot be used efficiently or effectively without the force of the whole body in terms of **strength** and **flexibility** and **coordination** and **endurance**:

- Strength and flexibility to perform the movements
- Coordination and endurance to perform the movements over a period of time without injury.

Strength, flexibility, coordination and endurance rely on **maintenance, good nutrition, posture** and **mobility**.

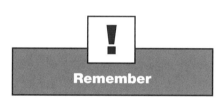

Remember

Care of the hands and arms denotes care for oneself, which in turn makes a person about to be massaged by you feel more confident in your ability to care for them! Lack of self-care may be interpreted by the client as potential lack of care for them.

Maintenance

Attention should be paid to the maintenance of the whole body and in particular the hands and arms. Hands and arms should be smooth, soft and free from cuts, grazes and bruises. Nails should be of a manageable length, clean and free of coloured enamel. It is important that hands are warm and inviting and therefore care should be given to their overall appearance and feel. When using machines for massage, these should be checked prior to use and be maintained to offer a hygienic appearance and an efficient working order. The tools of any trade require regular servicing and updating and you will be judged by the condition of your 'tools'.

An A–Z of common conditions that can affect the hands and arms

- ACROCYANOSIS – poor circulation of the hands and fingers (may also affect feet and toes). A harmless but persistent condition commonly affecting young women.
- ACROMEGALY – abnormal enlargement of the hands (may also affect the feet and face) accompanied by thickening of the skin caused by overproduction of the growth hormone by the pituitary gland.
- ACROPARAESTHESIA – intense tingling or prickly sensation in the fingers (may also affect the toes). May be caused by pressure on a nerve. More common in women, it is though to be associated with the chemical changes in the body caused by menstruation.

- ARTHRITIS – a general term for the inflammation of a joint.
- BUEGER'S DISEASE – progressive destruction of the blood vessels in the hands (and feet). Symptoms include pain, discolouration, numbness, burning and/or tingling and the area feels cold. It can be associated with heavy smoking.
- BURSITIS – inflammation of the bursa (sac-like extension of the synovial fluid) at a joint.
- CALLOUS – hard and thickened skin commonly found on the feet but may be present on the hands due to constant pressure or friction.
- CARPAL TUNNEL SYNDROME – a condition affecting the nerves from the wrist to the hand causing pain and loss of use.
- CHILBLAINS – sore purple swellings that affect the fingers (toes and ears) as a result of exposure to the cold. They may also be caused by poor circulation to the area.
- DIABETES – underproduction of insulin in the pancreas. Sensory nerves in the hands (and feet) may be affected resulting in pins and needles or numbness.
- DUPUYTREN'S CONTRACTURE – a fixed bending forward of the fingers due to the shortening and thickening of fibrous tissue in the palm.
- ECZEMA – a skin condition also known as dermatitis Commonly found on the hands, there are five different types, all of which have several symptoms including redness, swelling, itchiness and blisters.
- EGGSHELL NAILS – very thin nails resulting from defective circulation.
- FROZEN SHOULDER – a condition that develops gradually in the middle-aged and elderly resulting in a severe aching pain in the shoulder and upper arm that tends to get worse at night. Shoulder movements become increasingly restricted.
- FURROWS – ridges in the nails that may run transversely (Beau's lines) and are associated with temporary problems with the production of new cells, or longitudinally which are usually associated with age.
- GANGLION – a harmless swelling that often occurs at a tendon near a joint. Commonly found on the back of the wrist. Other sites include the palm of the hand and the fingers (may also affect feet and ankles).
- GANGRENE – a lack of blood supply will cause the extremities of the body, e.g. fingers and toes, to decay and die. Gangrene may also occur as a result of diabetes, frostbite, bedsores etc.
- GOUT – a disorder affecting the chemical processes of the body. Symptoms include severe pain, swelling and redness within a joint. The joint of the big toe is most commonly affected but ankles and wrists are also common sites. In

Tip

Many people bite or pick at the loose, dry skin associated with hangnails leaving the surrounding area untidy, sore and vulnerable to infection. Hangnails may be removed with cuticle nippers and the surrounding skin moisturised with a hand cream to maintain a neat and tidy appearance and safeguard against infection.

Remember

Tendons attach muscles to bones.

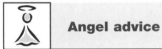

Angel advice

Imagine if a masseur/ masseuse approached you with bitten, picked at and flaky nails. How would this make you feel?

cases of chronic (long-term) gout, hard lumps may develop on the hands and feet.

- HANGNAIL (agnail) – the skin around the nail cuticle becomes loose, dry and ragged.
- HYPERHIDROSIS – excessive sweating affecting areas such as the hands and feet. May be congenital (present at birth) or hormonal.
- KERATOSIS – hard, dry, scaly, flat brown growths which often develop on the back of the hands as a result of long-term exposure to sunshine.
- KOILONYCHIA – spoon shaped nails commonly associated with a deficiency of iron in the diet.
- LEUCONYCHIA – white spots on the nail caused by a superficial knock.
- MALLET FINGER – a finger that cannot be straightened due to damage to the tendon.
- ONYCHATROPHIA – thinning of the nail.
- ONYCHAUXIS – thickening of the nail.
- ONYCHIA – inflammation of the skin under the nail often resulting in the loss of the nail.
- ONYCHOGRYPHOSIS – thickening and curving of the nail, causing it to become claw-like.
- ONYCHOLYSIS – separation of the nail from the underlying skin, the nail bed.
- ONYCHOMADESIS – complete loss of the nail.
- ONYCHOMALCIA – softening of the nail.
- ONYCHOMYCOSIS – fungal disease resulting in white, thickened nails that crumble easily.
- ONYCHOPHAGY – bitten nails.
- ONYCHOPTOSIS – shedding of the nail. May be associated with hair loss.
- ONYCHORRHEXIS – longitudinal splitting of the nail associated with dry, brittle nails and ageing.
- ONYCHOSCHIZIA – flaking nails.
- ONYCHOTILLOMANIA – neurotic picking of the nails.
- OSTEOARTHRITIS – gradual wearing away of cartilage at a joint causing pain, swelling and deformity. Commonly affects the joints of the fingers.
- OSTEOPOROSIS – weakening of the bones which may be caused by changing levels of the hormones oestrogen and progesterone.
- PARONYCHIA – bacterial or fungal infection affecting the skin at the sides of the nails.

Tip

Bacterial or fungal infections are highly contagious and can be passed from person to person.

Angel advice

A regular manicure can help prevent disorders that affect the hands and nails as well as improve circulation and joint mobility.

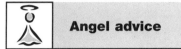

Angel advice

To avoid RSI a masseur/masseuse needs to vary their massage movements as well as the parts of the hands and arms they use. In addition they should ensure adequate resting time between treatments to avoid overuse.

!

Remember

Your hands and arms are the tools of your trade. Do not abuse them – they need care and attention in just the same way as a mechanical machine does i.e. regular servicing!

- PARKINSON'S DISEASE – a condition in which muscular stiffness and tremors develop as parts of the brain degenerate leading to a deficiency of dopamine which aids the transmission of nerve impulses.
- PTERYGIUM – overgrown cuticles that adhere to the nail.
- RAYNAUD'S SYNDROME – numbness and discolouration of the hands, fingers and feet affecting people who are unduly sensitive to the cold. May also be associated with circulatory disorders and/or smoking.
- REPETITIVE STRAIN INJURY (RSI) – excessive, prolonged and repetitive movements cause damage to the joints resulting in swelling, pain and loss of use. The wrist is commonly affected in massage therapists and this may be seen as an occupational hazard.
- RHEUMATISM – a general term used to describe pain affecting the muscles and joints.
- RHEUMATOID ARTHRITIS – progressive destruction of the joints, including those of the wrists and fingers resulting in stiff, swollen joints.
- TENNIS ELBOW – inflammation of the tendons that attach the muscles of the forearm to the elbow, following sudden excessive use of the forearm.
- TENOSYNOVITIS – inflammation of the sheath of tissue around a tendon where it passes over a joint. Commonly affected sites include the wrists and shoulders.
- WARTS – five types including common, plane, plantar, filiform and anogenital. They are all caused by viruses and are contagious. Common warts are rough, skin-coloured and are generally found on the hands.
- WHITLOW – an infection of the soft pad of the fingers or thumbs resulting in severe pain. Often confused with paronychia.

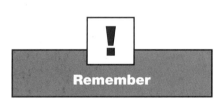

Activity

Book yourself a manicure or give yourself a home treatment. Notice the difference in your hands, nails and cuticles. Try to maintain this effect long term with regular manicures. Perhaps think about trading a body massage for a manicure when you are able!

Nutrition

Movement of the hands and indeed the whole body to perform massage relies on the production of energy within the muscles. This action needs glycogen (the end product of certain foodstuffs) and oxygen (from the air we breathe). Good nutrition results in the production of enough energy to maintain efficient massage over a period of time without suffering adverse effects. Poor nutrition results in weak, fatigued and aching muscles. Good nutrition depends on a well-balanced diet paying attention to recommended norms as well as efficient breathing.

Diet

The body needs a variety of food in order to stay alive including:

- **Carbohydrates** – which are broken down into glucose and taken by the blood to the liver. The liver sends some glucose to the muscles to be stored as muscle glycogen, which is then used with oxygen for the production of energy. The liver also stores some of the glucose itself in the form of glycogen to send to the muscles at a later date, and the rest of the glucose is circulated by the blood to be distributed to the cells with any excess being converted into fat for storage. There are 'fast releasing' carbohydrates such as sugar, sweets and most fast foods which provide us with a quick fix of energy and slow releasing carbohydrates such as whole grains, vegetables and fresh fruit which provide us with a more sustained flow of energy.

- **Proteins** – which are broken down into smaller particles called amino acids, provide the body with the means for growth and repair. The proteins that we eat in the form of eggs, cheese, meat, fish, soya, lentils, peas and beans etc. are broken down into different types of amino acids through the digestive process. These amino acids are then absorbed by the blood and taken to the liver where they are either sent out to be used by the cells of the body, used by the liver cells to form plasma proteins, transaminated – changed from one type to another – or deaminated – those that are not required are broken down further and formed into the waste product urea which is taken to the kidneys by the blood and eliminated from the body in the form of urine.

- **Fats** – which are absorbed into the lymphatic system via lacteals during the digestive process of emulsification before entering the blood flow at the lymphatic ducts, provide the body with another source of fuel. Fats are used to make parts of cells and to provide energy. Any excess fat is removed from the blood and stored until required. There are two main sources of fats including saturated fats or hard fats from dairy products and meat, and unsaturated fats or soft fats from vegetables, nuts and fish. Saturated fats are found in many processed foods and are not as useful to the body as unsaturated fats.

- **Vitamins** – A, B, C, D, E and K are absorbed by the blood from the digested foods from which they originate and are necessary for the help they provide to every process within the body. Excess vitamins can be stored in the body to be called upon in the event of deficiency, which may occur for

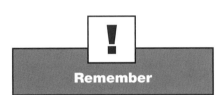

Remember

Any excess fat is stored in the body as fatty tissue forming the hypodermis, which lies between the dermis and the muscles. This fatty tissue may be used for energy in the event of lack of food e.g. dieting.

 Fascinating Fact

Cholesterol forms the waxy substance responsible for blocking arteries. It is essential in the body for the formation of cells and hormones and is formed in the liver as well as being present in our diet. Saturated fats contain cholesterol and eating an excess of this type of fat is one of the causes of heart attacks due to the clogging of vital arteries. It also contributes to the formation of gallstones in the gall bladder.

example during dieting. Vitamins A and B12 are stored in the liver and vitamins A, D, E and K, which are fat-soluble, are stored in the fat cells.

- **Minerals** – such as iron, calcium, sodium, chloride, potassium, phosphorous, magnesium, fluoride, zinc, selenium etc. are absorbed in much the same way as vitamins and are also necessary to assist the various processes that take place within the body. Surplus minerals are either not absorbed so lost from the body in faeces, or taken to the kidneys and lost through urine excretion.

- **Fibre** – is tough fibrous carbohydrate that cannot be digested. Insoluble fibre such as cellulose found in wheat bran, fruit and vegetables make it easier for faeces to pass along the large intestine by adding bulk. This bulk absorbs water making the faeces soft. The muscular layer of the large intestine is stimulated by the bulk and as a result, the waste leaves the body more quickly reducing the risk of constipation and infection.

- **Water** – is often referred to as the forgotten nutrient. Water is a necessary component of a good diet in order to maintain the body's fluid balance and prevent dehydration.

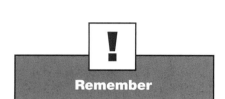

Remember

It is recommended that up to five portions of fruit and vegetables are included in your daily diet along with a balanced intake of the other nutrients. It is also important to drink between one and two litres of water a day.

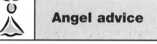

Angel advice

Ensure regular meals are eaten allowing adequate time for digestion to take place prior to giving or receiving massage.

Tip

It is best to ensure that a person has not *just eaten* or *not eaten for a long time* prior to giving or receiving any form of manual and/or mechanical massage. When a person has just eaten the blood is directed to the digestive organs and the giving and receiving of massage will redirect blood to the skin and muscles disturbing the digestive process. When a person has not eaten for a long time, the activity involved in giving and receiving massage will stimulate the body's need for food and initiate feelings of discomfort associated with hunger.

Breathing

The body can live a few weeks without food, a few days without water but only a few minutes without air. Poor breathing results in a reduction in the amount of oxygen available for each cell, causing the body to experience many problems including muscle cramps, headaches, anxiety, chest pains, tiredness etc. An awareness of the way in which we should breathe is crucial in avoiding such problems:

- **Lateral costal** – normal breathing, where the lungs take in enough oxygen to accommodate everyday activities.
- **Apical** – shallow and rapid breathing is used when the body wants to get maximum amounts of oxygen to the

muscles. Examples of those times include exercise, childbirth, stress, fear etc.

- **Diaphragmatic** – deep breathing associated with the period of relaxation that follows a period of activity and the associated shallow breathing.

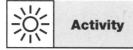 **Activity**

Take a few moments during the course of each day to concentrate on your own breathing. Try to learn to match your breathing to the needs of your body and ensure a period of relative inactivity follows a period of increased activity.

Posture

The body is maintained in an upright position through the amount of tone present in the core postural muscles. This tone should be balanced enabling us to stand straight and tall with shoulder and pelvic girdles centred, spine erect and head and limbs relaxed. All too often these muscles find themselves in an imbalanced state due to the stresses and strains exerted on them by poor posture, resulting in common figure faults such as rounded shoulders, protruding tummy etc. (see Chapter 8 for more details).

To avoid such figure faults and resulting pain and discomfort care should be given to maintain good posture generally:

- Weight should be evenly distributed between both legs and feet.
- Knees should be kept soft, never overextended.
- Pelvic girdle should be centred helping to keep the abdomen and buttocks tucked in.
- The curve of the waist should be even on both sides.
- Shoulder girdle should be centred with shoulders, arms and hands gently relaxed.
- Head should be held with the chin running parallel to the floor with even tone in the muscles at the front, back and sides of the neck.

Maintaining correct posture generally contributes to the overall well-being of the body in the following ways:

- It allows full, deep and unrestricted breathing to take place.
- Digestion is more efficient as organs are prevented from being compressed in the abdomen.
- Postural problems are avoided due to an even distribution of body weight.

- Figure faults are eliminated resulting in a more flattering body image.

In addition, it is of prime importance to maintain good posture whilst giving massage to prevent excessive strain and permanent injury. **Stride standing** and **walk standing** provide the basis for good posture whilst performing massage.

Stride standing

Used when working transversely i.e. across the area.

- Stand facing the couch with your feet hip distance apart
- Turn your feet out slightly.
- Keep knees soft and unlocked.
- Keep hips forward and bottom tucked in.
- Forearms should be at right angles to the body.
- Hands and wrists held loosely.
- Shoulders should be relaxed.
- When working on the nearside of the couch, bend your knees more to avoid straining your back.
- When working on the far side of the couch, straighten your legs as necessary to reach.

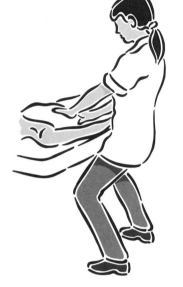

Stride standing

Angel advice

Your weight should be evenly distributed for stride standing enabling you to perform massage using the whole of your body without straining any one part.

Walk standing

Used when working longitudinally i.e. along the length of the area.

- Stand in line with the couch at one side facing forwards.
- Position your feet as if to form a lunge by placing the nearside leg behind you and the far side leg in front.
- The nearside foot should be turned out and the far side foot should be facing forward.
- Keep knees soft and unlocked.
- Keep hips forward and bottom tucked in.
- Shoulders, arms and hands should be relaxed.
- Work up the length of the body by transferring your weight from the back nearside foot to the front far side foot.

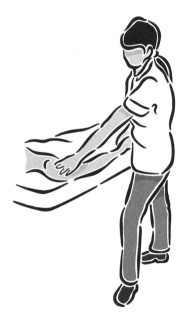

Walk standing

Activity

Practice these positions for yourself. Initially they may feel awkward and unnatural and you may even experience aching in certain muscles as a result. Your body needs to learn to adapt to the needs of the positions and in doing so will become stronger and more resilient.

Angel advice

You can learn to easily pivot between stride and walk standing as you change the direction of your massage.

Maintaining the correct body posture or stance helps to ensure an application of massage that is rhythmical and flowing and is applied with the correct amount of pressure suited to the needs of the area being treated. Correct posture therefore helps to ensure a safe treatment for both the client and the practitioner.

Posture is also important when receiving a massage and care should be taken to ensure that a person is correctly positioned prior to any massage treatment taking place. Most commonly a person lies on a specially prepared couch or sits in a chair for massage although variations to this may occur e.g. lying on a bed, sitting/lying on the floor.

Tip

It may be that you need to alter your standing position to accommodate the position of the person receiving the massage. This may incorporate you maintaining the stride and walk positions but from a kneeling position. Practice makes perfect!

Lying down for massage

This provides access to the whole of the body and is the most common position for the application of a full body massage. It may be necessary to give additional support in the form of pillows or rolled up towels to avoid discomfort when a person is lying on either their back or front depending on their natural posture. In some cases it may be necessary for a person to lie on their side for massage e.g. if they are unable to lie flat due to pregnancy, spinal problems etc.

Tip

When a person is lying on their back the position is known as **supine**. When a person is lying on their front the position is known as **prone**.

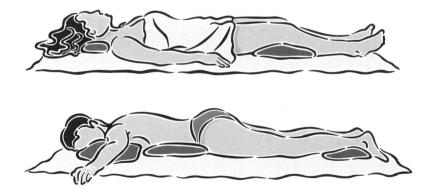

Laying down for massage – supine and prone positions

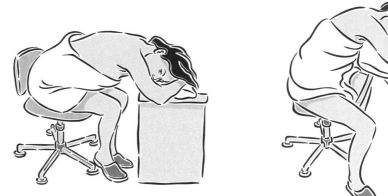

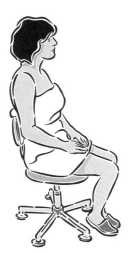

Sitting down for massage

Sitting down for massage

There are many ways in which a person's position sitting in a chair may be adapted for massage including:

- Sitting normally with the person's back being supported by the back of the chair. This position provides access to the hands and arms, feet and legs as well as upper back, shoulders, neck and head if the back support is low.
- Sitting in a low backed chair leaning forward and resting the upper body on a support e.g. couch, table or bed etc. This provides access to the back.
- Straddling the chair with a pillow resting on the back of the chair and the person resting their upper body for support. This provides access to the back.

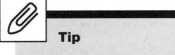

Tip

Special massage chairs are constantly being developed and re-developed to provide varied seated positions for the application of massage.

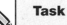

!

Remember

Any variations in the positioning of a person for massage should ensure that they are adequately supported, comfortable and safe and are free to move should they need to.

Task

Obtain brochures from at least three massage equipment manufacturers. Note the different variations of couches/chairs in terms of size, shape and function. Try to attend a trade exhibition, go to an equipment sales room and/or check out the couches and chairs available at your college, salon, or on the Internet etc. Make a report on at least three different couches/chairs outlining the pros and cons of each. Include in your report a free-standing and portable couch and at least one style of chair.

Mobility

Keeping the hands and arms mobile will contribute to the correct application of the massage techniques as well as improve the overall health and fitness of the parts.

Angel advice

It is also necessary to ensure that the rest of your body is fit and healthy by taking part in regular exercise. The recommended norm is to exercise for twenty minutes three times a week. Always seek professional advice before starting any exercise to ensure your personal safety and never exercise beyond your capability.

Angel advice

You may notice that the shoulder girdle feels tighter when you roll the shoulders backwards. Completing more backward rolls will help to rectify this. You may also experience greater stiffness in one shoulder than the other. Concentrate more on the stiff shoulder, taking care to avoid excessive strain until both sides feel more or less equal.

Strength, flexibility, coordination and endurance can be achieved through regular hand and arm exercises:

- Ensure you are neither hungry nor tired so that the body is able to cope with the increase in activity.
- Pay attention to good standing posture – this will ensure correct execution of exercises.
- Take three deep breaths, breathing in through the nose and breathing out through the mouth – this will start to relax you and prepare the body for exercise.
- Continue to concentrate on good breathing – this will ensure the cells receive adequate oxygen in order to complete the exercises.
- Relax by gently shaking your arms and hands to warm the area and stimulate the circulation.
- Mobilise the joints by rolling each shoulder forwards a few times and then backwards. Continue by working both shoulders alternately.
- With your arms by your side, continue to mobilise by turning each arm so that the palms face backwards and follow this movement by turning each arm so that the palms face forwards.
- Circle your wrists first one way and then the other.
- Circle your fingers and thumbs one way and then the other.
- Improve flexibility by making a fist and then straighten your fingers/thumbs.
- Aid coordination and endurance by tapping your fingers in the air as if playing a piano.
- Hold your hands out in front of you and try to separate the fingers one by one.
- Now sit down observing good posture as you do so – ensuring legs are kept uncrossed.
- Improve your hand and eye coordination by making a fist and striking it down gently on your legs (i).
- Lift your hands and isolate your thumbs before placing them down onto your legs (ii).
- Lift your hands and isolate the first two fingers before placing them down onto your legs (iii).

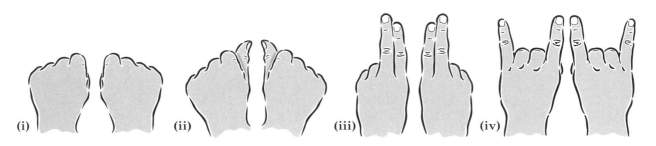

Hand exercises

- Lift your hands and isolate the index and little fingers before placing them down onto your legs (iv).
- Repeat this routine a few times until it becomes easy to do with both hands.
- Finish by standing up and gently shake your hands and arms.

It is useful to perform these hand and arm exercises regularly, especially when you are first learning massage. Once you are able to perform a massage treatment effectively these exercises are not as important although care should be taken to ensure that the shoulders, arms and hands are relaxed and warm prior to use. It may also be necessary to adapt the exercises post-massage in order to aid relaxation and prevent stiffness.

Techniques

Traditional manual massage (Swedish massage) incorporates the use of four basic techniques which may all be simulated by mechanical massage machines and are classified using their original French names: effleurage, petrissage, frottage and tapotement.

- **Effleurage** from the verb *effleurer* meaning 'to skim the surface by lightly stroking'.
- **Petrissage** from the verb *petrir* meaning 'to knead'.
- **Frottage** from the verb *frotter* meaning 'to rub'. Frottage is more commonly classified as **friction.**
- **Tapotement** from the verb *tapoter* meaning 'to tap'. Tapotement is often classified as **percussion** from the Latin noun *percutere* meaning 'to strike forcibly'.

Further classifications of massage have been identified since the introduction of the basic four including vibration, joint manipulation and holding:

- **Vibration** – a form of massage that creates rapid oscillation (movement to and fro).
- **Joint manipulation** – assisted movement performed to take a joint through its full range.
- **Holding** – a positive touch or hold involving the initial application of the hands onto the area to be treated and the final removal of the hands at the close of the treatment.

So how are massage movements performed?

Massage movements are traditionally performed with the palmar surface of the hands including the palm, thenar eminence and hypothenar eminence, palmar surface of the finger/thumbs and pads of the fingers/thumbs.

For each of the massage techniques there follows an introductory explanation and a method of application. Practice the methods by using your hands on an imaginary body first. This will help you to maintain the correct posture and appropriate execution of the movements. You may even try some of the movements on yourself. It is unadvisable to attempt any of the massage techniques on a person for the first time without supervision. A **suggested order of work** for each part of the body accompanies Part 4 of this book together with treatment considerations, adaptations and progression. Part 5 looks at the advanced massage techniques as well as complementary massage techniques.

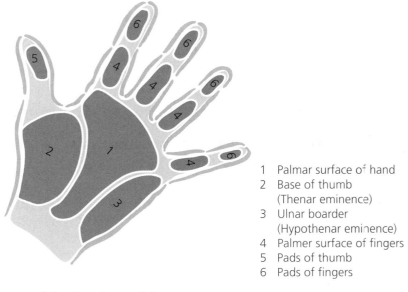

1 Palmar surface of hand
2 Base of thumb (Thenar eminence)
3 Ulnar boarder (Hypothenar eminence)
4 Palmer surface of fingers
5 Pads of thumb
6 Pads of fingers

Areas of the hands used for massage

Effleurage

Effleurage is a surface movement performed at the start, middle and end of a massage routine for each part of the body being treated. Effleurage is used to introduce the hands to the area being treated, to introduce the massage medium if used e.g. oil, cream/emulsion, gel or talc, to link other massage movements and to end the massage routine. Effleurage movements are gently stimulating and relaxing. Effleurage is performed with the palmar (palm side) surface of the hands either in **any direction** or with **directional pressure** towards the heart:

Effleurage in any direction – whole or part of the palmar surface of the hands and/or fingers/thumbs is used with equal pressure to stroke in any direction. Hands may be used together or alternately.

Method

- Ensure your hands and arms are relaxed and warm.
- Prepare the client making sure they are comfortable and warm.
- Isolate the area to be worked ensuring all other areas are adequately covered.
- Think about your posture in relation to the part to be massaged and get into the correct position i.e. walk or stride standing.
- Apply the massage medium to your own hands before making contact with the client.
- Stroke your hands gently over the area to be treated in any direction covering the whole of the area with an even application of massage medium.
- Try to apply a light, even, stroking pressure by moulding your hands to the surface of the area.
- Try using your hands together if the area allows and/or alternately making sure that as one hand finishes a stroke the other hand starts a stroke.

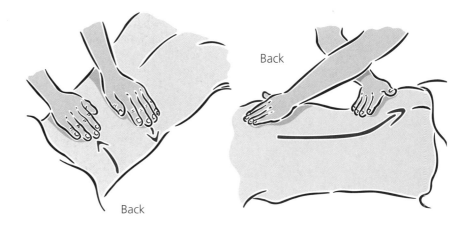

Back

Back

Hands

Feet

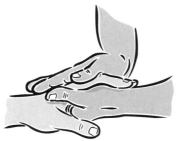

Effleurage in any direction

Directional effleurage – effleurage or stroking with pressure directed to the heart whereby the whole of the palmar surface of the hands and/or fingers/thumbs is used to cover the area being treated. The pressure builds as the stroke comes to an end, helping to direct the flow of venous blood towards the heart and flow of lymph towards the nearest lymph nodes and ducts. Hands may be used together or alternately.

Method

- On larger areas like the back place one hand next to the other and direct the strokes upwards either together or alternately.
- Gradually increase your pressure as you reach the top of the area.
- Slide your hands back to the beginning with *no* pressure.
- On smaller areas like the limbs place one hand above the other and direct your stroke upwards, once again returning with *no* pressure.
- On smaller areas still, support with one hand and use the other to gently stroke with pressure towards the heart.

Tip

Directional effleurage may also be referred to as **draining**. Deoxygenated blood is drained from the cells via veins towards the heart and lymph is drained from the cells towards the lymph nodes and ducts.

! Remember

Venous blood and lymph flow rely on movement to stimulate circulation – massage provides the necessary stimulation.

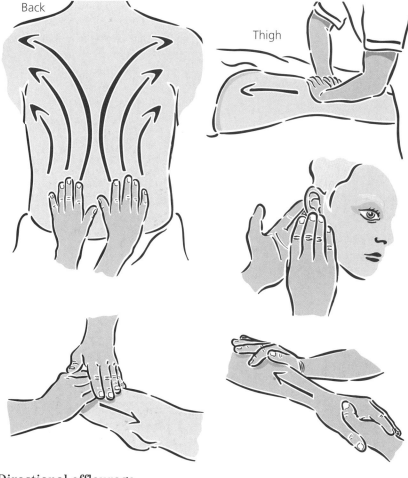

Directional effleurage

Effleurage should be used lightly to start, allowing the pressure to build as a rhythm is established. Pressure is gradually reduced at the end of a routine until only a light stroking pressure may be felt.

Task

It is important to note that no pressure should ever be applied over the soft underside of the elbow or knee joints, the groin and armpit areas and the middle of the neck. Knowledge of anatomy and physiology will help you to understand the possible adverse effects of applying excessive pressure on the underlying structures. Make an outline drawing of the whole body and pencil in the main veins, lymph nodes and lymphatic ducts. Use this diagram to remind you of the direction in which to apply directional effleurage and why.

Petrissage (foulage)

Tip

Shampooing and conditioning one's hair incorporates the use of kneading massage movements. As you work in the shampoo your hands/fingers/thumbs are performing *superficial kneading* and as you work in the conditioner pressing more firmly as you do so, you are performing *deep kneading*.

Petrissage involves a series of deep movements performed after effleurage movements when the area to be treated is warm and the person receiving the massage is accustomed to the feel and pressure of the touch. Petrissage is then used with varying amounts of pressure to manipulate the deeper tissues associated with the skin as well as the underlying muscles. Petrissage movements are deeply stimulating and relaxing. Petrissage may be performed with the whole of the hands and/or their parts i.e. fingers, thumbs or knuckles. Variations of petrissage massage include **kneading, picking up, wringing, rolling** and **knuckling**:

Kneading – the palmar surface of the hands, fingers and/ or thumbs are used to perform circular movements over the underlying tissue. The movements may be superficial and/ or deep with the pressure applied on the upward portion of the circular movement forcing the superficial tissue to move over the deeper tissue. Kneading may be performed as single, alternate, double and/or reinforced movements.

Single-handed palmar kneading – sometimes referred to as **flat-handed** kneading in which one hand performs singular circular movements. The other hand may be used to give support. Single-handed palmar kneading is used on small areas of the body.

Method

- Prepare the area with effleurage.
- Place one hand on the area to be treated and gently but firmly make a circle on the spot. Apply pressure on the

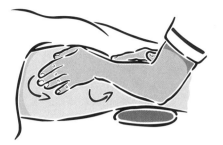

Single-handed palmar kneading

upward curve of the movement reducing the pressure on the downward curve.

- Feel the underlying tissues move under the pressure of your hands.
- Repeat a few times before moving to another area.

Alternate palmar kneading – both hands are used with one hand working before the other in a rhythmical manner. Alternate palmar kneading may be used on the limbs especially when working opposing muscle groups.

Method

- Prepare the area with effleurage.
- Place a hand on each muscle/muscle group to be treated.
- Apply single-handed kneading with one hand but as you complete the upward portion of the circle begin the movement with the other hand.
- Work both hands in this way for a few circles before moving onto another area.

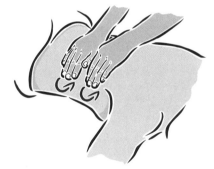

Alternate palmar kneading

Tip

The rhythm of this movement is similar to that which you would make if you were mimicking the movement of the wheels of a steam train.

Double-handed palmar kneading – both hands work side by side to cover a larger surface area e.g. back.

Method

- As for single-handed kneading but the two hands work together alongside one another to cover a larger surface area.

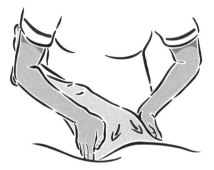

Double-handed palmar kneading

Reinforced palmar kneading – one hand is placed on top of the other hand to provide a deeper form of kneading often referred to as ironing.

Method

- As for single-handed kneading except that one hand is placed directly on top of the other so that greater depth of pressure may be applied.

Finger kneading – small circles are performed with the pads of the index, middle and/or ring fingers. Fingers may be used alone or together depending on the size of the area to be treated.

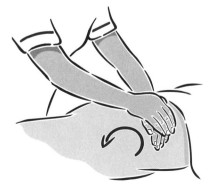

Reinforced palmar kneading

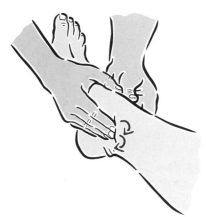

Finger kneading

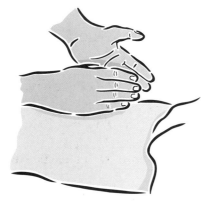

Thumb kneading

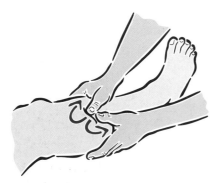

Border of the hand kneading

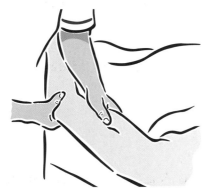

Single-handed picking up

Method

- Prepare the area with effleurage and whole hand kneading.
- Isolate a small area and apply a small circular movement using one or more fingers.
- Apply the pressure with the upward curve of the circle reducing the pressure with the downward curve.
- Do not allow the fingers to fully extend.
- Move rhythmically onto another area after each circle.

Thumb kneading – small circles are performed with the pads of the thumb in the same way as finger kneading.

Border of the hand kneading – the inner and/or outer pads of the palm of the hands, i.e. thenar eminence of the thumb border and hypothenar eminence of the little finger border, may be used for greater pressure in specific areas e.g. the temple area of the skull.

Method

- Turn the hand to either side and make circular on-the-spot movements.
- Ensure the pressure is applied with the upward curve of the movement, reducing the pressure with the downward curve.

Picking up – the palmar surface of the hands are used to pick up, hold and release the underlying tissue. Picking up may be performed single or alternate handed.

Single-handed picking up – one hand is used to support the area whilst the other hand performs the movement by placing the fingers under the tissue and the thumb above the tissue. The emphasis is placed on the movement of the fingers as the thumb provides support.

Method

- Prepare the area with effleurage and kneading if required.
- Using one hand to gently but firmly 'pick up' the bulk of the tissue, apply a squeeze of pressure and release.
- Move up to the next area.
- Move up the area in a rhythmical manner always directing the pressure upwards.
- Movements may be linked with effleurage.

Alternate handed picking up – both hands are used to alternately pick up the underlying tissue in a rhythmical manner i.e. as one hand starts a movement the other finishes. The pressure

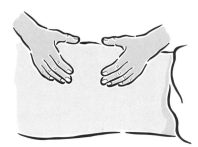

Alternate-handed picking up

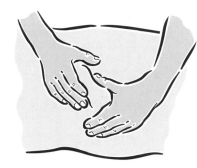

Wringing

is applied on the upward lift, increased on the squeeze and reduced on the downward release.

Wringing – the palmar surface of both hands are used alternately to gently lift the underlying tissue and work it against itself in a 'wringing' action.

Method

● Prepare the area with effleurage.

● The tissue is grasped with the palmar surface of both hands and lifted away.

● One hand lifts towards the body and the other hands lifts away from the body.

● This results in a wringing action.

● The hands repeat the action in the other direction.

Tip

This movement mimics the action you would make if wringing out a wet towel.

Rolling – the palmar surface of both hands is used to gently roll the underlying tissue. May be used superficially to roll the surface tissue i.e. skin and/or deeply roll the deeper tissue i.e. muscle.

Method

● Prepare the area with effleurage.

● When working the nearside of the body, press the tissue with the thumbs and extend the fingers.

● Move the fingers towards the thumbs rolling the underlying tissue.

● When working the far side of the body press the tissue with the fingers and extend the thumbs.

● Move the thumbs towards the fingers rolling the underlying tissue.

● When working the centre of a muscle/muscle group roll both ways.

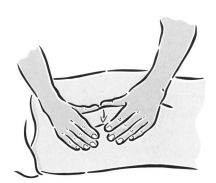

Rolling

Knuckling – the knuckles are used to apply small circular movements to an area. Hands may be used singly, alternately or together.

Method

● Curl your hands into loose fists.

● Using the middle section of your fingers circle each knuckle in turn starting with the little finger.

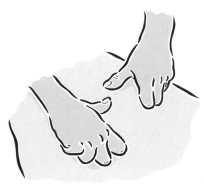

Knuckling

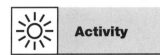

Tip

Greater depth can be achieved if the petrissage movements are performed slowly and rhythmically. The quicker the movement, the more superficial it becomes.

Activity

Practice the different petrissage movements on various parts of the body learning to adapt the choice of movement and depth of pressure according to the underlying tissue.

- Press the underlying tissue feeling it gently ripple beneath your fingers.

Petrisssage movements should be used with consideration for the underlying structures and the amount of pressure adapted to avoid any discomfort. Petrissage movements may be used in any order and combination as long as effleurage is used to precede, link and end the routine.

Task

Petrissage movements are deeper and more vigorous than effleurage movements and are therefore more stimulating to the underlying tissue. Using the anatomy and physiology section of this chapter for reference, write an essay about the ways in which the skeletal muscles are affected by poor posture, overwork, ageing and excessive strain. This will help you to appreciate the ways in which petrissage movements can be of benefit.

Friction (frottage)

Friction movements are the deepest of all Swedish massage movements. Frictions are used with a pressure that may remain constant throughout the movement or be progressively increased. Frictions work deeply to stimulate, relax and ease tense, fatigued and aching muscles. Frictions are generally performed with the fingers or thumbs and may be applied in a circular movement and/or transversely across the muscle fibres.

Circular friction – small circular movements performed in localised areas with the fingers or thumbs.

Tip

Localised areas of tension often feel hard and lumpy and painful to touch. Use your hands to sensitively seek out these areas by means of effleurage and petrissage movements before isolating them with the application of frictions.

Method

- Prepare the area with effleurage and petrissage movements.
- As result of this localised areas of tension may be identified and worked on with frictions.
- Use the pads of the fingers or thumbs to apply localised circular pressure.
- Press more firmly and more deeply into the tissue as you continue to circle.
- Take care not to overextend the joints of the fingers or thumbs.
- Do not use beyond a person's tolerance.

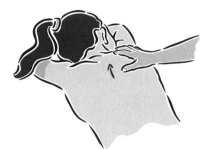

Circular friction

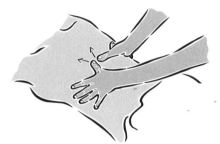

Transverse friction

● Release the pressure completely before moving onto another localised area of tension.

Transverse friction – thumbs or fingers are used to work *across* a localised area of tension.

Method

● Prepare the area with effleurage and petrissage movements as appropriate.

● Isolate the localised area of tension and using the pads of the thumbs or fingers apply even pressure backwards and forwards.

● Take care not to strain the fingers or thumbs by overextending their joints.

● Fingers/thumbs may be used singly or alternately.

Friction movements should not be confused with finger/thumb kneading which aims to apply pressure in the upward curve of circular movements. Friction movements are used to apply localised pressure only and may be used quickly and superficially to generate surface stimulation and/or slowly and deeply to stimulate more deeper level stimulation.

Tip

The pads of the index, middle, ring fingers and thumbs are commonly used for frictions although the borders of the hands may also be used. The index finger offers the most amount of pressure and the ring finger the least. Thumbs offer even more pressure. The index finger may be reinforced with the middle finger for greater depth of pressure.

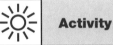

Activity

When performing frictions the fingers or thumbs do not glide over the area; instead they stay stationary and 'rub' the underlying layers of tissue which have become knotted and tight with increasing pressure as the movement progresses. Take care when finding these localised areas of tension as once found it is easy to 'fall off' them, which in turn causes discomfort. Try to locate areas of tension in your own body by gently feeling over the area along the top of your shoulders. As you locate a lumpy area stop and apply friction movements. Do not worry if you do not have any lumpy areas – this means you have little or no tension in your shoulders! Learn to become sensitive in your approach to the needs of the body and learn to match the application of massage movements accordingly. Remember this will not happen overnight. Instead it requires hours of experiential learning, which will never come to an end!

Tapotement/percussion

Tapotement and percussion movements are movements that involve a repetitious tapping or striking of the body. Tapotement and percussion movements are used to stimulate and invigorate and may be applied with varying amounts of pressure. They are performed briskly and rapidly after the area being treated has first been warmed by effleurage and petrissage movements. Tapotement movements include **butterfly, flicking, plucking/snatching, whipping, hacking, cupping, pounding** and **beating**:

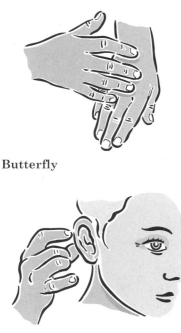

Butterfly

- **Butterfly** – the tips of the fingers and thumbs are used to gently tap the surface tissue. The light pressure may be likened to the gentle fluttering of butterfly wings against the skin. Commonly used on the face and scalp.
- **Flicking** – the index finger and thumb are used together to lightly flick the surface tissue. Commonly used on the ears.
- **Plucking/snatching** – the tips of the fingers and thumbs are used to gently pluck or snatch the surface tissue. Commonly used on the fingers and toes.
- **Whipping** – the whole of the hands are used to gently roll over the surface tissue in a whipping action. Commonly used on the fingers and toes.

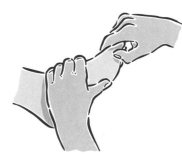

Flicking

Tip

Butterfly, flicking, snatching and whipping are all applied with light pressure and may be classified as being more **tapotement**-type movements as they involve a form of **'tapping'**.

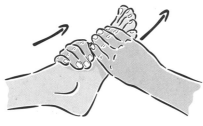

Plucking/snatching

Percussion movements involve greater pressure and stimulation and as such are generally used on fleshier areas of the body only. They include:

- **Hacking** – the hands are held over the body with the palms facing one another. The lateral sides of the hands (little finger side) are used alternately to gently strike the surface tissue. Hands are relaxed; fingers are open and elbows bent outwards with the movement coming from the wrist.

Whipping

Tip

When hacking is applied correctly, the fingers should gently flop against one another making a slight slapping sound as they come into contact with each other. If done incorrectly the fingers will remain static and perform a movement similar to a karate chop! This will be painful for the receiver and likely to cause bruising.

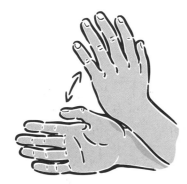

Hacking

● **Cupping** – the hands are cupped and used alternately to gently strike the surface tissue so that the underside of the 'cup' makes contact. Suction is produced as the hands are raised creating a stimulating effect.

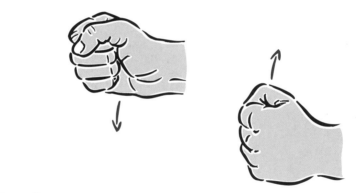

Cupping

● **Pounding** – the hands are made into loose fists, which are used alternately to gently strike the surface tissue. The lateral (little finger side) side of the hand makes contact before springing back up with a slight flick, making this a firm but bouncy movement.

Pounding

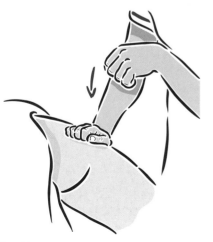

● **Beating** – similar to pounding except the knuckles of the fist strike the surface tissue. Like pounding, the hands are used alternately with brisk, bouncy pressure and lifted with a slight flick.

Beating

Tip

Hacking, cupping, pounding and beating are all applied with a firm pressure and may be classified as being more **percussion**-type movements as they involve a form of '**striking**'.

The use of tapotement and percussion movements should be avoided over bony areas of the body and must always be linked with effleurage movements to re-establish relaxation.

☀ Activity

It is useful to practice tapotement and percussion movements on a pillow first! This will help you to perfect the techniques without causing damage to yourself or another person. Monitor your progress by gradually trying the techniques on yourself.

- Try the butterfly movements on your face. They are especially good when used to 'stipple' toners or moisturisers into the skin.
- Try the flicking movements over your ears to warm and stimulate.
- Try the plucking/snatching and whipping movements on your feet to encourage the blood flow to the tips of the toes.
- Try cupping, hacking, pounding and beating on the fleshy parts of your upper thigh. Practice equally on both legs to get used to different positions but also to avoid overstimulation of one area.

Notice when and why a movement feels right. Notice also how it feels if the movement is incorrectly applied and learn to correct it. If in any doubt always ask for further supervision.

Vibration

Vibration movements produce tremors in the underlying tissues. Vibrations are used to gently shake the skin and muscles freeing them of built up tension. Vibrations are performed with the palmar surface of the hands, fingers or thumbs and include **static, moving** and **shaking**:

Static vibration – the underlying tissue is vibrated using the hands/fingers or thumb in a static position.

Method

- Prepare the area with effleurage and petrissage movements as appropriate.
- Place the hands/fingers/thumbs onto the area to be treated.
- Tense the arm so that you cause it to gently vibrate.

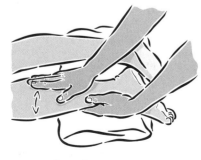

Static vibration

- The tremors travel down the arm to the hands/fingers/thumbs having an effect on the underlying tissue.

Moving vibration – the underlying tissue is vibrated using the hands/fingers or thumbs in a moving action running up or down the area being treated.

Method

- Performed as for static vibrations but instead of keeping the hands/fingers/thumbs still they are moved up or down the area being treated.

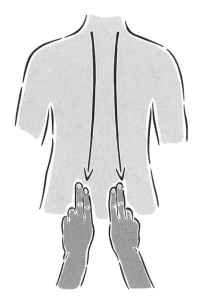

Moving vibration

Shaking – a more vigorous form of vibration in which the muscles are physically grasped and then shaken. Shaking can be performed with one hand whilst the other hand acts as support or alternatively may be performed two-handed.

Method

- Prepare the area with effleurage and petrissage movements as appropriate.
- Grasp and lift smaller muscles with one hand whilst using the other hand for support.
- Grasp and lift larger muscles/groups with both hands.
- Ensure that the muscles are relaxed before gently shaking from side to side.

Vibrations should be used with care and knowledge of the underlying muscle structure.

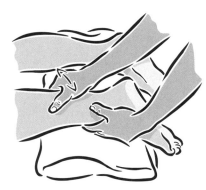

Shaking

Joint manipulation

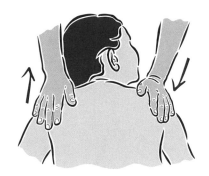

Rocking

Joint manipulation movements are movements which when performed assist the range of movement possible where bone meets bone at a synovial (freely moveable) joint. Joint manipulation movements are performed after the area has been warmed with effleurage, petrissage and friction movements to encourage greater ease of movement and include **rocking, rotation, stretching** and **twisting**:

- **Rocking** – a body part is rocked rhythmically from side to side or back and forth e.g. shoulder girdle to encourage correct alignment.
- **Rotation** – a supported movement taking a joint with rotational functions through its natural range of movements. The part is rotated first one way and then the other e.g. wrists, ankles, fingers and thumbs.

Feet Hands

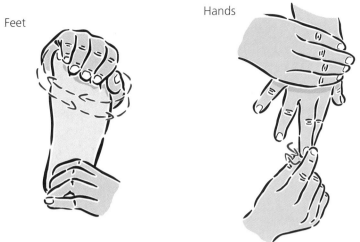

Rotation

● **Stretching** – involving a gentle pull to the area to relieve pressure in joints and ligaments, muscles and tendons.

Feet Hands Ears

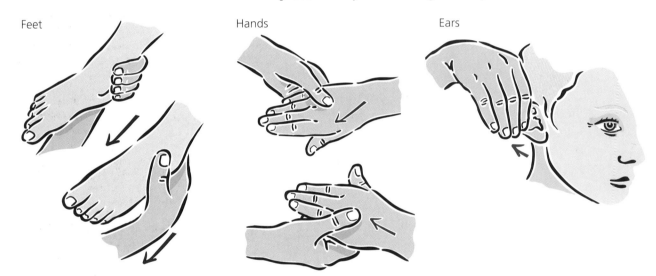

Stretch

● **Twisting** – both hands are used in a twisting motion over the area to be treated to ease tightness e.g. feet and hands.

Feet Hands

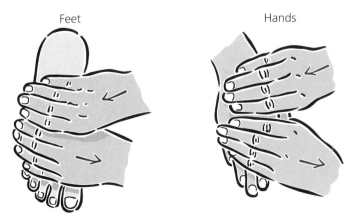

Twist

Joint manipulation movements should be followed by effleurage movements to re-establish relaxation.

✎	**Task**

Make a chart of the body listing the names of the bones that make up each area, the classification of the associated synovial joints and the actions of the corresponding muscles/muscle groups. This will assist in the application of joint manipulation movements.

Holding

Holding is often referred to as a 'greeting' and formally introduces the practitioner's hands to the area being treated as part of a specific treatment e.g. the feet, hands or ears in reflexology. This technique may also be used to close the treatment and precipitates the final releasing of the hands.

Holding movements may be used to maintain contact during discussion, to offer comfort and support and to express an emotion without the need for words.

📖	**Fascinating Fact**

Mechanical massage machines simulate manual massage in the following ways:

- Vibratory massage machines including percussion and audio sonic machines simulate manual vibration movements.

- Gyratory massage machines including hand-held and free-standing G5 machines and brush cleanse machines simulate manual effleurage, petrissage, friction, and tapotement/percussion movements with the use of different applicators.

- Vacuum suction massage machines including intermittent and continuous suction simulate manual petrissage and tapotement/percussion movements.

It is worth noting that a massage treatment may be likened to an exercise routine from which it took its origins involving:

- Warm up – effleurage
- Aerobics – petrissage and frictions

- Muscular strength and endurance – tapotement/percussion and vibrations
- Stretching – joint manipulations
- Cool down – effleurage.

Holding may be used to greet at the beginning and end of the routine.

Remember

A massage routine, just like an exercise routine, should always include a warm up and a cool down but the middle section may be varied to suit the needs of the individual.

Indications and contraindications

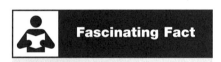
Everybody is potentially **indicated** for massage and adaptations may be made to accommodate varying ages, cultures and conditions.

There are however times when a person may be unsuitable to give and/or to receive a massage and this includes situations where the application of manual and/or mechanical massage may worsen an existing condition and/or cause cross-contamination and/or cross-infection. The common term used to describe such conditions is **contraindication**.

Contraindications may be classified as being **restrictive**, **preventive** and **referred**:

- Restrictive contraindications include localised conditions such as those that have an adverse effect on an isolated area e.g. bruise etc. A massage treatment may take place avoiding the affected area.
- Preventive contraindications include systemic conditions i.e. those that have an adverse affect the whole body e.g. flu etc. A massage treatment may not take place until the condition has cleared.
- Referred contraindications include conditions that are already being treated by another professional i.e. doctor, physiotherapist, chiropractor etc. A massage treatment may not take place until approval has been sought from the specialist involved.

Indications and contraindications to massage must never be based on the diagnosis of conditions by the masseur/masseuse. Only the medical profession can offer a diagnosis. Instead decisions as to the suitability of massage for an individual are based on knowledge and common sense:

- Knowledge of the body through anatomy and physiology.
- Common sense to determine when a condition may be improved or worsened by the application of massage.

Tip

Further information relating to **indications** and **contraindications** accompany the suggested **order of work** for each treatment area in Part 4.

How does the body respond to massage?

The response of the body to massage may be viewed as being a **reaction** and can be further classified as being either an **action** or **contra action:**

- Action – physical and psychological process which may be seen as being a positive reaction to massage.
- Contra action – a contrary process which may be seen as being a negative reaction to massage.

Action

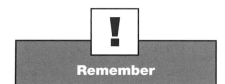

Remember

Remember the actions of the different massage techniques:

The application of massage has an action on both the giver and the receiver affecting their physical and psychological well-being. Massage has the potential to provide a whole body workout with the emphasis being on **stimulation** for **relaxation** and vice versa depending on the actions associated with the individual body systems.

- Effleurage provides gentle, surface stimulation and draining.
- Petrissage, frictions and vibrations provide deep tissue stimulation.
- Tapotement and percussion provide brisk and invigorating stimulation.
- Joint manipulation provides stimulation to the individual joint formations.

System sorter

MASSAGE

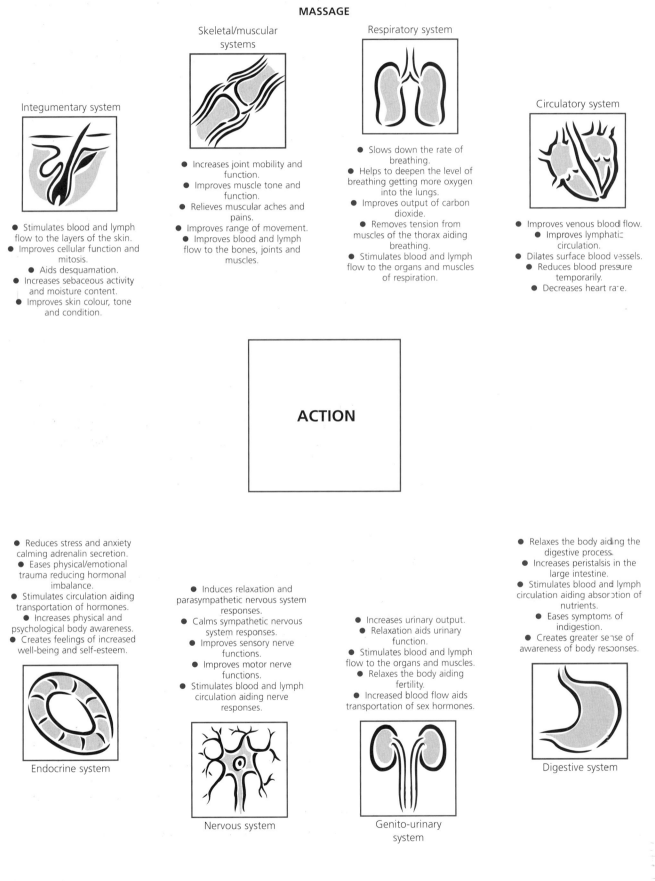

Integumentary system

- Stimulates blood and lymph flow to the layers of the skin.
- Improves cellular function and mitosis.
- Aids desquamation.
- Increases sebaceous activity and moisture content.
- Improves skin colour, tone and condition.

Skeletal/muscular systems

- Increases joint mobility and function.
- Improves muscle tone and function.
- Relieves muscular aches and pains.
- Improves range of movement.
- Improves blood and lymph flow to the bones, joints and muscles.

Respiratory system

- Slows down the rate of breathing.
- Helps to deepen the level of breathing getting more oxygen into the lungs.
- Improves output of carbon dioxide.
- Removes tension from muscles of the thorax aiding breathing.
- Stimulates blood and lymph flow to the organs and muscles of respiration.

Circulatory system

- Improves venous blood flow.
- Improves lymphatic circulation.
- Dilates surface blood vessels.
- Reduces blood pressure temporarily.
- Decreases heart rate.

ACTION

Endocrine system

- Reduces stress and anxiety calming adrenalin secretion.
- Eases physical/emotional trauma reducing hormonal imbalance.
- Stimulates circulation aiding transportation of hormones.
- Increases physical and psychological body awareness.
- Creates feelings of increased well-being and self-esteem.

Nervous system

- Induces relaxation and parasympathetic nervous system responses.
- Calms sympathetic nervous system responses.
- Improves sensory nerve functions.
- Improves motor nerve functions.
- Stimulates blood and lymph circulation aiding nerve responses.

Genito-urinary system

- Increases urinary output.
- Relaxation aids urinary function.
- Stimulates blood and lymph flow to the organs and muscles.
- Relaxes the body aiding fertility.
- Increased blood flow aids transportation of sex hormones.

Digestive system

- Relaxes the body aiding the digestive process.
- Increases peristalsis in the large intestine.
- Stimulates blood and lymph circulation aiding absorption of nutrients.
- Eases symptoms of indigestion.
- Creates greater sense of awareness of body responses.

Massage has the potential to affect every living cell through the interrelation of body systems: if each body system relies on another for its well-being then massaging one system must automatically affect the others.

The physical effects of massage on the action of the body systems therefore have a 'knock on' effect on the psychological well-being of a person. Physical well-being helps to promote a feeling of emotional well-being and vice versa: as a person becomes more in tune with their emotions they may experience a spiritual awareness. This may help to encourage a more balanced connection between the body, mind and spirit. Massage is therefore an holistic way of treating each of the three stages of the General Adaptation Syndrome (GAS) associated with stress helping to **alleviate**, **maintain** and **prevent**:

- Alleviate symptoms of stress at the alarm, resistance and exhaustion stages.
- Maintain homeostasis in order to cope more effectively with fluctuating stress levels.
- Prevent physical, psychological and spiritual problems associated with fluctuating stress levels.

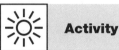

Activity

Have a body massage and think about the effects the treatment can have on your mind. Make a list of the ways in which the treatment affects your emotional well-being. This will help you to appreciate the psychological effects of massage.

Task

Make a chart highlighting the different massage techniques and the different body systems. Fill in the chart by stating the effects each technique has on each body system. This will help you to appreciate the physical effects of massage.

Contra action

The application of massage can sometimes bring about a 'disturbance of state' in the form of a contra action.

Common contra actions may be classified as being related to the **output** and **input** functions of the body and may be experienced up to 24–48 hours post-treatment:

Contra actions relating to **output** include:

- Increased need to urinate as the body releases excess waste.
- Increase in bowel movements with accompanying flatulence, especially if the abdomen has been massaged.
- Skin breakouts as a result of stimulation to the skin.
- Aching muscles and headaches may occur as a natural reaction to the release of excessive physical tension and emotional stress.
- Heightened feelings of emotions e.g. weeping.

Contra actions relating to **input** include:

- Increase in feelings of hunger and/or thirst as a more relaxed mind is alerted to the body's need for nutrients.

- Feelings of tiredness through to extreme exhaustion as the body attempts to make a person aware of its need for rest.

- Feelings of emptiness often accompany the release of extreme emotions and this may highlight the body's need for loving care.

Tip

An allergic reaction is classified as a contra action. The skin responds by becoming red, hot and itchy. This response is part of the alarm reaction is a defence mechanism alerting the body to potential attack.

Knowledge review

1   List the bones that make up the wrists, hands/fingers and thumbs.

2   Which types of joints are formed between the individual bones of the fingers and thumbs?

3   Where is the thenar eminence located and what hand action does it contribute to?

4   Which massage medium is most commonly used and why?

5   Which massage medium was traditionally used for the application of Swedish massage?

6   What does the term arthritis describe?

7   What is the disorder onychophagy more commonly known as?

8   What is a whitlow?

9   Name the seven different types of nutrients needed to keep the body alive.

10   What are the differences between lateral costal, apical and diaphragmatic breathing?

11   Which standing position is used when working transversely?

12   Which standing position is used when working longitudinally?

13   What do the terms prone and supine refer to?

14   Which massage technique starts, links and ends a massage routine?

15   Name four different petrissage techniques.

16   Name the two types of frictions.

17   List five different tapotement/percussion movements

18   Name the three different types of vibrations.

19   Name two joint manipulation techniques.

20   When might holding techniques be used and why?

Part 3
Massage preparation

Learning objectives

After reading this part you should be able to:

- Recognise the need for massage preparation.

- Identify the processes involved in preparing for a professional massage treatment.

- Understand the importance of each stage of massage preparation.

- Be aware of the legal, professional and personal aspects of massage preparation.

- Appreciate the links between massage preparation and the effectiveness of the massage treatment.

As we have seen in previous chapters, the art of massage is an intuitive skill that comes primarily from within and as such is bound by the personal and cultural boundaries set by each individual. However with the advances associated with the science of massage, and the development of professional treatments, there exists a more formal set of boundaries that have to be adhered to.

The following chapters aim to outline the boundaries associated with massage preparation whilst at the same time addressing the following key learning points:

- What must be considered when *preparing* for the provision of massage treatments?
- How is a client *prepared* for massage treatments?
- How can a masseur/masseuse *prepare* themselves to give a massage treatment?

7

Preparation of the working area

What must be considered when preparing for the provision of massage?

Preparation for the provision of massage should be conducted in a professional and caring manner. Care should be taken in the first instance of the preparation of the working area, the client and the masseur/masseuse with reference to **legislative requirements** and **professional codes of ethics.**

Whether working from home, from a salon or clinic or offering massage treatments in a person's home or workplace, legislative requirements and professional codes of ethics must always be considered and adhered to as appropriate.

- Legislative requirements form a general set of rules laid down by a government department to safeguard the health, safety and welfare of the general public (clients and practitioners – employed and self-employed).

- Professional codes of ethics form a specific set of rules laid down by a regulatory body to safeguard the welfare of the massage client and the masseur/masseuse.

Legislative requirements

It is important to have a working knowledge of the legislative requirements and to keep up to date with the changes and developments that might occur over time. The following list outlines those legislative requirements relevant to the provision of massage treatments.

- The Health and Safety at Work Act 1974 (HASAWA) – the environment in which the massage treatment is to take place must conform to certain guidelines including provision and use of safe equipment and safe systems of work, safe handling, storage and transport of substances, safe place of work with safe entrance and exit, adequate facilities and protective equipment. European directives include the protection of non-smokers from tobacco smoke and the provision of rest facilities for pregnant and nursing mothers.

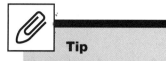

Tip

The working temperature of a room should be maintained at approximately 16°C or 61°F. The amount of moisture in the air (humidity) should be between 30%–70% and there should be sufficient exchange and movement of circulating air.

Remember

First aid training needs to be regularly updated. Seek advice from the British Red Cross or St John's ambulance for details of first aid training and updates in your area.

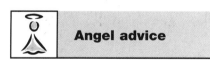

Angel advice

Better to be safe than sorry!

Fascinating Fact

In addition to the British Acts of Parliament, working practices are also governed by European law. Fifteen countries form the European Union and follow the same legislation which is decided upon through the European Courts in Brussels.

- The Work Place (health, safety and welfare) Regulations 1992 – this relates to the maintenance of the workplace and equipment in terms of ventilation, temperature, lighting, cleanliness, sanitary and washing facilities, supply of drinking water and safety of personal belongings.

- Health and Safety (first aid) Regulations 1981 – employers should provide adequate facilities for administering first aid. When working alone it is good practice to have access to a first aid box for minor first aid problems and to be a trained first aider in the event of more serious problems.

- The Working Time Regulations 1998 – regulates the number of hours worked by an employed person. Self-employed people have no such restrictions but should monitor their working time in accordance with their stress levels and health.

- The Management of Health and Safety at Work Regulations 1999 – recommends the assessment of the risks to staff and clients whilst undertaking or receiving treatment. Such assessments should thereby reduce the risks and at the same time have procedures in place in the event of a problem occurring.

- Control of Substances Hazardous to Health Regulations 1999 (COSHH) – any substance that can be inhaled, ingested and/or absorbed into the skin must be identified and assessed for risks to health. As a result, substances should be appropriately labelled, effective measures employed to reduce any risks and any possible risks regularly reviewed.

Tip

Potential hazards relating to the provision of massage treatments include those products that may be classified as **irritants** e.g. massage oils containing nut extracts etc. and **flammable** e.g. alcohol sterilising solutions etc.

Tip

Always check the ingredients in any product you purchase or use to ensure that they comply with these regulations. If in doubt – avoid use!

- The Dangerous Substances and Preparations (nickel) Regulations 2000 – this prohibits the use of products containing nickel or nickel compound which may come into contact with the skin unless the rate of nickel release is less than 0.5 microgrammes per week.

- Employers Liability (compulsory insurance) Act 1969 – if you employ staff it is your responsibility to ensure that you are insured against liability for injury or disease sustained in the course of employment. An employer must insure for at least £5 million for any individual claim and a certificate of insurance must be displayed. This ruling applies to work experience students also.

- Electricity at Work Act 1989 – it is necessary to list all electrical items used as part of the supply of any treatment including CD players, kettles etc. These items should be checked prior to use, adequately maintained and tested by an outside contractor yearly. Results of electrical testing must be recorded.

- The Reporting of Injuries, Diseases and Dangerous Occurrences Regulations 1995 (RIDDOR) – notification of major injury or disease must be made to the Incident Contact Centre. In addition, an accident report book should be available to record accidents and injury.

- The Fire Precautions Act 1971 – a fire certificate is required if more than twenty people are employed on one floor, or more than ten people on different floors at any one time. All premises should have adequate fire fighting equipment and access to escape in the event of a fire. Fire extinguishers should be checked annually and training provided for safe use.

- The Environmental Protection Act 1990 – care should be taken in the safe disposal of waste by following manufacturer's guidelines. It is good practice to dispose of waste such as couch roll and tissues in a double bin bag.

- The Provisions and Use of Work Equipment Regulations 1992 – all equipment must be suitable for use, properly maintained and appropriate training undertaken prior to use.

- Personal Protective Equipment at Work Regulations 1992 – personal protection should be considered when using products or equipment that expose a person to any possible risk.

- The Health and Safety Display Screen Equipment Regulations 1992 – it is commonly recognised that excessive computer work can lead to eyestrain, mental and physical stress. To avoid this, use should be limited to safe timings. This is useful advice for clients who may not have employers to monitor safe use as well as for ourselves.

- Manual Handling Operations regulations 1992 – safety procedures for manual handling to prevent injury. Care should be taken to: avoid lifting anything that is too heavy, ensure that any lifting is carried out with bent knees and a straight back and not to carry heavy loads too far or for too long.

- Trade Descriptions Act 1968 and 1972 – to avoid making any false allegations (verbally and/or in written form) as to the effects and benefits of the treatments and/or products used.

- The Consumer Protection Act 1987 – to safeguard against the sale and use of unsafe products and services.

- The Cosmetic Products (Safety) Regulations 1996 – form a part of the Consumer Protection Act and refer to the composition, description and marketing of products as well as the labelling of ingredients.

- The Sale and Supply of Goods Act 1994 – prevents the sale of goods and/or services that are defective and do not meet recognised standards.

- Data Protection Act 1984 and 1998 – any business that stores information relating to staff and/or clients on a computer must register with the Data Protection Registrar.

- Sex Discrimination Act 1975 and 1986 – ensures equal opportunities for all employees. Good practice ensures that clients of differing sexual orientation are not disadvantaged in anyway.

- Race Relations Act 1976 – ensures equal opportunities relating to race. Good practice ensures that clients of all races are treated with sensitivity and tact and that care is taken to respect any cultural differences.

- The Disability Discrimination Act 1995 – the working environment should provide adequate access and facilities to prevent staff and clients with disabilities from being disadvantaged.

- Copyright, Design and Patents Act 1988 – under this act it is illegal to play copyrighted music in an area open to the general public unless a fee is paid annually to the Performing Rights Society (PRS). Some companies supply non-copyrighted music which is exempt from such requirements.

- Local Government (Miscellaneous Provisions) Act 1982 – relates to local authorities and the registration of practitioners who pierce the skin e.g. epilation, acupuncture etc.

- Local authority by-laws – it is necessary to register your business with the local council and abide by any bylaws they enforce and which often differ from region to region.

Professional codes of ethics

It is important to have a working knowledge of the appropriate professional codes of ethics and to keep up to date with any changes and developments that might occur over time. The following list outlines the areas for concern:

- Conduct – professional working methods observing client confidentiality and privacy whilst maintaining moral and hygiene codes of practice.

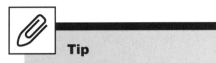

Tip

Contact the Data Protection Registrar, Springfield House, Water Lane, Wilmslow, Cheshire, SK9 5AX.

Tip

Before setting up a business offering massage treatments, contact your local authority or borough council to check out the existing by-laws and make sure you are able to abide by them.

Tip

When treating members of the opposite sex it is important not to do so alone. Ensure someone else is within earshot to safeguard both you and the client against any possible misinterpretation of treatment.

- Practice – professional working area and practice should be maintained at all times adapted to suit the circumstances e.g. working within a client's home/workplace etc.

- Referral – clients with conditions beyond the limits of the practitioner's expertise should be referred to a suitable and reputable specialist and any subsequent massage treatment should be with the appropriate specialist's approval.

- Record keeping – information collected from the client should be dealt with sensitively and securely. Access to record cards should be restricted to the practitioner although clients are able to read their own records upon request.

- Insurance – public liability (refers to damage to the client whilst in your establishment) and professional indemnity (refers to damage caused to a client during treatment) are not statutory requirements but are necessary when a practitioner joins a regulatory body.

- Qualifications – recognised qualifications are a requirement of all responsible regulatory bodies and demonstrate that a certain level of competency has been achieved. Providing clients with access to view your qualifications is good practice as is inclusion in recommended lists forwarded to clients from recognised organisations.

- Continued Professional Development (CPD) – there is a constant need to update and progress the direct skills associated with massage and the indirect skills associated with other beauty/holistic treatments, business management etc. Lifelong learning is the key to any treatment provision and time should be allocated to ensure that this takes place on a regular basis. Activities may include sharing experiences with other practitioners, attending trade fairs, exhibitions and reading trade magazines, experiential learning through giving and receiving treatments, formal training for recognised qualifications, informal workshops, staff meetings etc.

Tip

It is useful to get involved with local initiatives associated with small businesses that may be able to provide additional support and access to information and in some cases funding e.g. local business clubs, the Prince's Trust etc.

As well as adhering to legislative requirements and industry codes of ethics it is also good practice to have a prepared policy statement for each of the following:

- Health and safety – general guidelines that demonstrate the thought and action given to the welfare of clients and staff.

- Hygiene – a checklist for clients and staff to measure performance.

- Equal opportunities – a formal commitment to fair provision of service.

- Complaints procedure – a formal means by which clients and staff can address any problems they may encounter.

Task

Research your responsibilities under the legislative requirements and professional codes of ethics. You can obtain further information from your college, workplace, local authority or regulatory bodies such as HABIA (Hairdressing And Beauty Industry Authority). Alternatively review the codes of practice in your workplace and make suggestions for improvement where appropriate.

Bearing in mind the legislative requirements and the professional codes of ethics, attention should be paid to the preparation of the *environment* in which the massage is to take place, the *equipment*, *products* and *tools* to be used for massage:

Massage environment

The massage environment should be one that is conducive to the expected outcomes of the treatment and every attempt should be made to ensure that this is achieved in terms of:

- Hygiene – maintenance of the working environment to protect against possible risk of cross-infection through the processes of sterilisation and sanitisation i.e. creating an environment where possible whereby micro-organisms are destroyed (sterilisation) and creating an environment pertaining to health (sanitisation).

- Privacy – greater levels of relaxation may be achieved the more private the working area.

- Decor – colour, style and image play an important part in creating an environment suitable for massage. Care should be taken to create an image in which everyone feels comfortable without excluding anyone.

- Lighting – the autonomic nervous system responds to changes in light by preparing the body for activity in sunlight and preparing the body for rest in moonlight. Artificial lighting can be used to simulate either sunlight or moonlight and attention should be paid to the possible effects our choice of lighting may evoke. Thought should also be given to the type of lighting a person is going to be exposed to after their massage treatment. Ideally it is most effective to dim the lights or draw the curtains during a relaxing massage and return the lighting to normal at the close of the treatment.

- Heating – the working temperature of a room should be maintained at approximately 16° Centigrade or 61° Fahrenheit. During a massage treatment the body temperature of the masseur/masseuse increases with the increased activity involved with giving a massage and that

Angel advice

Candlelight is a very effective way of creating a pleasant ambiance that is conducive to relaxation.

Tip

The use of towels, blankets and duvets may be incorporated to ensure client warmth and comfort throughout the massage treatment.

Fascinating Fact

Sight is a sense controlled by the activity in the left hemisphere of the brain whilst hearing is controlled by the right hemisphere of the brain. It has been found that each person is either left or right brain dominant, which means that they respond more readily to either visual images e.g. colour or sound e.g. music.

of the client decreases due to the prolonged levels of inactivity.

- Ventilation – there should be adequate exchange and movement of circulating air to ensure that it is fresh and free from fumes and odours that may be detrimental to health e.g. chemical fumes etc. and/or offensive e.g. body odour etc.

- Sound – differing levels of sound evoke differing feelings within a person. Loud noises can be disruptive whilst repetitive noises may be irritating. The massage environment should generally be a quiet, peaceful and noise-free zone. Soft music may be played to aid relaxation.

Massage equipment, products and tools

A variety of equipment, products and tools are available for the provision of massage treatments ranging from massage couches and specially adapted chairs to trolleys, stools, mechanical massage machines and specialist massage mediums. The following considerations should be taken into account prior to purchase:

- Safety – does the choice of equipment, product or tool conform to safety requirements e.g. legislative requirements?

- Suitability – is the choice of equipment, product or tool suitable for the job it is to perform e.g. correct height couch etc?

- Cost – value for money e.g. brightly coloured couches tend to be more costly than plain white couches – if the couch is permanently covered with blankets and towels does the extra cost involved provide good value?

- Fit for use – does the choice of equipment, product or tool meet the requirements of its intended use e.g. is a portable couch easily transported etc?

The priority with reference to the provision of any form of massage treatment in terms of equipment is the massage couch or chair, which should met the following criteria.

Flat massage couch

- Correct height – when standing up against the couch you should be able to extend your arms, placing the palms of your hands flat onto the surface of the couch without strain.

- Sturdy, secure and safe – portable couches should be correctly assembled and free-standing couches correctly positioned ensuring the floor beneath is even.

- Height adjustable couches should have their mechanisms regularly checked to avoid potential problems.

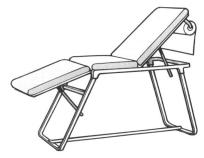

Massage couch/chair

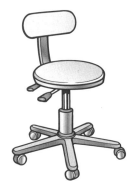

Adjustable stool

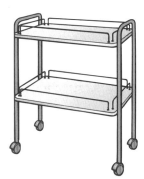

Trolley

- Cushioning should provide adequate thickness to ensure comfort.
- Head rests and/or air holes are a useful addition to any couch for added client comfort.

Massage chairs

- A variety of massage chairs are now available ranging from conventional chairs to specially adapted chairs.
- Care should be taken to ensure that the chosen chair is suitable for use and offers maximum client comfort.
- Thought should also be given to the position of the masseur/masseuse when treating a client seated in a chair to avoid any excess strain.

Additional equipment may include:

- **Footstool** – to assist a client when getting on and off a high couch.
- **Adjustable stool** – preferably on casters and with a backrest. A stool may be used by the masseur/masseuse when the massage is conducted from a seated position e.g. facial massage.
- **Trolley** – preferably multi-shelved and on castors. Used to hold products, tools and mechanical machines.
- **Sterilising equipment** – the use of an autoclave which works in a similar way to a pressure cooker ensures that small metal tools e.g. tweezers can be made sterile prior to use.
- **Portable screen** – may be used to ensure an element of privacy in a public area.

Tip

In a situation where a client comes to you for treatment, it is useful to also provide access to a consultation area that is equipped with a table and two chairs. When visiting a person's home or workplace this may not be readily available and a compromise may have to be considered, paying particular attention to health and safety.

- **Mechanical massage machines** – including vibratory machines e.g. percussion and audio sonic, gyratory machines e.g. free-standing and hand-held and vacuum suction machines. These machines are available for the face and/or body and can be used to simulate and/or complement manual massage.

Massage products and tools

The choice of products and tools for the provision of massage treatments should reflect the needs of the clients in terms of:

- **Massage products (mediums)** – including oils, creams/emulsions, gels and powders.
- **Sanitising products** – used to cleanse equipment and tools prior to and after use as well as a means to cleanse skin pre-treatment e.g. chemical soaps/wipes/sprays used to cleanse areas such as the feet and hands etc.
- **Pre-massage products** – including facial/body cleansers, toners and exfoliators or scrubs used to prepare the skin ready for massage.
- **Post-massage products** – including cologne sprays to remove excess massage medium, specialist masks to aid specific skin problems e.g. acne and self-tanning products providing an additional service.
- **Consumables** – including tissue roll used to provide a hygienic cover for the surfaces of couches/chairs, which is changed for each client, tissues and cotton wool used for skin preparation pre- and post-massage.
- **Containers, bowls and spatulas** – for hygienic storage, use and removal of products and consumables. These should all be sanitised prior to use.
- **Blankets/ duvets, towels, gowns and flannels** – to maintain client modesty, protection of clothing, comfort and warmth throughout the massage treatment; should be clean for each client.
- **Disposable slippers** – it is unhygienic for a client to walk around barefoot and care should be taken to ensure that slippers are used at all times.
- **Waste disposal** – including lidded, pedal *waste bins* lined with plastic bin bags for the disposal of waste related to each treatment e.g. soiled cotton wool, and tissue etc. and *refuse bins* lined with heavy duty liners for the disposal of tied waste bin bags at the end of the day.
- **Storage for client belongings** – including coat hangers, containers for jewellery and storage boxes for shoes and handbags etc.

The preparation of the environment for the provision of massage should be a process that is rigorously followed in the initial setting up of the environment, checked prior to the commencement of any massage treatment and regularly updated.

Tip

A bactericide is a chemical that destroys bacteria, a fungicide destroys fungi and a virucide destroys viruses. Sanitising products are often referred to as being detergents and disinfectants or antiseptics meaning they destroy or inhibit the growth of micro-organisms generally. It is important to follow the manufacturer's guidelines for use as these products may include chemicals that may be irritants and/or flammable.

Tip

It is important to check with your local authority for their rulings on the safe disposal of waste.

Knowledge review

1   What does HASAWA stand for?

2   What is the meaning of COSHH?

3   How often should electrical equipment be tested by an outside contractor under the Electricity at Work Act 1989?

4   What approximate temperature should the working area be maintained at?

5   What is the difference between public liability and professional indemnity insurance?

6   Under the Employers Liability Act 1969 what should be always be displayed?

7   What do the initials RIDDOR stand for?

8   When lifting heavy objects what are the postural considerations for the knees and back?

9   Which act is concerned with the avoidance of any false allegations (verbal and/or written) being made about a product or service offered to members of the public?

10   What type of data is the Data Protection Act concerned with?

11   What is illegal under the Copyright, Design and Patents Act 1988?

12   What is the meaning of the initials CPD?

13   What is the difference between sterilisation and sanitisation?

14   What is the correct height of a massage couch?

15   When could an adjustable height stool be used in the provision of a massage treatment?

16   Describe the uses for a waste bin and a refuse bin.

17   Give an example of a pre-massage product.

18   Give an example of a post-massage product.

19   Give an example of a consumable product used in the provision of massage treatments.

20   What may be used to ensure the client is kept warm throughout a massage treatment?

8

Consultation

The preparation of the client for a massage treatment should take into account the appropriate legislative requirements as well as the professional codes of ethics as outlined in the previous chapter and is conducted in the form of a **consultation**.

A consultation consists of three main stages:

- **Stage one** is predominantly paper-based whereby the practitioner takes a full client case history.
- **Stage two** involves a practical assessment and analysis of the area to be treated.
- **Stage three** is associated with treatment outcomes and recommendations for further treatment and home care.

The consultation process begins from the moment a client makes an initial enquiry about massage and is a continuous and progressive process that forms the basis of every subsequent treatment. An effective consultation relies on effective **communication**.

Communication is a two-way process that incorporates the use of the whole of our being to receive and convey messages between other beings by:

- Detecting and receiving messages through the sensory organs with sensations of touch, smell, sight, hearing and taste.
- Interpretation of these messages by the brain.
- Responding with verbal and non-verbal methods of communication

Verbal communication

Speaking is the art of *verbal communication* and ensures messages are communicated through the use of **sound, speed, articulation** and **emphasis**:

- Sound – the volume, pitch and tone of your voice will relay a mixture of messages e.g. anger is often communicated with a loud voice etc.
- Speed – the rate at which one talks communicates the feelings associated with the message e.g. a message conveying urgency would be spoken quickly etc.
- Articulation – the use of words to communicate a clear and specific message e.g. a teacher speaking to a student should communicate clearly to ensure understanding and learning etc.
- Emphasis – the force with which the words are being expressed helps to communicate the importance of the message e.g. 'I *really* think you should come in from the rain' etc.

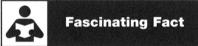

Fascinating Fact

Eye contact is usually broken if a person is attempting to lie!

Fascinating Fact

Some eye movements are uncontrollable yet send out very strong messages e.g. our pupils dilate when we see something or someone that attracts us!

Non-verbal communication

Body language is art of *non-verbal communication* and ensures messages are communicated through the use of **facial expressions, eye contact, eye movement, posture, gestures, appearance** and **proximity**:

- Facial expressions – smiling with pleasure, grimacing with distaste, frowning with confusion etc. are all examples of how our facial expressions communicate what we are feeling.
- Eye contact – looking a person in the eye communicates interest and care. Lack of eye contact is often associated with lack of self-esteem.
- Eye movements – moving the eyes helps to synchronise speech and to communicate interest.
- Posture – the way a person stands or sits communicates the true message behind their words e.g. if a person sits facing a person, their posture communicates interest. However, if they sit with their legs facing in another direction it clearly communicates disinterest etc.
- Gestures – the use of hand movements help to communicate strong messages. 'Talking with your hands' is an example of such gestures.
- Appearance – physical grooming e.g. hairstyle and make-up, together with our choice of clothes, helps to communicate the messages associated with image.

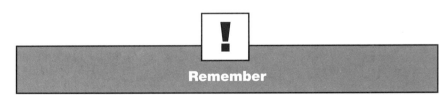

!

Remember

First impressions count therefore a masseur/masseuse needs to pay particular attention to the type of image their appearance communicates to their clients.

Remember

Touch is a two-way method of communication and consideration should be given to permission and pressure. Any form of touch requires agreement and pressure of touch should meet agreed needs.

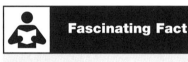

Fascinating Fact

Extra sensory communication refers to those methods of communication for which we can find no logical explanation. Think about the times when the telephone rings and the person on the other end is the person you have just been thinking of.

- Proximity – the distance maintained between people communicates the type of relationship they have e.g. *public* over 4 metres distance between people, *social* from 1.25–4 metres, *personal* from 0.5–1.25 metres and *intimate* from 0.5 metres to actually touching.

Other methods of non-verbal communication include **tactile** and **thought** messages:

- Tactile messages – are messages communicated through touch e.g. care, sympathy etc.
- Thought messages – non face-to-face communication e.g. written messages.

These methods of communication are never used in isolation but instead form a part of a variety of related and non-related factors including: *personality, emotions, language, stereotyping* and *perceptio*n. As a result, mixed messages are often communicated and barriers are formed between people giving rise to misinterpretation and confusion. A balanced use of communicating skills helps to break down such barriers and is an important factor in conducting an effective consultation.

Task

Make a list of the possible barriers to effective communication and think about ways in which you would attempt to resolve them.

Consultation – stage one

The main aim of the first stage of the consultation process is to ascertain whether or not the proposed massage treatment is suitable for the client's needs. As a result, this stage of the consultation can be a very personal and potentially invasive and intrusive process. It is important therefore to ensure that the consultation is conducted in a sensitive and thoughtful manner paying particular attention to the client's *reasons for* and *expectations of* the treatment.

In order to ascertain whether or not a client is suitable for a massage treatment a number of checks need to undertaken with the client's consent including:

- **Personal check**: including full name, address and telephone number. This information enables a practitioner to contact their client in the event of having to cancel or rearrange an appointment. It is also useful to get other personal information with the client's permission such as date of birth, doctor's details, profession, marital status, whether or not they have children, height and weight, their reasons for seeking treatment and their general expectations. This information provides an initial insight that goes beyond first impressions helping to paint a picture of the client, their personal situation and their needs.

- **Medical health:** including details of pregnancy, medication, surgical operations and any other complaints that have in the past or currently require medical attention e.g. illnesses, allergies, hereditary diseases etc. This information helps to determine the suitable areas for treatment. It is also useful at this stage to ask the client how they view their general state of health and to include questions relating to whether or not they are or have been a smoker. This helps to lead onto the more detailed questions of the consultation as well as provide greater access to the client's individual needs as they see them.

- **Physical health:** including questions relating to the physical well-being of the body as a whole and of the individual body systems e.g. skeletal, muscular, circulatory etc. This information helps to target the possible stresses associated with each individual body system as well as highlight the links with the other systems of the body through the accompanying signs and symptoms.

- **Emotional health:** including details of how the client relates to stress, tension, anxiety and depression. This information helps to ascertain how the client views themselves in terms of their emotional welfare and how much support they are going to need in terms of their quest for well-being. This information helps to highlight the links between emotional and physical well-being and the knock-on effect one has on the other.

- **Lifestyle:** including details relating to work, leisure, diet and exercise. This information helps to ascertain the likely causes of stress-related symptoms e.g. overwork, lack of free time, poor eating habits and lack of exercise are all associated with stress. There may be additional personal or professional stresses involved contributing to a short-term problem which if not addressed have the potential to create medium and even long-term physical and/or emotional problems.

The way in which the questions relating to these factors are asked is a crucial part of the consultation process, providing the key to gaining a person's trust and respect. Care should be taken to present questions that can be seen as being justifiable (the client needs to understand the reasons why you are asking such questions) and that are:

- Open – questions that encourage the client to answer with a sentence rather than with a positive or a negative e.g. 'How are you?' instead of 'Are you well?'

- Follow-up – questions that help to gain more specific information e.g. 'How often do you experience these symptoms?' and 'How do you cope with them?' etc.

Tip

Sometimes it may be necessary to ask a *closed question*. This type of questioning requires one word answers e.g. 'Are you currently taking any medication?' Closed questions do not encourage free conversation – they just confirm or eliminate information.

CONSULTATION FORM – STAGE ONE

Name .... Date ....

Address .... Tel. No work ....

.... Tel. No home ....

....Tel. No mobile ....

Date of birth ....

Doctors' details ....

Marital status .... Children .... ages ....

Height .... Weight ....

Reason for treatment ....

Expectation of treatment ....

Medical health

- Pregnancy ....
- Medication ....
- Operations and dates ....
- Major illnesses and dates ....
- Allergies ....
- Hereditary illness ....
- Smoker .... Frequency .... Amount ....
- Client's view of general state of health ....

Physical health – condition of and/or problems associated with:

Integumentary system

- Skin ....
- Hair ....
- Nails ....

Muscular/Skeletal system

- Bones .... Muscles ....
- Neck .... Back ....
- Shoulders .... Hips ....
- Knees .... Elbows ....
- Ankles .... Wrist ....

Respiratory system

- Hay fever .... Ashma ....
- How many times a year do you get a cold? ....

Which part(s) does it affect –

Head .... Chest .... Throat .... Sinuses .... Ears .... Eyes .... Nose ....

CONSULTATION FORM – STAGE ONE *(continued)*

Circulatory systems

- Blood pressure .... Pulse rate ....
- Varicose veins .... Tired legs ....
- Fluid retention .... Cellulite ....

Digestive system

- Teeth .... Taste ....
- Eating .... Drinking ....
- Indigestion .... Bloated ....
- Constipation .... Diarrhoea ....

Urinary system

- Kidneys ....
- Bladder ....

Reproductive system

Females:

- Regular periods .... Date of last period ....
- Period now? .... Day .... Flow ....
- Contraception .... Pregnancy ....

Males:

- Prostate gland ....

Nervous system

- Headaches .... Migraine ....
- Pins and needles .... Numbness ....
- Cold hands and feet ....
- Eyesight ....

Endocrine system

- PMT ....
- Menopause .... HRT ....
- Mood swings? ....

Emotional health – rate 1–10 (1 = low, 10 = high)

- Stress levels .... details ....
- Anxiety .... details ....
- Tension .... details ....
- Depression .... details ....

CONSULTATION FORM – STAGE ONE *(continued)*

Lifestyle

Work

- Profession ....
- Typical working hours ....
- Breaks? .... Frequency .... Length ....

Leisure

- Ability to relax .... Activities ....
- Hobbies .... Interests ....
- Sleep pattern .... Energy levels ....

Diet

- Preferences (vegetarian, vegan etc) ....
- How many meals per day .... Supplements ....
- Fresh fruit/veg per day .... Protein ....
- Carbohydrate .... Fats ....
- Dairy products .... Additives (salt, sugar etc.) ....
- Water per day .... Tea/coffee/cola per day ....
- Fruit juice per day .... Alcohol per day. ....
- Herbal tea per day .... Type .... Reason ....
- Details of food/fluid intake today ....
  ....
  ....

Exercise

- Type .... Frequency ....

Additional info

- Use of sunbed .... Sunscreen ....
- Posture check ....
- Anything else client would like to discuss ....
- Any questions ....
  ....
  ....

The information I have given is correct to the best of my knowledge.

I have been fully informed about contraindications.

I am happy to proceed with the treatment.

Client signature ....

Practitioner signature ....

Remember

A masseur/masseuse is not a doctor and as such is not expected to know every medical detail so do not be afraid to ask.

Remember

Your tone of voice will contribute to the way in which the questions are interpreted.

Tip

A consultation usually takes place in the same area as the massage treatment.

- Unthreatening – questions that make a client feel 'safe' so that they can be free to answer honestly e.g. 'It is amazing how little exercise the average person gets. Do you find you get much exercise?' instead of 'We should all exercise three times a week. Do you?'

- Jargon free – questions that avoid the use of technical terms that a client may not know the meaning of and which have the potential of making them feel uncomfortable and lacking in knowledge e.g. 'How often do you find that you have aching shoulders?' instead of 'Do you often suffer with fatigue in the trapezius muscle?'

- Non-judgemental – questions that do not offer an opinion or criticism e.g. 'How would you describe your alcohol intake?' instead of 'Don't you think that drinking a bottle of wine a day is a bit excessive?'

- Clarifying – questions that allow you to check details e.g. to clarify a type of medication you may not have heard of and do not know what it is for or to clarify the spelling of a word you are unfamiliar with.

- Linking – questions that help you to link systems and symptoms e.g. 'You have said that you have problems with aching muscles in your shoulders. Do you find that you hold your shoulders tense whilst you are working?' etc.

The first stage of the consultation process may be divided into five distinct phases – **preparation, introduction, case history, explanation** and **confirmation**:

Preparation

A means to become ready. An effective treatment relies on an efficient consultation, so thought should be given to:

- Environment – this should be private and out of sight and earshot of other clients. It should be comfortable and inviting, safe and warm. Seats for the practitioner and client should be of equal height facing one another at an appropriate angle and distance. This ensures eye contact at an equal level, which in turn sets the level of the relationship, which should also be equal. Avoid sitting behind a desk or table as this creates a physical and psychological barrier between the practitioner and client. Heating, lighting and ventilation should be checked and it is necessary to ensure that there is adequate access and provision for disabled clients e.g. wheelchair, guide dog etc.

- Tools and equipment – a consultation form and pen should be ready for use together with any other resources you may want to use to supplement your consultation e.g. charts showing the bones, joints and muscles of the body. It is useful to have sight of a clock in order to check the timing of the consultation. A box of tissues should be on hand (a consultation can in some cases evoke an emotional response) and antiseptic wipes should be available in the event of having to check the area to be treated.

- Masseur/masseuse – attention should be paid to the way in which you present yourself to the client. All aspects of your personal appearance should be considered in order to convey a professional image appropriate to your workplace. In particular care should be taken to ensure that your outfit is appropriate, hands are clean and soft, nails are enamel free and short and hair is tied back away from the face. Jewellery should be kept to a minimum for safety reasons and due to the fact that it can impede energy flow if tight and restrictive. In addition, all thoughts of previous clients and personal situations should be cleared from your mind to be able to focus your full attention.

- Client – removal and safekeeping of coats, jackets, briefcases, shopping etc. keeping valuables e.g. handbags or wallet with them at all times.

Task

Draw up a checklist for personal presentation appropriate to your job role. Think about the importance of each aspect of the checklist.

Introduction

A means to become acquainted. An effective massage treatment relies on the interconnection between the client and masseur/masseuse so thought should be given to:

- Greeting – it is important to introduce yourself to the client positively making full eye contact and speaking clearly and concisely using your tone of voice, choice of words and general body language in a welcoming manner.

- Reference – ensure that you are using the client's correct name and title checking pronunciation as appropriate. If a

Tip

If you feel comfortable shaking hands when you meet a new client ensure that your handshake is firm and positive and your hands are clean and dry.

Tip

It is common practice in some establishments to adopt a more casual approach to clients often referring to them by popular terms of endearment e.g. darling, sweetie etc. and greeting them with a kiss and a hug etc. It is important to bear in mind that such terms and methods of greeting may be open to misinterpretation.

client has booked an appointment as Mr Fred Bloggs do not presume to call him Fred, especially if he is older than you. It is more politely correct to refer to him as Mr Bloggs until such time as you feel that it is appropriate to ask the client if he would mind you calling him Fred, or if he asks you to call him by his first name.

- Process – a first time client will have little or no knowledge of the treatment or of the consultation that precedes it. It is therefore necessary to spend a few moments discussing this to ensure that the client is comfortable with the processes and happy to proceed. Even regular clients need reminding of the process!

Case history

A means to gain information and knowledge. An effective massage treatment relies on the efficient use of our senses and the examination may be classified as being **visual, oral, aural, olfactory, perceptive** and **tactile**:

- Visual – observe your client from the moment you greet them to the moment you leave them, taking note of what you see. Note a client's posture, general demeanour and body language – what does this tell you about them? Note the way in which they walk to the treatment area and sit themselves down – was it difficult? Did they need assistance? Are they showing visual signs of nervousness? What is their breathing like? Do they visibly calm down during the consultation or are they fidgety? This visual information will prove to be a vital aid to the development of the consultation.

- Oral – it will be necessary to ask questions and take note of the answers given. Be aware of the sensitivity of what is being said and reassure the client using your tone of voice as well as your choice of words. When discussing more personal information a lack of embarrassment on your part will encourage the same attitude in the client. If the client is making a telephone enquiry, it may be necessary to take certain personal details from them other than their name and telephone number. If this is the case, check that the person is able to talk, as they may feel inhibited if they are making the call from work etc.

- Aural – ensure that you are engaged in active listening i.e. that you are both 'hearing' and 'listening' to what is being said. Use your body language to demonstrate to the client that you are listening actively. Nod to confirm acknowledgement, smile to convey care, maintain eye contact to show interest etc.

- Olfactory – use your sense of smell to 'pick up' further information from your client. The odour associated with the body generally, the feet and breath specifically may alert you to the way in which a person applies care to themselves. Be aware of the impression created with your own personal odour. Avoid the use of strong, heavy perfumes that may be off-putting for clients paying particular attention to all aspects of your personal hygiene.

- Perceptive – you will intuitively get a sense of your client just as they will you. Be aware of your gut feeling – this will allow you to adapt your skills to suit the needs of the client more effectively. Be respectful of the client's sense of you. It may be that you are not the person to treat them – a consultation will provide them with the opportunity to decide this for themselves.

- Tactile – the use of touch is a necessary tool in advancing your consultation skills. It may be appropriate to touch the client to demonstrate that you empathise with them. It may be that the client's words 'touched' you. Use the feelings that this evokes to create greater empathy, understanding and awareness of your client. Use touch sensitively and appropriately to get a feel for the person within.

Explanation

A way of conveying a meaning. An efficient massage treatment relies on the increasing knowledge and awareness on the part of the client. This encourages them to take an active role in the development of their own well-being, so thought should be given to providing the client with:

- Treatment procedure – a client needs to know what the treatment entails e.g. which part of the body you are going to be treating, whether or not they need to remove any clothing, do they sit or lie down, that you may leave them to fetch a glass of water, wash your hands etc.

- Effects and benefits – it is important to make the client aware of what you can and cannot do. The information given should be realistic and accurate ensuring that you dispel any unrealistic expectations the client may have.

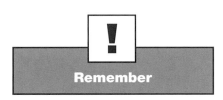

Remember

You will be comfortable with every aspect of the treatment and know exactly what will happen and when. Do not forget that the client does not have access to this information unless you tell them!

Remember

You cannot make a medical diagnosis unless qualified to do so and you cannot cure a disorder. What you can do is provide a complement (with doctor's approval) and in some cases an alternative (for minor disorders e.g. stress related) to medical treatment as well as help to stimulate the body's own healing and coping mechanisms.

Confirmation

A means to agree a course of action i.e. a treatment plan. When the necessary information has been discussed and recorded it is then possible to make a recommendation for a massage treatment based on the client's needs. This recommendation is dependent on client approval and agreement and time must therefore be allocated within the consultation for client questions prior to the client's formal agreement to the proposed treatment. The treatment may then be booked for a specific date and time or, as in most cases take place immediately after the consultation. Finally, both the client and the practitioner sign the consultation form:

- The client signs to agree the treatment but to also confirm that the information they have given is correct to the best of their knowledge and that they understand the implications of giving false information.

- The practitioner also signs to agree the treatment as well as to confirm that they have given correct information and recommendations regarding treatment to suit the client's individual needs as a result of the consultation process.

Tip

This information is important in the unlikely event of legal action being taken against the practitioner. A thorough consultation, which has been recorded and signed by both parties, demonstrates professionalism and is a sign of good practice.

Activity

Practice conducting stage one of the consultation on a partner using the consultation form as a guide. Adapt the form to provide yourself with a more personally user-friendly version.
Experiment by talking to each other when you are both seated at different heights. The person seated at the higher level automatically assumes a superior position and the person in the lower seat automatically feels inferior. Discuss with your partner how each position makes you feel and think of ways in which you can use your verbal and non-verbal communication skills to perform an effective consultation. Think about the relevance of the questions you are asking with reference to the massage you are about to give. Adapt your questioning and length of consultation time accordingly.

Consultation – stage two

The second stage of the consultation involves a physical **assessment** of the body as a whole, and/or a physical **analysis** of the area to be treated. A client may be conducted to a changing area and asked to remove the necessary items of clothing in order to perform the treatment. It is usual practice for both male and female clients to leave their lower underwear on.

CONSULTATION STAGE TWO
PHYSICAL EXAMINATION

Back   Notes ....
                        ....
                        ....
                        ....
                        ....
                        ....
                        ....

Arms and   Notes ....
hands   ....
                        ....
                        ....
                        ....
                        ....
                        ....
                        ....

Buttocks, legs   Notes ....
and feet   ....
                        ....
                        ....
                        ....
                        ....
                        ....
                        ....

Abdomen   Notes ....
                        ....
                        ....
                        ....
                        ....
                        ....
                        ....

Upper body   Notes ....
                        ....
                        ....
                        ....
                        ....
                        ....

Tip

Always ensure that the client is aware of *exactly* what items of clothing they are to remove and which you require them to leave on – this prevents any misunderstanding later on.

Tip

It is important to ensure client privacy is maintained whilst a client gets changed – both at the start and close of the treatment.

This stage of the consultation forms a continuation of the fact-finding process that is carried out in stage one. This physical assessment and/or examination is generally conducted as part of the treatment and is predominantly *visual* and *tactile* incorporating **palpation** techniques.

Tip

Palpation means the examination of a part by touch or pressure of the hand.

Aural, olfactory and perceptive skills are also associated with stage two relating to what you hear, smell and sense. In addition, it may also be necessary to ask questions as well as discuss with the client the details of the examination. The information gained from this part of the consultation helps to confirm the information received during stage one.

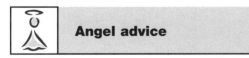

Angel advice

Sometimes information that was not mentioned during stage one may come to light during stage two.

Physical assessment

When conducting a physical assessment it is useful to follow certain guidelines in terms of what to look for and the interpretation of such findings.

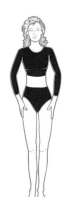

Ectomorph

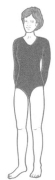

Mesomorph

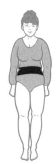

Endomorph

Useful guidelines include: **body types, posture** and **postural faults.**

Body types

Known technically as *somatotypes* this refers to particular types of body build including:

- Ectomorph – long limbed, slim, lean and angular. People with this body type tend to have little body fat and muscle bulk and do not easily gain weight.
- Mesomorph – broad, stocky, muscular and athletic. People with this body type tend to gain weight slowly and are able increase muscle strength through exercise easily.
- Endomorph – short, curvaceous, stocky and plump. People with this body type tend to gain weight easily and find weight loss is difficult.

Most people are predominantly of one particular body type but may share some characteristics of another. These characteristics are inherited and as such an individual who is predominantly an endomorph body type will never be able to achieve an ectomorph body type etc.

☀ **Activity**

Assess your own body type and that of other members of your group/family etc. Learn to be more aware of the characteristics of your own body type and accept those aspects you cannot change. Encourage this awareness and acceptance in others.

Posture is influenced by many physical and psychological factors including:

- Height – tall people often round their shoulders in an attempt to make themselves appear shorter.
- Weight distribution – uneven body weight causes uneven body alignment e.g. heavy breasts puts strain on the upper back and shoulders, pregnancy puts strain on the lower back etc. Carrying extra weight in the form of heavy bags, children etc. can create imbalance as one side of the body is under greater strain than the other.
- Tension – physical and psychological stress are contributory to many postural problems. A tense body results in muscle strain and associated postural problems e.g. aching shoulders, eye strain etc.
- Fatigue – it is difficult to maintain good posture when the body and mind are tired. The body has a tendency to droop

when tired and the mind becomes filled with negative thoughts.

- Health and well-being – good posture is very much associated with being well and happy – body and mind are uplifted. Poor posture is often a direct result of physical and mental illness – pressure that brings a person down both physically and psychologically.

- Ill-fitting and high heeled shoes – cause the body to adjust its standing position and the alignment of muscles often contributing to knee, hip and back problems.

- Poor standing and sitting positions – become a matter of habit eventually causing the muscles to become permanently realigned in order to accommodate the changes in body positions. Subsequent changes in terms of adopting good posture are often accompanied by aching muscles as they learn to realign.

Postural faults

These occur as a direct result of excessive stress and strain on the body including:

- Kyphosis – exaggerated concave curvature of the spine in the thoracic region (mid back) creating a hump back and rounded shoulders. The chin protrudes forward shortening and extending the neck.

- Lordosis – exaggerated convex curvature of the spine in the lumbar region (lower back). The pelvis is tilted forward creating a hollow back. Often associated with the painful condition lumbago.

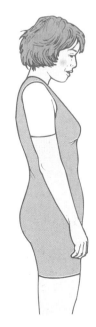

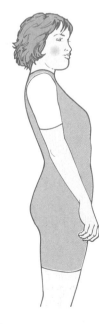

Kyphosis   **Lordosis**

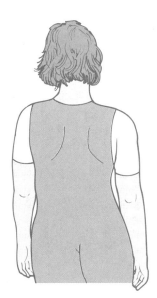

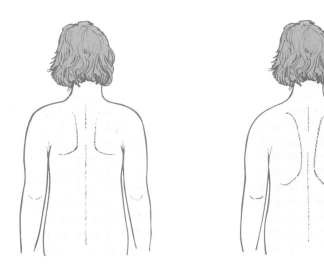

Scoliosis   **Flat back**   **Winged scapula**

- Scoliosis – a lateral (away from the mid line) curvature of the spine associated with overuse of one side of the body or other. This condition results in uneven levels of the shoulders and hips.

- Flat back – little or no curvature of the lumbar region of the spine. The pelvis is tilted backwards and the shoulders are often rounded.

- Winged scapula – the middle border and lower angle of the shoulder blades (scapulae bones) protrude away from the ribs making it difficult to lift the arms above shoulder level and to push the arms forward.

Postural faults are common, can occur at any age and can be treated. Improving general posture along with simple realigning exercises and massage treatment offer a useful way of treating such problems (see Part 4 for details relating to each part of the body).

Physical analysis

When conducting a physical analysis it is useful to follow certain guidelines in terms of what to look for and the interpretation of such findings:

Useful guidelines include **skin types** and **skin conditions**.

Skin types

When analysing skin types it is useful to consider the general colour, texture, temperature, age, imperfections and moisture content of the skin.

Colour – the colour of the skin is determined by the amount of melanin produced in the epidermis, the levels of carotene present and the blood circulation.

Tip

Carotene is a yellow pigment stored in the skin from the foods we eat e.g. carrots, tomatoes and fats.

Texture – the skin feels uneven for two main reasons. First when there is an *excess* of natural moisture (sebum) preventing natural exfoliation from taking place and dead skin cells get trapped in the sebum making the skin feel bumpy and congested. Second, the skin feels uneven when there is a *lack* of natural moisture making the surface skin cells dry and flaky.

Temperature – a hot skin is associated with excessive stimulation whilst a cold skin denotes a general lack of stimulation. A warm skin is a sign of general good health and well-being.

Age – skin ages at different rates and does not always reflect a person's age in years. Overexposure to the elements especially the sun, cigarette smoke, poor diet, illness, lack of care etc. all contribute to premature ageing which can be seen in a general lack of tone when the skin is gently pinched together between the forefinger and thumb. A young skin will bounce back quickly when released. This reaction slows with the effects of ageing as the skin and underlying muscles lose their tone.

Imperfections – including areas of open and blocked pores, papules and pustules (skin blemishes), comedones (blackheads) and milea (whiteheads). Areas of broken capillaries, hyperpigmentation (excess colour e.g. age spots) and hypopigmentation (lack of colour) may also be classified under this heading.

Moisture content – the skin and indeed the body as a whole is made up of a large percentage of water. The moisture content of the skin can be judged in two ways – surface moisture and internal moisture. Surface moisture relates to the skin's natural oil in the form of sebum which is in turn made up of a large percentage of water. Internal moisture relates to the amount of water in the body and thus the skin. Surface moisture contributes to the dryness or oiliness experienced in some skin types whilst internal moisture contributes to general hydration and dehydration.

The skin type may then be judged as a direct result of analysing the skin in this way. General classification of skin types include:

- **Mature** – skin that shows visible signs of the ageing process in terms of uneven colour, texture, temperature and moisture content. The skin is subsequently dull, wrinkled and generally lacking in tone.
- **Young** – skin that does not yet show signs of the ageing process.
- **Normal** – even colour, texture, temperature and moisture content and generally associated with a younger skin
- **Dry** – dull in colour, uneven and flaky in texture, warm in temperature, lacking in moisture and generally associated with an ageing skin.
- **Oily** – sallow in colour, uneven and congested in texture, cool in temperature, excessive sebum (oil) and generally associated with puberty.
- **Sensitive** – pink in colour, fine texture, warm temperature, usually slightly lacking in moisture and generally associated with pale skins of any age.

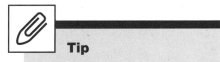

Tip

Oily skin is often referred to as **seborrhoeic**.

- **Combination** – an oily type on the skin of the forehead, nose and chin (centre panel) with normal to dry/sensitive type on the skin of the cheeks and neck. This skin type is the most common skin type amongst all ages.

In addition the skin may exhibit other characteristics including:

- **Hardness** – often develops over areas of the body for added protection and is usually associated with excessive pressure in a particular area e.g. hard skin on the feet is often caused by the added pressure associated with poor posture, on the hands with hard manual work and on other areas of the body with piercings and injury.
- **Tightness** – often associated with tension in underlying muscles and joints.
- **Flaking and peeling** – may signify a disorder e.g. athlete's foot.
- **Cracked** – may be caused by overexposure to harsh weather and unsuitable products and/or signify a skin disorder e.g. eczema etc.
- **Puffiness** – indicates general congestion associated with disorders such as cellulite, acne etc.

Skin conditions

It is not the job of a masseur/masseuse to ever make a diagnosis when conducting a skin analysis. However, it is necessary to ascertain whether or not a condition can be treated with massage. When analysing skin conditions it is useful to consider the **specific** types of conditions in terms of being **genetic, degenerative** and those caused by **microbes.**

- **Genetic** – these include inherited conditions. TREAT WITH CARE obtaining medical approval first.
- **Degenerative** – these include conditions associated with the effects from overexposure to extreme elements, the overuse of incorrect and harsh products and in some cases the side effects of certain medications. TREAT WITH CARE obtaining medical guidance.
- **Microbes** – these include infectious conditions that are caused by either viruses e.g. cold sores (Herpes Simplex), bacteria e.g. impetigo, fungi e.g. athlete's foot and parasites e.g. head lice. DO NOT TREAT until condition has cleared.

Analysis of the accompanying symptoms will provide additional guidelines. Possible symptoms include:

- **Inflammation** – redness, heat, swelling, pain and loss of function. DO NOT TREAT.
- **Fever** – an increase in normal body temperature. DO NOT TREAT.
- **Oedema** – swelling as a result of an excessive amount of fluid in the tissues. TREAT WITH CARE.

Tip

Different skin types may be treated with massage paying attention to depth of pressure and choice of medium (product).

Tip

Do not treat any area of undiagnosed swelling – instead refer the client to their GP for diagnosis.

- **Allergic reaction** – extreme sensitivity to a substance (allergen) that is normally harmless. DO NOT TREAT.
- **Tumours** – abnormal growth of tissue, which may be benign (not serious) or malignant (tendency to become progressively worse resulting in death). DO NOT TREAT.

These conditions and accompanying symptoms may be classified as being either *local* or *systemic*, *congenital* or *acquired* and *acute* or *chronic*.

- **Local** – affecting one part or a limited area of the body.
- **Systemic** – affecting the whole of the body or several of its parts.
- **Congenital** –present in the body from the time of birth.
- **Acquired** – developed since birth.
- **Acute** – sudden and severe but short in duration.
- **Chronic** – long in duration.

The condition of the skin of the body will also reflect care and attention. If lack of care of a part of the body is evident then there is likely to be a lack of attention to the whole of the body and vice versa! The possible causes of this will help to determine a person's mental state e.g.

- A lonely person may feel that as no one appears to care for them why should they care for themselves.
- A person who has experienced physical/verbal abuse may have been made to feel that they do not deserve any care and so are afraid to care for themselves.
- A person who dislikes themselves or a part of themselves may feel that they are not worthy of care.

It is also worth noting that perhaps a person is not aware of how to take care of a certain part of their body and so needs specific advice on general aftercare e.g.

- Ensure the area is kept clean and dry.
- Exfoliate regularly using a product appropriate to the part e.g. facial/body scrubs.
- Moisturise daily to hydrate and protect the surface skin.
- Drink plenty of water to hydrate and protect from within.
- Pay attention to diet to ensure adequate nutrients are available for repair and maintenance.
- Pay attention to breathing to ensure that cellular respiration is efficient.
- Protect the area from the elements with suitable clothing as appropriate.

Client care is therefore of primary importance during a consultation and can be a vital tool in encouraging the client to care for themselves.

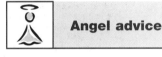

Angel advice

What a person thinks about their body often reflects the way they think about themselves as a whole.

Remember

The level of care given to a client must be professional – it is not a practitioner's job to befriend – and within the scope of your individual skills e.g. refer a client who needs specialist help.

System sorter

CONTRAINDICATIONS

Any medical condition, abnormality or change in the body should be checked and medical advice sought if in doubt as to the suitability of massage.

Skeletal/muscular systems

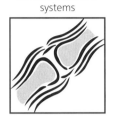

Respiratory system

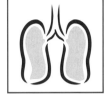

Integumentary system

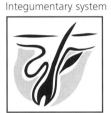

Circulatory system

- Open and infected areas of skin may cause cross-infection if massaged.
- Skin diseases and disorders may be irritated and worsened through massage.
- Bruising, sunburn and windburn will be painful and skin may be further damaged by massage.
- Recent scar tissue may be irritated and painful if massaged, thus hindering healing.
- Large, hairy or inflamed moles may be stimulated through massage.

- Bone fractures may be prevented from setting if massaged over.
- Painful or swollen joints may be further irritated by massage.
- Injured muscles, tendons and/or ligaments should be avoided to allow healing to take place.
- Severe arthritis, rheumatism and/or osteoporosis as massage may cause pain and damage.
- Undiagnosed pain e.g. back pain in the case of serious damage.

- Severe asthma needs medical approval and care over the chest area.
- Laboured breathing requires medical attention prior to massage.
- Shortness of breath requires medical attention prior to massage.
- Influenza may cause cross-infection.
- Severe coughs and colds may cause cross-infection and be irritated by the massage.

- Heart conditions should be checked as massage stimulates the circulation.
- High blood pressure requires medical attention if not already controlled.
- Low blood pressure requires medical attention as massage may lower blood pressure further.
- A blood clot (thrombosis) or a history of circulating blood clots (embolism) as massage may dislodge the clot causing it to travel through the system and block a vital organ.
- Inflammation of the veins (phlebitis) and varicose veins causing pain and discomfort and may accompany thrombosis.

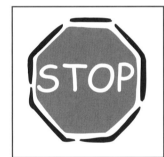

- Diabetes requires medical advice.
- Problems prior, during and post pregnancy require medical advice.
- Abnormal changes in skin colour require medical attention.
- Transsexualism requires medical advice during hormone treatment.
- IVF (*in vitro* fertilisation) requires medical advice during hormone treatment.

- Inflammation of the nerves (neuritis) as massage will cause further irritation.
- Trapped or pinched nerves need medical advice prior to the application of massage.
- Paralysis due to loss of function and loss of feeling.
- Epilepsy requires medical advice.
- Migraine headaches as massage may worsen the effects.

- The first trimester of pregnancy as the stimulation of massage may initiate a miscarriage.
- Leading up to and during menstruation as massage may irritate and increase blood flow.
- Kidney infections as massage may cause further discomfort.
- A full bladder which will be irritated by massage.
- Gynaecological infections.

- Full stomach as massage stimulates the circulation to the skin and muscles and away from the digestive system, delaying digestion.
- Empty stomach as massage will increase hunger levels.
- Under the influence of drugs or alcohol as massage will speed up absorption and circulation around the body.
- Undiagnosed pain in the abdominal organs.
- Diarrhoea and stomach cramps.

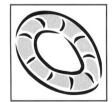

Endocrine system

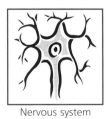

Nervous system

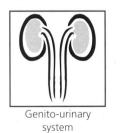

Genito-urinary system

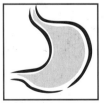

Digestive system

NB. Cancer may affect any system of the body and in some cases more than one system. In any situation a client suffering with cancer requires medical attention and a masseur/masseuse needs ongoing medical advice and guidance if treatment is agreed.

Once stages one and two have been completed the treatment itself may take place, and this forms a natural progression with the use of the massage techniques discussed in Chapter 7 (see Part 4 for a suggested order of work for each part of the body).

However, fact finding continues to take place through the tactile methods associated with manual massage as well as by using specific **palpation techniques** in order to be able to detect differences in the texture and tone of the tissues i.e. skin, muscles, ligaments, tendons and bones as well as identify areas of damage.

Palpation techniques involve the use of the hands, fingers and/or thumbs to gently feel over the area. A level of sensitivity is required in the hands/fingers/thumbs that is often not present in someone new to massage. Practice and experience leads to greater levels of sensitivity and simple tasks can help including:

- Try differentiating between a grain of rice, sea salt and sugar through touch alone (eyes closed). Gradually repeat this exercise with smaller particles e.g. different grades of sand.

- Place a strand of hair on a hard surface and with your eyes closed run your fingers over the surface trying to detect the position of the hair. Now try this exercise with a strand of hair on a soft surface and/or an uneven surface.

- Slide your hand/fingers/thumbs over your own skin with varying amounts of pressure and try to detect the various changes in texture and tone. Think about the underlying structures and learn to identify changes that are normal and those which may be caused by tension, overwork and/or damage.

Consultation – stage three

The third stage of the consultation takes place at the close of the massage treatment, providing the opportunity to discuss **outcomes**, **reactions**, **aftercare**, **home care** and **further treatments.**

Outcomes

The result of the treatment. Giving and obtaining feedback is a vital part of the massage treatment, providing the practitioner and the client with the means to find out more about how the treatment relates to the individual.

- It is necessary to discuss your findings with the client relating them to the information gained at each stage of the consultation e.g. amount of physical tension in the part etc.

- It is also useful to obtain feedback from the client with reference to how they felt during the treatment e.g. depth of pressure etc. as well as how they are feeling post-treatment e.g. relaxed, increased well-being etc.

CONSULTATION STAGE THREE – TREATMENT CLOSE

Treatment date: ....

Outcomes: ....

....

....

Reactions: ....

....

....

Aftercare: ....

....

....

Homecare: ....

....

Further treatments: ....

....

....

Any other comments: ....

....

....

....

....

....

Tip

Prior to the giving and receiving of feedback it is advisable to move the client into a seated position (if not already) ensuring that they are well covered and warm.

● It is useful for subsequent treatments to ask the client to take note of their feelings both physically and emotionally over the next 24–48 hours.

Reactions

What may happen as a result of the treatment in terms of *actions* and *contra actions*. A client needs to be aware of the type of the positive reactions to treatment (actions) – increased well-being etc. – as well as the possible negative reactions to treatment (contra actions) – increased emotions etc. – they may realistically expect to experience as a result of the treatment they have received (see Chapter 6 for details).

Aftercare

Advice relating to the reactions experienced as a result of the treatment. It is important to alert a client to the likely reactions to treatment and to what action they should take e.g.

Angel advice

How many times have we heard people saying that they haven't had the time to go to the loo during the course of a day? Think about the accumulative adverse affects this has on the body and mind as the body fills up with unreleased waste! This thought alone is enough to remind us to go!

- Respond to the releasing requirements of the body i.e. fulfil the urge to urinate, defecate etc. Allow time for the body to activate its healing mechanisms and consider ways in which the coping mechanisms may be enhanced by avoiding excesses.

- Respond to the replenishing requirements of the body i.e. natural, uncarbonated spring water and a light meal is recommended post-treatment. The avoidance of caffeine, alcohol and difficult to digest foods is advisable. A period of rest is recommended post-treatment with any further activity monitored to ensure that any excess is avoided where possible.

Aftercare is usually basic common sense but nonetheless should be reinforced as part of the consultation process for all clients.

Tip

Justification of a proposed course of aftercare promotes greater understanding and in turn more action!

Home care

Advice relating to the practice of self-help procedures. In addition to basic aftercare advice, information should be available for the client to continue caring for themselves between treatments. This advice should be relevant to the information gained during the consultation and treatment, achievable for the client and within the limits of the practitioner's expertise. Home care advice may include information on the following (see Part 4 for more details relating to each part of the body):

- Nutrition – basic advice relating to healthy breathing, eating and drinking.
- Ageing – information on the effects of the ageing process and realistic techniques to help to counteract and accept.
- Rest – the importance of time out.
- Exercise – the use of simple exercises to aid postural problems.
- Awareness – listening to the body and responding accordingly.
- Special care – realistic self-help techniques to de-stress e.g. self-massage, meditation, the effects of positive thinking with the use of visualisations and affirmations.

Angel advice

Visualisations incorporate the use of a positive visual image and affirmations incorporate the use of a spoken word or phrase. Both techniques can help to reinforce positive thinking.

Home care should be individual to each client and form the basis for continued self-development, remembering to refer a client to a specialist when recommendations are out of the realms of your expertise. This encourages clients to take responsibility for their own well-being.

Further treatments

Advice on subsequent and complementary treatments. All forms of massage treatments offer cumulative effects over a period of time and care should be taken to explain this to a client relating the timing to the nature and severity of their condition.

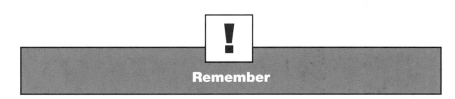

Remember

It often takes people a long time to become stressed and/or ill. In the same way it will also take time for a person become de-stressed and/or well. Neither situation happens over night.

There is no limit to how often a massage treatment may be carried out but attention should be paid to all aspects of the consultation as well as the outcomes and reactions of the treatment. This ensures that recommendations may be made in terms of individual adaptations for the area to be treated, and the length and depth of subsequent treatments.

Task

It may be necessary to provide a client with advice on other treatments that complement massage. Make a list of the treatments you feel would be a complement to massage. Remember that if you are unable to perform these treatments, suitable recommendations and referrals should be made.

The close of the consultation provides the time for any final client questions and confirms the ending with the client getting dressed, completion of payment and subsequent booking details.

Finally, a consultation may be seen as a **connecting** process between the client, practitioner and treatment and as a result has the potential be either **effective** or **non-effective**.

- An effective consultation involves intuitive practice set amongst a backdrop of theory (rules, regulations and guidelines) to ensure health, safety and welfare resulting in an open dialogue between client and practitioner for the good of the treatment.
- A non-effective consultation is one that ignores the balance between theory and practice, becoming either impersonal and automated or too personal and inappropriate.

Massage provides an holistic treatment which has the potential to affect the whole of the body, mind and spirit and care should be taken to ensure that there is balance and harmony between the theory and the practice of the consultation process. Paying attention to the theory ensures that the consultation is carried cut correctly and being aware that the practice can be adapted ensures that the consultation feels right.

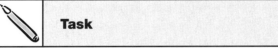

Task

Devise a client questionnaire to be used by the client post-treatment. Include questions relating to the treatment as well as how they felt over the next 24–48 hours. Think about how you can use the information gained in subsequent treatments.

Task

Devise a general aftercare sheet that may be given to the client during stage three of the consultation.

Task

Start to compile a portfolio of evidence to demonstrate your commitment to provision of service. Include all paperwork that may be used during the consultation e.g. consultation forms, information sheets, client questionnaires, aftercare sheets. Also include information relating to the health, safety and welfare of the clients with regard to the code of ethics and legislative requirements e.g. qualification certificates, insurance documents, policy statements etc. This portfolio can be added to as you progress and provides a focal point for client information.

Knowledge review

1   How many stages make up a consultation?

2   When does a consultation begin?

3   Give two ways in which verbal messages are communicated.

4   Give four examples of non-verbal communication.

5   How are tactile messages communicated?

6   What is the main aim of the first stage of the consultation process?

7   List the five areas for checking during stage one of the consultation.

8   What are 'open questions'?

9   What is jargon?

10   What do clarifying questions do?

11   What are the six senses used to aid stage one of a consultation process?

12   Who signs the consultation form?

13   What is palpation?

14   Name the three body types.

15   Which figure fault is recognised by a hump back and rounded shoulders?

16   Which figure fault is recognised by a hollow back?

17   List the six guidelines associated with skin analysis.

18   What is an oedema?

19   What is a benign tumour?

20   What is the term given to a condition that affects the whole of the body or several of its parts?

Part 4
Massage treatment

Learning objectives

After reading this part you should be able to:

- Recognise the anatomy and physiology of the parts of the body indicated for massage treatment.

- Identify the needs of the whole of the body as well as the parts in terms of massage treatment.

- Understand the principles and practice of manual massage treatment.

- Be aware of the considerations and adaptations to massage treatment.

- Appreciate the holistic links associated with massage treatment.

The continuous practical, theoretical and spiritual research into the art and science of massage over many hundreds of years, spanning all corners of the world has led to the introduction of many variations of massage treatment. As discussed in previous chapters, massage is primarily an intuitive skill that takes its origins from the art of touch – the birthright of each and every individual. As such, massage requires no formal introduction or study because we can all do it. To lose sight of this fact and focus too much attention on learning defeats the object of massage. The following chapters aim to focus the emphasis on creating a balance between the theory and practice of massage. Drawing from the research, development and experience of our forefathers (and mothers) but never losing sight of the inbuilt, intuitive skill that is our own, the next chapters will provide treatment suggestions and insights to be interpreted, used, adapted and changed to suit the needs of each individual masseur/masseuse and each individual client within the boundaries of recognised standards.

Massage really is a journey of discovery in the greatest sense of the word. As you discover more about yourself and your client you will subsequently discover more about massage and vice versa.

The back

The back is an amazing place to start when learning to apply the art of massage as a treatment.

- The back is a large, relatively flat expanse of tissue that is excellent to practice all massage movements on.
- It avoids the need for eye contact as the client faces away from the masseur/masseuse, so making the treatment less daunting to perform and to receive.
- You will never be short of people to practice on because everyone needs and wants a back massage!

However, before attempting to treat members of the public, the theory of massage needs to be considered in order to ensure a safe and professional treatment including:

- Anatomy and physiology of the back – exactly what you are working on.
- Considerations – specific guidelines for the safe treatment of the back.
- Treatment tracker – tracking the treatment from start to finish.

Anatomy and physiology of the back

The back forms the posterior surface of the trunk. It extends longitudinally from the top to the base of the spine. As such the back incorporates the neck, shoulders, upper, middle and lower back.

Bones and joints of the back

The bones and joints of the back include:

- The spine – a central column consisting of irregular bones forming the cervical, thoracic, lumbar, sacrum and coccyx

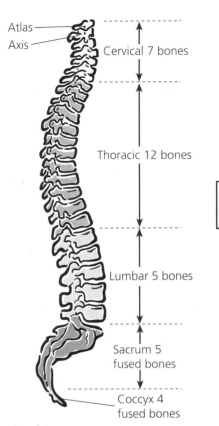

Atlas

Axis

Cervical 7 bones

Thoracic 12 bones

Lumbar 5 bones

Sacrum 5 fused bones

Coccyx 4 fused bones

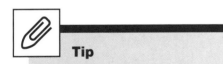

The spine

regions. There are seven cervical bones, twelve thoracic bones, five lumbar, five sacrum and four coccyx bones. The top two bones are known as the atlas and axis and contain synovial (freely moveable) joints. The next five bones of the cervical region form cartilaginous joints (limited movement) together with the bones of the thoracic and lumbar regions. The bones of the sacrum and coccyx regions are fused together to form fibrous joints (no movement).

Tip

The lower body is protected by the **pelvic girdle** of which the sacrum and coccyx form the attachment at the base of the back with a synovial gliding joint. This allows for slight movement between these bones during pregnancy.

- Twelve pairs of ribs – long bones forming the rib cage.
- The shoulder blades – two flat bones called the scapulae bones.
- The collar bones – two long bones called the clavicle bones.

Tip

The upper body is protected by the **thorax** which is made up of the twelve pairs of ribs which attach to the twelve thoracic vertebrae at the back. The ribs curve around to form the ribcage with the seven upper pairs attaching to the sternum (breast plate) at the front of the body. The next three pairs of ribs attach themselves to the upper seventh pair of ribs leaving two pairs of floating ribs having no attachment at all at the front of the body.

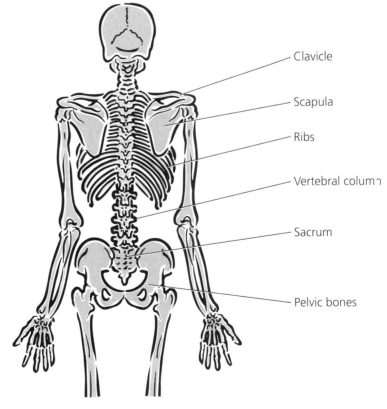

Clavicle

Scapula

Ribs

Vertebral column

Sacrum

Pelvic bones

Bones of the back

Muscles of the back

The muscles of the back include:

- **Trapezius** – large triangular muscle of the upper back.
  - Position – extending from the base of the skull at the occipital bone along the cervical and thoracic vertebrae to the clavicle bones and scapulae.
  - Action – aids in movements of the head i.e. nodding and movement of the shoulders i.e. lifting, rotating and adducting the scapulae.
- **Erector spinae** – a group of three deep muscles lying in layers including the **iliocostalis** (outer layer), **longissimus** (middle layer) and **spinalis** (inner layer).
  - Position – extend along the spine at the centre of the back from the neck to the pelvis.
  - Action – responsible for maintaining upright posture, lateral flexion and extension of the spine.
- **Rhomboids** – major and minor muscles which lie *under* the trapezius muscle.
  - Position – major extends from the 2nd–5th thoracic vertebrae to the scapula. Minor extends from the 7th cervical and 1st thoracic vertebrae to the scapula.
  - Action – aids in shoulder movements i.e. adduction and upward rotation of the scapulae.

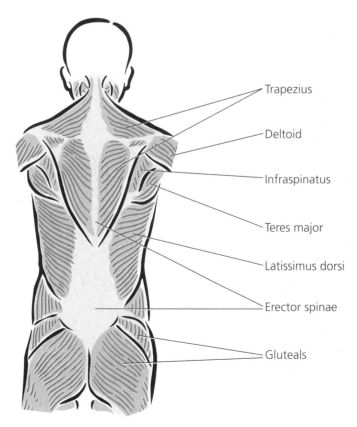

Muscles of the back

- **Latissimus dorsi** – large muscle of the mid back.
  - Position – extends from the lower six thoracic, lumbar and sacral vertebrae to the humerus bone of the upper arm.
  - Action – aids in shoulder movements i.e. rotation, adduction, extension and helps to lower shoulders when raised.
- **Leveter scapulae**
  - Position – extends from the first four cervical vertebrae to the scapula.
  - Action – aids in raising the shoulder.
- **Serratus anterior**
  - Position – extends from the borders of the upper eight to nine ribs to the scapulae.
  - Action – aids in shoulder movements i.e. abduction and upward rotation of the scapulae.
- **Teres** – major and minor muscles.
  - Position – extend from the scapula to the humerus.
  - Action – aids in shoulder movements i.e. extension, adduction and rotation of the shoulders.
- **Infraspinatus**
  - Position – extends from the scapula to the humerus.
  - Action – aids in shoulder movements i.e. rotation, abduction and extension of the shoulder.
- **Deltoid** – contains anterior, middle and posterior fibres.
  - Position – extends from the clavicle to humerus bones at the front, middle and back of the shoulder.
  - Action – aids in shoulder movements i.e. abduction, flexion, adduction and rotation of the shoulder.

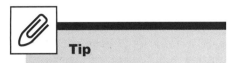

Tip

The serratus anterior muscle helps in the actions associated with pushing and punching.

Tip

Parts of the waist and buttocks are included in a back massage. The **oblique** muscle group form the waist and the **gluteal** muscle group form the buttocks.

Blood and lymphatic vessels

The main vessels associated with the circulatory systems are located within the trunk of the body for which the back as a whole provides a protective posterior surface. The lungs, heart and main arteries and veins are located in the upper region of the trunk. Blood and lymphatic capillaries are situated throughout the back draining into the **axillary** lymph nodes in the armpits, the **inguinal** lymph nodes in the groin and the **thoracic** and **right lymphatic ducts** before entering the right and left **subclavian veins** in the upper chest (see Chapter 5 for details).

Nerves

The spinal cord, which forms part of the central nervous system together with the brain, lies beneath the vertebrae of the spine.

Thirty-one pairs of spinal nerves radiate out from the spinal cord in between the vertebrae to all parts of the body. These nerves are part of the peripheral nervous system and are arranged in the following way:

- 8 pairs of cervical nerves
- 12 pairs of thoracic nerves
- 5 pairs of lumbar nerves
- 5 pairs of sacral nerves
- 1 pair of coccyx nerves.

These spinal nerves intermingle to form networks or groups called *plexuses* from which they divide and branch out to provide nerves to all parts of the body. The nerves of each area of the spine form plexuses except for the thoracic region. The thoracic nerves provide individual nerve supply specifically to the muscles of the chest and abdomen.

The main plexuses include:

- **The cervical plexus** – containing the first four cervical nerves which branch out to supply the skin and muscles of the neck and shoulder. The **phrenic** nerve is associated with this plexus and it stimulates the contraction of the diaphragm during respiration.
- **The brachial plexus** – containing the remaining four cervical nerves and part of the first thoracic nerve which branch out to supply the skin and muscles of the upper limbs. Nerves from this plexus include the **radial** and **ulnar** nerves that affect the triceps and biceps muscles of the upper arm as well as the skin and muscles down the arm to the fingertips.
- **The lumbar plexus** – containing the first three lumbar nerves and part of the fourth which branch out to supply skin and muscles of the lower abdomen, groin and part of the lower limbs.
- **The sacral plexus** – containing part of the fourth lumbar nerve, the fifth lumbar nerve and the first four sacral nerves which branch out to supply the skin and muscles of the pelvis, the buttocks and part of the lower limbs. The **sciatic** nerve is one of the nerves that branches out from this plexus.

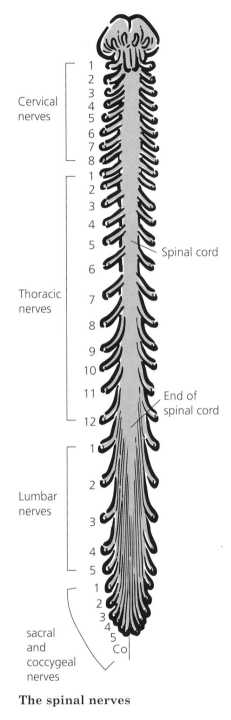

Cervical nerves
1
2
3
4
5
6
7
8

Thoracic nerves
1
2
3
4
5
6
7
8
9
10
11
12

Spinal cord

End of spinal cord

Lumbar nerves
1
2
3
4
5

sacral and coccygeal nerves
1
2
3
4
5
Co

The spinal nerves

Fascinating Fact

The sciatic nerve is the longest nerve of the body and is responsible for the pain associated with the disorder sciatica. The nerve supply becomes impeded by excess pressure or damage and pain is experienced in the hips and buttocks down through the knee to the ankle.

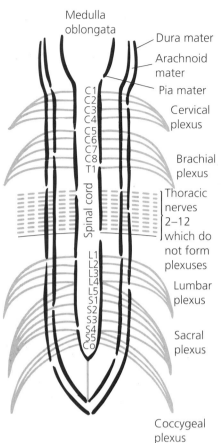

Medulla oblongata

Dura mater

Arachnoid mater

Pia mater

C1
C2
C3
C4
C5
C6
C7
C8
T1

Cervical plexus

Brachial plexus

Spinal cord

Thoracic nerves 2–12 which do not form plexuses

L1
L2
L3
L4
L5
S1
S2
S3
S4
S5
Co

Lumbar plexus

Sacral plexus

Coccygeal plexus

The spinal plexuses

- **The coccygeal plexus** – containing part of the fourth and fifth sacral nerves and the coccygeal nerves which branch out to supply the muscles and skin of the external structures of the digestive and reproductive organs.

The peripheral nervous system contains both sensory (afferent) nerves allowing impulses to be sent from the body to the spine and brain and motor (efferent) nerves allowing impulses to be sent from the brain and spinal cord to the various parts of the body.

In addition, the autonomic nervous system provides a network of nerves that lie in front of the vertebrae from the thoracic to the lumbar region branching out to supply the organs of the body.

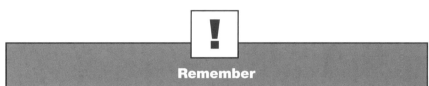

!

Remember

The peripheral nervous system is responsible for **voluntary** actions e.g. movement and the autonomic nervous system is responsible for **involuntary** actions e.g. breathing, digestion etc.

Associated organs

The back provides a protective external posterior covering for most of the major organs of the body. Knowledge of their position and function is vital when treating the back (see Chapter 5 for details).

Considerations

In order to ascertain the suitability for massage treatment of the back, the preferred choice of massage medium and the specific contraindications it is necessary to consider the following:

Skin type and condition

The skin of the back is often poorly cared for because of its location and as a result tends to suffer the extremes of skin conditions, for example:

- Oily skin prone to enlarged and blocked pores, papules, pustules and comedones. Oily skin is usually associated with a young skin type. Powder or gel is the preferred choice of massage medium.

- Dry skin prone to flakiness and tightness due to lack of natural moisture in the form of sebum. Dry skin is usually associated with ageing skin. Oils or creams/emulsions are the preferred choice of massage medium.

- Dehydrated skin caused by lack of internal moisture in the form of water. Dehydrated skin is associated with all ages and skin types. Oils or creams/emulsions are the preferred choice of massage medium.

Other considerations pertaining to the skin of the back include:

- Hair is often present on the backs of men. Powder may be the preferred choice of massage medium to prevent hair from tangling and any accompanying discomfort.

- Moles may be present and changes often go undetected as a person cannot always see their back. Record moles on the record card and inform the client of any changes.

Remember

Any changes in the appearance and texture of moles may denote an underlying serious problem that needs urgent medical attention.

- Tattoos are increasingly popular and often found on the back. Recent tattoos will be contraindicated to massage and the skin may only be treated when the area is completely healed.

- Fatty deposits are often found at the base of the neck (referred to as a Dowager's hump) which may cause problems with maintaining correct head position as the head is pushed forward. Massage can help to ease the tension associated with such a build-up.

- Fatty deposits are often found at the waistline and below requiring more stimulating massage.

Muscle tone and condition

The muscles of the back work together with the muscles of the front of the body to maintain an upright position. As such, the muscles of the back exhibit a certain amount of tone at all times except when the body is at rest. Muscle tone should be equal between the muscles at the front and back of the body but all too often imbalance exists as muscles are held excessively tight for long periods of time due to poor posture – sitting at a computer for long hours, carrying a heavy child, briefcase etc. resulting in muscle strain and aching muscles. Muscles can only maintain tone for limited periods of time before they need replenishing with rest and nutrients. Failure to meet these basic needs means that the muscles perform at a less than optimum level resulting in muscle fatigue; they feel tight and sore to touch and in extreme cases postural figure faults including kyphosis, lordosis and scoliosis occur. In addition, muscle fibres become knotted in an attempt to maintain tone and this can be felt as hard, painful lumps (often referred to as *nodules*) when the muscles are pressed against bone. Massage can help to loosen tight and knotted muscles, easing the nodules, stimulating the circulation and improving overall tone and condition. Care must be taken to ensure that the pressure is not too great at the start of the massage treatment, increased slowly and with care to prevent undue discomfort.

Activity

Feel your own shoulders with your fingers. Do they feel tight? If you press a little more firmly can you feel hard lumps that move around? These are nodules and may be quite painful so touch with care. Notice how you can slowly increase your pressure as you get used to the feel of your fingers on the area. Remember this when you start to massage other people.

Joint mobility

Tight muscles result in tight joints and the temporary loss of the full range of movement in the joint. This is often apparent in the neck and shoulders. Head movements become strained and painful and shoulder movements restricted. Joint movements become easier when the surrounding muscles are relaxed and the synovial fluid that bathes the joints is warm. Massage to the neck and shoulders has the potential to achieve this and so is a useful aid to improving joint mobility in the upper body generally. Care must be taken never to force any movement in a joint.

Stress

A stressed body shows itself in the overall condition of the back resulting in tight muscles and joints which in turn impedes blood and lymphatic circulation as well as the flow of electrical impulses through the nerves. Massage to the back will stimulate the circulation and help to free the neuro-muscular pathways.

Tip

The peripheral nerves pass from the spinal cord in between the vertebrae and branch out to the rest of the body through muscles. Their route is referred to as neuromuscular pathways.

This has the effect of improving the activity within the whole of the body making a back massage a necessary component in the quest for stress relief.

Contraindications

Always conduct a consultation checking general contraindications pertaining to the body as a whole – refer to Chapter 8 for more details.

Specific contraindications to back massage include:

- Undiagnosed back pain – DO NOT TREAT, refer to GP for advice.
- Lung disorders where lying on the front inhibits breathing – reduce pressure over the lungs or avoid completely.
- Kidney disorders where massage to the lower back would be painful. DO NOT TREAT, seek medical advice.

Ask the client if they need to visit the toilet prior to having their back massaged as lying in a prone position being massaged will put pressure on the bladder!

- Early stages of pregnancy due to the risk of miscarriage caused by excessive stimulation to the lower back. DO NOT TREAT.
- Later stages of pregnancy as the client cannot lie prone – TREAT WITH CARE, an alternative position should be sought e.g. lying on their side etc.
- Just prior to and during menstruation as massage to the lower back may cause discomfort and stimulate blood loss. TREAT WITH CARE with guidance from client (some people gain comfort from gentle massage to the back prior to and/or during menstruation).

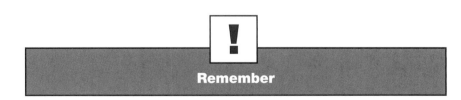

Common sense is needed when assessing a client for massage. If in doubt always seek confirmation from a more senior colleague if possible and/or obtain medical advice prior to any massage taking place.

Suggested order of work – the back

The back massage commences with a simple **hold**, as the hands are gently placed on the top or bottom of the back, and the application of a suitable massage medium with non-directional effleurage movements. This allows for the gentle introduction of the product and the practitioner's hands which may both be a little cold and strange at first.

The massage continues with:

1 **Directional effleurage**
   - Both hands together – start at the base of the back. Place a hand on either side of the spine. Stroke upwards, with pressure, towards the shoulders using the whole of the palmar surface of the hands. Bring the hands back down to the base of the back easing off the pressure. Repeat 3–6 times.
   - Alternate hands – as above using the hands alternately.
   - Figure of eight – place one hand on top of the other at the base of the back. Stroke up one side of the back until you reach the scapula. Continue moving the hands around first one scapula and then the other in a figure of eight pattern. As you do so walk around to the head of the couch.
   - Reverse effleurage – starting at the top of the back, effleurage with both hands. Effleurage down to the base of the back with no pressure and back up with pressure.

Tip

Reverse effleurage may be carried out with the hands pulling up the lateral (outer) sides of the back or with the hands pulling up the centre either side of the spine. The former promotes good posture and the latter relieves tension in the erector spinae muscles.

Moving back to stand at the base of the back using figure of eight effleurage, the back massage continues with:

2 **Petrissage**
   - Flat-handed kneading – three to four movements over the length of each side of the back to gently ease the tension in the muscle fibres.
   - Thumb or finger kneading – small circles up the sides of the spine and around the scapulae feeling for the knots of tension.
   - Alternate-handed picking up – both hands used alternately to pick up the flesh in three rows along the length of the back working both sides of the spine.

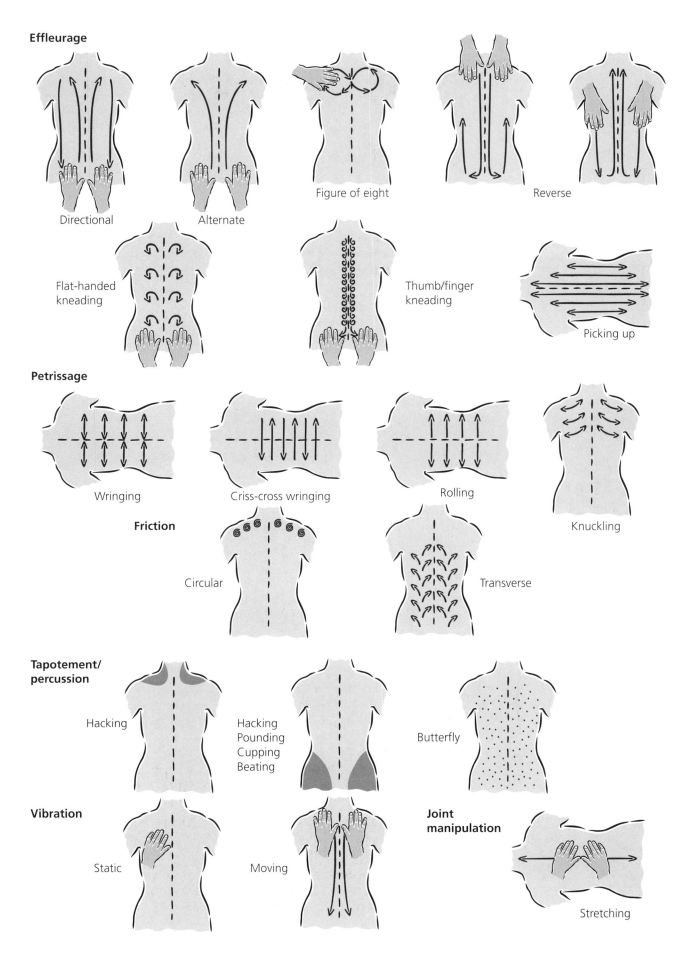

Effleurage

Directional

Alternate

Figure of eight

Reverse

Flat-handed kneading

Thumb/finger kneading

Picking up

Petrissage

Wringing

Criss-cross wringing

Rolling

Knuckling

Friction

Circular

Transverse

Tapotement/percussion

Hacking

Hacking
Pounding
Cupping
Beating

Butterfly

Vibration

Static

Moving

Joint manipulation

Stretching

- Wringing – across the length of both sides of the back in turn. This may be followed with a criss-cross wringing over the entire back.
- Rolling – along the length of both sides of the back in turn.
- Knuckling – along and into the shoulders and around the scapulae.

3   **Friction**

- Circular friction – paying particular attention to localised knots of tension (nodules) perform circular friction with the fingers or thumbs.
- Transverse friction – may be performed up the length of the back in rows easing out the underlying muscle tension.

4   **Tapotement/percussion**

- Hacking – may be used with care over the fleshy areas of the upper back and shoulders avoiding the scapulae and vertebrae.
- Hacking, cupping, beating and pounding – may be used over areas of fatty tissue at the base of the back and waist with care.
- Butterfly – over the entire back provides gentle stimulation.

!

Remember

Always link tapotement/ percussion movements with effleurage.

Tip

Tapotement/percussion movements can be noisy to perform and may disrupt relaxation simply because of the sound!

5   **Vibration**

- Static vibration – can be used over each scapula in turn with the whole of the palmar surface of the hands.
- Moving vibration – can be used with the fingers moving up or down the spine.

6   **Joint manipulation**

- Stretching – place both hands across the centre of the back (fingers facing the far side of the back) and gently stretch one hand towards the base of the neck and the other towards the base of the back.

7   **Effleurage**

- Directional – over the entire back as performed at the start of the routine.
- Figure of eight – to move to the head of the couch.
- Reverse – as before.
- Non-directional – finishing off the treatment with gently strokes.

8   **Holding** – ending the treatment with a gentle hold at the top of the back or shoulders and lift off to close.

Treatment tracker

THE BACK

A back massage may be carried out as an isolated treatment – treatment time 30–45 minutes including consultation.

A back massage may be carried out as part of a full body massage – treatment time 1 hour with 10–20 minutes for the back.

If part of a full body massage, the back is generally treated at the close of the treatment.

Preparation

- Conduct a full consultation.
- Check general and specific contraindications.
- Agree treatment and preferred massage medium with client.
- Removal of upper clothing – females may leave their bra on if they prefer and just have it unclipped for treatment.
- Removal of lower body clothing if necessary to avoid creasing.
- Skin may be cleansed with appropriate cleanser.
- Exfoliation may be performed as appropriate to skin type and condition.

Babies/children – stroking effleurage and gentle petrissage movements may be applied to the back to ease tension and encourage relaxation at times of stress. This is particularly beneficial if performed by a parent as it has the effect of soothing both parties. Massage may be performed on a baby without or without clothes.

Elderly – the skin and muscle tissue tends to be thin and fine and may have adhered to the underlying bones due to loss of movement. Massage movements need to be gentle and the length of massage time shortened to ensure discomfort is avoided.

Male – muscular tissue tends to be bulkier and stronger in male clients and as such requires a greater depth of pressure. This may be more apparent along the top and base of the back.

Female – special care needs to be given during menstruation and pregnancy i.e. a non-contraindicated pregnant client may choose to lie on their side and consideration should be given to the use of pillows to ensure adequate support. In addition, massage chairs may also be used for back massage and when used, a position should be sought that takes into account comfort and safety of both the client and masseur/masseuse.

Position

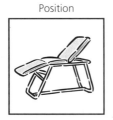

Client – the usual position for a back massage is with the client lying prone on a flat couch with their head either:

- To the side resting on a towel or pillow.
- Centred with their face resting through a face hole in the couch.
- Centred with their forehead resting on their hands.

Masseur – the usual position is standing to one side of the couch and:

- Moving around to the head of the couch to work the upper back.
- Moving around to the opposite side of the couch if necessary.

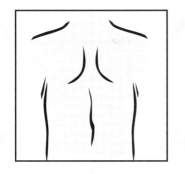

Lymphatic drainage – draining movements will help to remove the toxins associated with tense muscles. Movements should be directed to:

- Upper back – axillary lymph nodes under the arms.
- Lower back – inguinal lymph nodes in the groin.

Posture – should be checked and advice given for correction:

- Shoulders should be centred.
- Pelvis should be centred.
- Waist even.
- Weight evenly distributed through back.

Client care

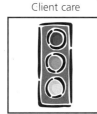

Considerations for client comfort when having a back massage include:

- An extra pillow may be needed under the chest to support the thoracic curve associated with *kyphosis*.
- An extra pillow may be needed to put under the abdomen to support the lumbar curve associated with *lordosis*.
- Rolled up towels may be used under the top of the feet to support the ankle if needed.
- A blanket, duvet or towel may be used to ensure modesty and warmth.
- Ensure hair is out of the way of the area to be treated.
- Necklaces, dangling ear rings etc. should be removed.
- Clients should be reminded that they may move as and when they feel they need to.
- Skin with little underlying fatty tissue will be more sensitive to touch and temperature. Take care to warn the client that you are about to start the massage and try to warm your hands before doing so.

- A few moments should be allowed for the client to come to gradually.
- Removal of excess massage medium may be carried out with cologne wipes and/or spritzers.
- Post-treatment procedures may be carried out as appropriate i.e. masks, self tan etc.
- Client should turn over and assume a seated position slowly if not already seated.
- Offer the client a glass of water to refresh and purify.
- Obtain feedback and offer aftercare, homecare and further treatment advice.

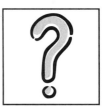

Adaptations

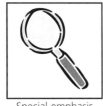

Special emphasis

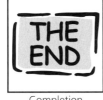

Completion

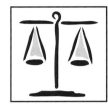

Holistic harmony

The back is a precious part of the body that suffers greatly from neglect and misuse. It is an area of the body that quickly tells us when we are stressed. Research has shown that the most likely reason for someone taking time off work is because of back problems. It is therefore not enough for someone to seek a back massage or indeed perform a back massage with the expectation that all aches and pains, stresses and strains will miraculously disappear. Becoming stress-free is a way of life just as becoming stressed soon develops into a way of life! Holistic harmony presents the means to increase awareness and understanding of the body's quest for balance. A balanced state between body, mind and spirit is the key to coping with the stresses of life and such a state is complementary to the effects of massage. Massage should not be viewed in isolation, it is in fact a small part of a much bigger picture that if viewed as a whole has the potential to be much more effective in maintaining a healthy state. As such, thought should be given to the following.

Pre-treatment procedures

It is quite common for many people to seek a back massage as a last resort i.e. when their back really aches and their shoulders are so tight they are almost reaching their ears! It is however useful to encourage clients to think about their activity prior to having a massage as well as procedures the practitioner can put into place to enhance the effectiveness of the massage including:

- Exercise – a visit to the gym can help to de-stress the mind and body in preparation for massage.

- Cleansing – a shower can help to physically cleanse the body but also provide the time to cleanse the mind of the day's stresses. Power showers can focus the spray of water on particularly tight muscles and the warmth of the water provides a soothing preparatory effect.

- Communal heat treatments – sauna, steam and spa treatments are a pleasant way of de-stressing the mind and body after a long day. The heat helps to relax tight muscles and the social interaction helps to distract and energise the mind.

- Individual heat treatments – the use of a paraffin wax, steamer, heat lamp or hot towels prior to massage taking place can target specific trouble spots on the back providing warmth and relaxation.

Tip

Paraffin wax treatments are particularly beneficial in aiding joint mobility as well as providing a nourishing treatment for the skin.

- Exfoliation – body scrubs massaged vigorously onto the skin can be both mentally and physically stimulating. Negative thoughts are sloughed away as the surface skin cells desquamate leaving the mind clear and the body smooth!

Tip

Massage mediums are more readily absorbed into the skin if it has been previously prepared with exfoliation.

Additions

Mechanical massage treatments may be used in addition to the manual massage including:

- Audio sonic vibrator – may be used on areas of extreme tension. The vibrations penetrate deeply into the tissue making this an ideal additional treatment to back massage.
- Brush cleanse – a gyratory treatment that may be used in two ways:
  1 As a preparatory treatment to deep cleanse the area. This is especially beneficial for congested and blemished skin types.
  2 As a means to encourage greater absorption of product. This is especially useful for dry skin types.
- Gyratory – hand-held or free-standing gyratory machines have the benefit of simulating all types of massage movements and are particularly useful if a client is nervous of being touched. A machine often seems less personal. It is also useful if a deep massage is needed as different heads can be applied with different speeds.
- Vacuum suction – used specifically to aid the removal of static lymph from congested areas of the body and to stimulate lymphatic drainage. This is particularly useful in areas where there is an excess of fatty tissue which often contributes to sluggish circulation e.g. sides and base of the back. Movements would be directed to the inguinal lymph nodes in the groin.

Post-treatment procedures

It is always advisable to leave the client for a few moments post-treatment to allow them to 'come to'. In addition thought can be given to providing post-treatment procedures to enhance the effects of the massage including:

- Mask – a pre-prepared mask e.g. gel or cream mask, a specially prepared mask e.g. clay mask or a thermal mask may be applied to suit the skin type in much the same way as one would treat the face as part of a facial. This is often referred to as being a 'back facial'.

- Self-tan – it has become increasingly popular for clients to request the application of self-tanning products that can be applied after the skin has been exfoliated and moisturised taking care to ensure an even application.
- Spritz – a final spray with cologne is a pleasant way to end the treatment, remove any excess massage medium and refresh and reawaken a client.

Self-help

It is important to provide aftercare advice that encourages a person to take greater responsibility for their own well-being both generally and specifically. General aftercare procedures should be followed after any form of massage treatment (please refer to Chapter 8 stage 3 of the consultation process).

In addition specific information may be given including:

Nutrition

Nutritional advice should be realistic, progressive and achievable. A good starting point is to recommend that a person drinks in the region of one and half litres of water daily. People often find this difficult, especially if they are not used to drinking water. In the short term it may therefore be advisable to encourage a person to drink just one glass of water in addition to their other drinks each day or alternatively replace one of their daily drinks with a glass of water until the next time you see them. If they have managed this successfully, you will be able to encourage them to gradually increase their daily water intake and decrease their intake of tea, coffee etc. until it is at a more acceptable level for health and well-being.

Remember

Drinks that contain caffeine, e.g. tea and coffee, are *diuretics*. This means that they encourage the body to lose water rather than conserve it. This contributes to dehydration. Alcohol is also a diuretic.

Ageing

The skin and muscles of the back age at the same rate as the skin and muscles everywhere else on the body. However, lack of care contributes to the speeding up of the ageing process and the back is a notoriously difficult area of the body to apply self care. Regular massage treatments together with pre- and post-treatment procedures can help to establish a care routine that will provide long-term benefit. Self massage to the neck and shoulders will contribute to anti-ageing and well-being. We cannot prevent the ageing process but with care and attention we can help to delay it and learn to live with it more effectively.

Rest

The back is responsible in part for maintaining an upright posture and as such, the muscles are in a constant state of tone. In order to maintain this tone and prevent muscle fatigue, it is important to allow the muscles of the back time to rest. Resting the muscles allows replenishment of vital nutrients in the form of oxygen from breathing and food and water from the diet. When at rest the back should be well supported with a firm mattress for sleeping and a comfortable chair for relaxing.

Exercise

Exercise is of particular benefit for maintaining the health of the back. Posture checks and postural corrections should be applied prior to any form of exercise and attention to maintaining correct posture should be paid throughout.

Specific exercises for postural figure faults include:

- **Kyphosis** – the aim is to **strengthen** the trapezius and rhomboid muscles and **stretch** the pectoral muscles helping to draw the shoulders backwards.
  - Circle shoulders backwards.
  - Circle arms backwards.
  - Clasp hands behind the back, pulling the arms up and the shoulders back.
- **Lordosis** – the aim is to **stretch** the erector spinae muscles and to **strengthen** the abdominal muscles.
  - Lying face up on the floor with the knees bent, pressing the lumbar region of the spine into the floor.
  - Lying face up on the floor with knees bent, chin in the chest, raising the head and shoulders to look at the knees.
  - Kneeling on all fours, arching the back.
- **Scoliosis** – the aim is to restore balance between the muscles on the sides of the back e.g. the muscles on the outside of the curve will need **strengthening** and the muscles on the inside of the curve will need **stretching**.
  - Standing with feet hip distance apart, reaching up with the hand on the concave side of the curve, reaching down towards the floor with the other hand.
  - Standing with feet hip distance apart, bending to the convex side where the muscles are stretched.

- Lying on the floor face up, stretching one arm above the head and opposite leg along the floor to stretch and raising opposite arms and legs to strengthen.

- **Flat back** – the aim is to **strengthen** the erector spinae muscles.

  - Lying face up on the floor lifting the legs alternately.
  - Kneeling on all fours, lifting alternate legs up and back.
  - Kneeling on all fours alternately arch and hollow the back.

- **Winged scapula** – to **strengthen** the muscles of the scapula.

  - Kneeling on all fours, bending and straightening the elbows.
  - Press ups with bent or straight legs depending on muscle strength.
  - Punching a punch bag.

General exercises such as swimming, yoga, pilates etc. are of particular benefit to the care of the back.

Awareness

Massage takes its origins from many cultures and times throughout history. Developing an awareness of the many cultural differences surrounding massage is a useful tool in self development as well as the development of our own massage treatments. Eastern cultures focus heavily on the effects of massage on energy. The Chinese refer to this energy as 'chi' or 'Qi', the Japanese as 'ki'; both cultures believing that energy flows through meridians or channels in the body. The Ayurvedic beliefs of India describe energy as 'prana' and refer to seven **chakras** which they believe are energy stores, points where the male Yang energy and the female Yin energy meet. They act as transformers, collecting and storing energy so that it can be used effectively within the body. The Ayurvedic belief is that the chakras are located along the central nervous system in the brain and spinal column and include:

- The first chakra located in the coccyx region of the spine.
- The second chakra located in the sacral region of the spine.
- The third chakra located in the lumbar region of the spine.
- The fourth chakra located in the thoracic region of the spine
- The fifth chakra is located in the cervical region of the spine.
- The sixth chakra is located in the brain at centre forehead.
- The seventh chakra is located in the brain in the middle of the head.

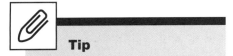

Tip

Exercise should only be attempted when the muscles are warm.

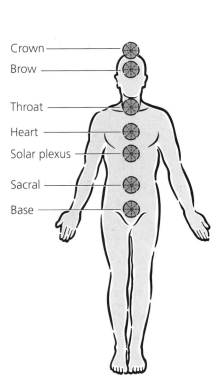

Crown
Brow
Throat
Heart
Solar plexus
Sacral
Base

The chakras

Massage treatment to the back is believed to have a positive effect on the energy within these chakras which in turn has a positive effect on the rest of the body. And as a person is made up of more than just a body and is body, mind and spirit, this produces an holistic effect i.e. affects the whole person.

Special care

The whole body will reap the benefits of any special care given to the back. Affirmations and visualisations provide a useful means of reinforcing this care. They are easily done, do not cost anything and if they instil a sense of positivity then they have achieved a great deal!

Examples for the back include:

- Affirmation – 'My life is whole, I am supported, I am flexible and I am able to move freely.'
- Visualisation – visualise the rays of the sun bathing the back in warmth. Imagine the feeling as the tight muscles soften and loosen. Now visualise a cool breeze maintaining just the right temperature as you continue to bask in the afterglow.

Tip

An affirmation is a thought or phrase to affirm positive intent. A visualisation is a positive image in which one feels safe and secure.

 Activity

Practice the order of work with a partner who is also studying massage if you can. Discuss the treatment with each other highlighting one another's strengths and weaknesses i.e. how does the massage feel? Does it flow? Is the pressure suitable? etc.

Task

Imagine you had a client for a back massage and during the treatment you noticed that they had two large dark moles on their back. What action would you take and why?

Knowledge review

1   What are vertebrae?

2   Name the individual regions of the spine.

3   How many bones make up each region?

4   Which two regions of the spine contain bones that are fused together?

5   How many pairs of ribs make up the rib cage?

6   What are the collar bones and shoulder blades called?

7   What is the name of the large triangular muscle of the back?

8   Name the muscle that contains three layers that is located along the spine.

9   Where is the latissimus dorsi muscle located?

10   How many pairs of spinal nerves make up the peripheral nervous system?

11   What is a plexus?

12   What is the name given to the longest nerve of the body?

13   What are the names of the lymph nodes situated in the underarms and groin?

14   Name the two lymphatic ducts.

15   What is a neuro-muscular pathway?

16   What can changes in the colour and texture of a mole on the back signify?

17   Which massage medium is most suited to treat a hairy back?

18   Why is the early stage of pregnancy a contraindication for back massage?

19   Which massage movements start and end a back massage as well as link other movements?

20   Which massage movement enables the masseur/masseuse to move from the side of the couch to the head of the couch without losing physical contact with the client?

The arms and hands

The arms and hands are classified as the *upper limbs* whilst the legs and feet constitute the *lower limbs.* As such, the arms and hands are a popular site for massage either as part of a manicure treatment or as part of a full body massage.

Anatomy and physiology of the arms and hands

The arms and hands attach to the body at the shoulder joint forming external separate limbs that extend down to beyond the hip joint.

Bones and joints of the arms and hands

The arms and hands form part of the appendicular skeleton and consist of the:

- Humerus – long bones forming the upper arms.
- Ulna and radius – long bones forming the forearm.

These three bones join to form the elbow joint at which there are two separate joints:

- Hinge joint between the humerus, ulna and radius allowing movements of flexion and extension.
- Pivot joint between the ulna and radius allowing rotational movements i.e. supinate – turn so that the palm faces up – and pronate – turn so that palm faces down.

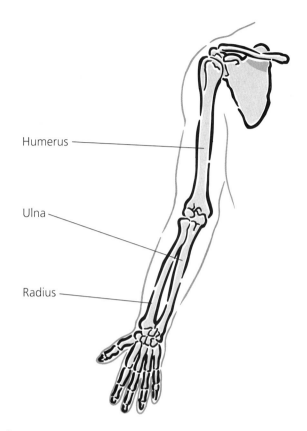

Humerus

Ulna

Radius

Bones of the arm

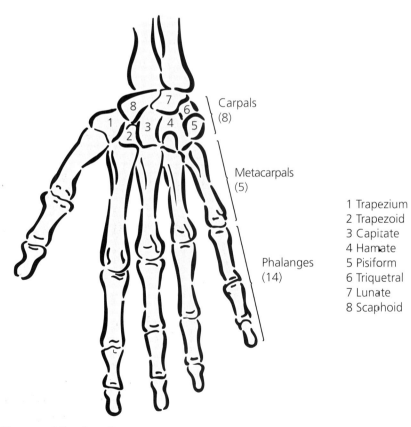

Carpals
(8)

Metacarpals
(5)

Phalanges
(14)

1 Trapezium
2 Trapezoid
3 Capitate
4 Hamate
5 Pisiform
6 Triquetral
7 Lunate
8 Scaphoid

Bones of the hand

Remember

The prominence of the elbow joint forms the olecranon process.

The wrist is made up of eight individual short bones:

- Trapezium
- Trapezoid
- Capitate
- Hamate
- Pisiform
- Triqutral
- Lunate
- Scaphoid.

The joint at the wrist between the radius and the carpal bones is an ellipsoid allowing movements of flexion, extension, abduction and adduction.

Plane joints exist between the individual carpal bones offering a gliding movement.

The hand and fingers are made up of:

- Metacarpal bones – five miniature long bones forming the length of the hand.
- Phalange bones – fourteen miniature long bones – two to each thumb and three to each finger.

The thumb forms a saddle with the carpal and metacarpal bones allowing an almost full range of movement.

The fingers form condyloid joints where the phalange bones meet the metacarpal bones allowing slightly less movement.

The joints between the bones of the fingers and thumbs are all hinge joints, allowing flexion and extension only.

Muscles of the arms and hands

Muscles of the upper arm include the **deltoid, biceps, triceps** and **brachialis:**

- **Deltoid** – contains anterior, middle and posterior fibres.
    - Position – extends from the clavicle to humerus bones at the front, middle and back of the shoulder.
    - Action – aids in shoulder movements i.e. abduction, flexion, adduction and rotation of the shoulder.

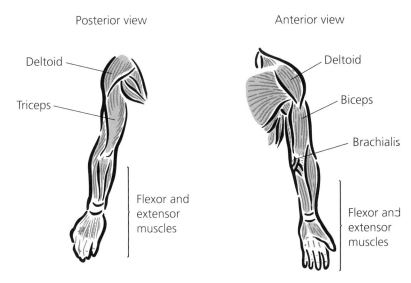

Posterior view   Anterior view

Deltoid
Triceps
Flexor and extensor muscles

Deltoid
Biceps
Brachialis
Flexor and extensor muscles

Muscles of the arms

- **Biceps brachii**
    - Position – extends from the scapula at the shoulder joint to the radius bone at the elbow joint at the front of the upper arm.
    - Action – aids in the flexion of the arm at the elbow, supination of the forearm and hand (turning the palm upwards).

- **Triceps brachii**
    - Position – extends from the shoulder joint to the elbow joint at the back of the upper arm.
    - Action – works in opposition with the biceps to extend the arm.

- **Brachialis**
    - Position – situated at the front of the arm extending from the lower part of the humerus bone to the upper part of the ulna bone.
    - Action – works with the biceps to flex the arm at the elbow.

Muscles of the lower arm and hand include **flexor and extensor** muscles of the forearms and hands:

- **Flexor muscles of the forearms**
    - Position – extend from the radius and ulna bones at the elbow to the metatarsal bones at the base of the fingers.
    - Action – flex the wrist.

- **Extensor muscles of the forearms**
    - Position – extend from the radius and ulna bones at the elbow to the metacarpal bones at the base of the fingers.
    - Action – extend the wrist.

- **Flexor muscles of the hand**
    - Position – extend from the base of the humerus at the elbow to the phalange bones of the fingers and thumb.
    - Action – flex the fingers and thumb.

Tip

The small muscles of the palm of the hand form the *thenar eminence* at the base of the thumb and the *hypothenar eminence* at the base of the little finger. These can be felt as fleshy protrusions.

- **Extensor muscles of the hand**
  - Position – extend from the base of the humerus at the elbow to the phalange bones of the fingers and thumb.
  - Action – extend the fingers and thumb.

Tip

Abductor and adductor muscles are present at the sides of the forearm and hand allowing the hand to move from side to side.

Blood and lymphatic vessels

Oxygenated blood is circulated to the arms and hands from the heart via the aorta which branches out to form the subclavian, axillary and brachial arteries.

Deoxygenated blood is circulated from the arms and hands via the brachial, axillary and subclavian veins before draining into the superior vena cava and finally the heart.

Lymphatic capillaries drain waste in the form of lymph from the cells for filtering in the nodes:

- Supratrochlear nodes – situated in the crook of the elbow.
- Axillary nodes – situated in the armpit.

The remaining lymph is circulated to the lymphatic ducts:

- Right lymphatic duct drains lymph from the right arm and hand.
- Thoracic duct drains lymph from the left arm and hand.

These ducts drain into the subclavian veins (see Chapter 5 for details).

Nerves

The brachial plexus contains four cervical nerves and part of the first thoracic nerve which branch out to supply the skin and muscles of the upper limbs. Nerves from this plexus include the **radial** and **ulnar** nerves that affect the triceps and biceps muscles of the upper arm as well as the skin and muscles down the arm to the fingertips.

Associated organs

There are no specific organs associated with the arms and hands as all of the organs of the body are located within the trunk and head.

Considerations

Tip

The skin of the arms may be hairy especially in men, in which case powder may be a preferred choice of massage medium.

Tip

Nail problems often accompany dry skin e.g. flaking, peeling, thin and/or brittle nails.

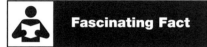

Fascinating Fact

Just as many people are now seeking laser treatment to remove tattoos as are having tattoos!

Remember

Masseurs/masseuses are likely to develop well toned muscles in their arms and hands due to the nature of their work.

As with other areas of the body, it is necessary to give thought to certain considerations prior to the application of massage to the arms and hands including:

Skin type and condition

The skin of the arms and hands is generally normal to dry and as such the preferred massage medium is generally oils or creams/emulsions. Specific conditions affecting the arms and hands include:

- Sun damage – the hands in particular are constantly exposed to the effects of the sun's rays and are often forgotten when it comes to the application of sun screening products (think about the times we wash our hands after applying sunscreen to the rest of the body!). Overexposure to the ultra violet rays will result in pigmentation marks, dry, rough and wrinkling skin.

- Wear and tear – the hands again tend to suffer the most from everyday wear and tear because of the continuous physical stress and strain they are under. The constant use of water, especially extreme temperatures together with detergents of any kind, tends to dry out and irritate the skin contributing to signs of premature ageing.

- Fatty deposits – are common on the upper arm. Massage can help to break down these fatty deposits for utilisation by the body as energy as part of a calorie controlled diet.

- Tattoos – are popular on the whole of the arm and may even extend onto the hands and fingers. Care should be taken to ensure they have healed completely prior to massage taking place.

- Pressure marks – from jewellery e.g. rings, watches etc may be present. It is advisable to remove all jewellery prior to a massage treatment taking place.

Muscle tone and condition

Muscle tone associated with the arms and hands is generally good due to the fact that the upper limbs are in constant use. A common site for the weakening of muscle tone is the upper arms. The triceps muscle is less used than the biceps and tends to become slack with lack of use resulting in loose, sagging upper arms.

Joint mobility

Due to the many joints associated with the arms and hands as well as the amount of stress and strain this area of the body is under on a daily basis the general mobility can be greatly affected. Areas most commonly affected include:

Fascinating Fact

Frozen shoulder is a condition affecting the middle-aged and elderly whereby severe aching pain is experienced in the shoulder joint and is accompanied by restricted mobility.

- Shoulder – many problems may be experienced associated with the upper arm where it joins the shoulder girdle resulting in partial or complete loss of mobility.
- Wrist and hands – repetitive strain injury (RSI) is a common disorder affecting the joints of the wrist and hands resulting in pain, loss of strength and partial or complete loss of mobility. Excessive joint use can also result in inflammation associated with conditions such as *arthritis*.

Fascinating Fact

Repetitive strain injury is a common complaint with masseurs/masseuses. Care should be taken to ensure movements are performed correctly and hands are treated well, e.g. adequate resting time between treatments, hand exercises etc.

Stress

Stress manifests itself in the arms and hands in a two-way process:

- Tension from the head, neck and shoulders is carried **down** through the length of the arms.
- Tension from the fingers and hands is carried **up** the length of the arms.

Working long hours at the computer and long distance driving are common causes of stress that affects the arms and hands. Tension tends to travel from the head and neck *down* the arms through poor sitting positions as well as being carried *up* the arms through the excessive use of the hands when typing or holding onto the steering wheel of a car.

The build-up of tension in this way will eventually result in muscle fatigue, partial or complete loss of mobility and accompanying pain. Massage provides an ideal means of helping to counteract the effects of stress.

Contraindications

A full consultation should be carried out prior to any form of treatment to the arms and hands. Specific contraindications pertaining to the arms and hands include:

- Any undiagnosed pain and/or swellings. DO NOT TREAT, seek medical advice.
- Complete loss of mobility and associated pain. DO NOT TREAT, seek medical advice.
- Warts are commonly found on the hands and may be contagious. AVOID AREA by covering with a plaster. Refer to GP for advice.

Remember

Common sense must also be used with regard to contraindications – if in doubt, leave it out!

Suggested order of work – the arms and hands

The arm and hand massage commences with a simple **hold** allowing the practitioner's hands to make contact with the area to be treated. The appropriate massage medium can then be applied using effleurage movements in any direction.

The massage treatment continues with:

1 **Directional effleurage to the arm and hand**
   - Support the client's arm with one hand. With the other hand stroke (a) **under** the length of the arm and hand with pressure and (b) stroke **over** the length of the arm and hand with no pressure. Change hands and repeat. Repeat using both hands twice more.
   - Place the arm down on the couch and work with one hand directly above the other to effleurage **up** the hand and arm with pressure and **down** without pressure. Repeat twice more.

2 **Directional effleurage to the upper arm**
   - As above starting from the elbow and working up to the shoulder.

3 **Petrissage to the upper arm**
   - Alternate palmar kneading working the triceps and biceps.
   - Single-handed picking up starting at the elbow and (a) working up to the shoulder on the outside of the arm, and (b) change hands and repeat on the inside of the arm.
   - Alternate-handed picking up from the elbow to shoulder.
   - Wringing starting at the elbow and working up to the shoulder.

4 **Tapotement/percussion to the upper arm**
   - Hacking may be applied to the upper arm with care.

5 **Vibration to the upper arm**
   - Shaking may be used if necessary by supporting the arm with one hand and gently shaking the muscles (biceps and triceps) in turn with the other hand.

6 **Directional effleurage to the upper arm**
   - Direct effleurage strokes from the elbow to the shoulder using alternate hands in an under and over motion, i.e. under the arm with pressure and over the arm without pressure.
   - Direct effleurage strokes from the elbow to the shoulder using two hands, i.e. up with pressure and down without pressure.

7 **Directional effleurage to forearm**
   - As above working from the wrist to the elbow.

8 **Kneading to the elbow**
   - Thumb or finger kneading in small circles around the elbow.

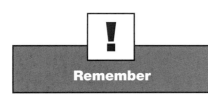

Remember

Always link tapotement/percussion movements with effleurage.

Directional effleurage

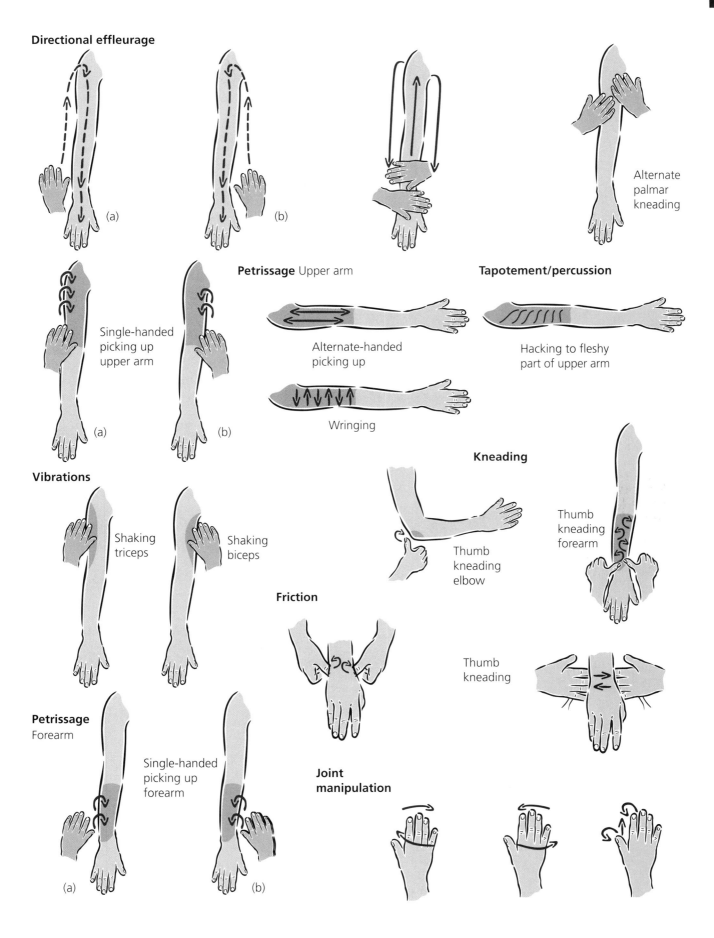

(a)   (b)

Alternate palmar kneading

Single-handed picking up upper arm

(a)   (b)

Petrissage Upper arm

Alternate-handed picking up

Wringing

Tapotement/percussion

Hacking to fleshy part of upper arm

Vibrations

Shaking triceps   Shaking biceps

Kneading

Thumb kneading elbow

Thumb kneading forearm

Friction

Thumb kneading

Petrissage
Forearm

Single-handed picking up forearm

(a)   (b)

Joint manipulation

Tip

Tapotement/percussion movements are generally *avoided* when working the forearm, hands, fingers and thumbs due to the lack of fatty tissue.

9 **Petrissage to the forearm**
- Thumb kneading up the forearm.
- Support the arm with one hand and apply single-handed picking up to (a) the lateral (outer) border of the forearm, change hands and apply to (b) medial (inner) border.

10 **Petrissage to the wrist/hand/fingers/thumb**
- Thumb kneading to the wrist, palm and back of the hand and up each finger and thumb.

11 **Friction to the wrist**
- Transverse friction applied superficially and quickly can be used to warm the wrist joint.

12 **Joint manipulation to the wrist**
- Support the arm and apply assisted rotation taking the wrist joint around gently in one direction and then the other.

13 **Joint manipulation to the fingers/thumb**
- Support the arm and hand and apply assisted rotation taking the fingers and thumbs around gently in one direction and then the other. Note that the thumb has more rotational movement than the fingers.

14 **Directional effleurage to the whole arm and hand**
- As for the start of the treatment.

15 **Hold**
- A gentle hold at the end of an effleurage stroke placing the hand and arm under the towel/blanket to end the treatment.

Treatment tracker

ARMS AND HANDS

The arms and hands may be massaged as part of a manicure, in which case the hands and arms are treated up to and including the elbow – total treatment time 45–75 mins including consultation. Massage time approximately 10 mins.

The arms and hands may be massaged in their entirety as part of a full body massage – treatment time 1 hour with 5 mins for each arm and hand.

If treated as part of a full body massage the arms and hands are generally massaged first.

Preparation

- Conduct a full consultation.
- Check for general and specific contraindications.
- Agree the treatment and preferred massage medium with the client.
- Remove clothing down to underwear for a full body massage. For an isolated arm and hand massage it is enough to roll up the sleeves.
- Skin may be cleansed with an appropriate cleanser.
- Exfoliation may be carried out appropriate to skin type.

Position

The position for a client to be in for an arm and hand massage depends on the nature of the treatment:

- As part of a manicure – the client would normally be in a seated position with their arm supported on a table and/or cushion.
- As part of a full body massage – the client would normally be lying in either a flat or semi-reclined supine position.

The position of the masseur/masseuse is at the side or opposite the client for a manicure and at the appropriate side of the couch for a treatment during a full body massage.

Client care

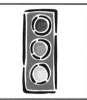

Considerations for client comfort when having an arm and hand massage in a lying down position include:

- Pillow behind the head for support if necessary.
- Blankets, duvets and towels for warmth, comfort and modesty.
- Watches, bracelets and rings should be removed.
- Hand and arm fully supported throughout massage treatment.
- A client should be reminded that they are free to move about if they wish.

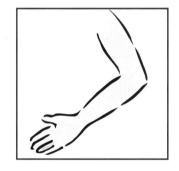

Babies/children – stroking effleurage and gentle petrissage movements may be used bearing in mind that certain areas of the hand and arm may be sensitive to touch i.e. palm of the hand and inside of the arm. This may cause a ticklish sensation in the young.

Elderly – loose flesh and stiff joints are commonly associated with the arms and hands of the elderly. Petrissage movements should be more superficial and joint manipulation movements performed with extreme care.

Male – firmer massage is generally needed especially over the large biceps and triceps muscles of the upper arm where tapotement/percussion movements may be more indicated than when treating a female client.

Female – looser muscle tone especially on the triceps of the upper arm requires additional toning treatment in the form of exercise which may be given as part of the after care advice.

Lymphatic drainage – drainage movements may be used to remove toxins associated with tense muscles. Movements should be directed to:

- Hands and lower arms – supratrochlear lymph nodes in the crook of the elbow.
- Upper arms – axillary lymph nodes under the arms.

Posture – the weight of the arms can easily pull the shoulder out of line if care is not taken to adopt correct posture:

- Shoulders centred.
- Arms held loose and free.
- Hands and fingers held loose and free.

- Remove excess massage medium if necessary.
- Move onto next procedure if part of a manicure.
- Apply post-treatment procedures e.g. masks, self tan etc.
- Cover the arm and hand to ensure warmth and comfort.
- Move onto next arm or next area of the body in a full body massage.

Adaptations

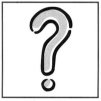

Special emphasis

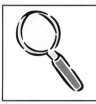

Completion

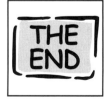

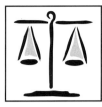

Holistic harmony

Forming part of the appendicular skeleton, the hands and arms are very much taken for granted. We forget to realise the very real contribution they make to everyday tasks. The arms and hands perform many varied and vital functions during the course of a day and require a certain amount of care in return if they are to maintain these functions in the long term. Specific areas for concern are often highlighted during a consultation and subsequent massage treatment and the close of the treatment is an ideal time to make recommendations for future treatments as well as home care.

A manicure generally incorporates treatment of the hand and forearm with the emphasis on the condition and appearance of the hands and nails.

Pre-treatment procedures

As part of a manicure the arms and hands are often treated to pre-massage treatments in the form of:

- Cleansing – antiseptic wipes may be used as a matter of course to ensure the area is clean and to check for contraindications. In addition, the use of foaming, perfumed cleansers and hot flannel mitts adds a touch of luxury to the treatment.

- Exfoliation – may be used as part of the cleansing process ensuring the removal of dead surface skin cells so that any nourishing product is more easily absorbed. This has the effect of livening up the skin leaving it fresh and smooth.

- Individual heat treatments – oils may be used as part of a 'hot oil manicure' to nourish the nails and cuticles through soaking before being used to massage the hands and arms. Heated mitts may also be applied to encourage further absorption. Paraffin wax is a popular pre-massage treatment for the hands and is often incorporated as part of a luxury treatment to aid joint mobility prior to massage.

All of these treatments, although primarily part of a traditional manicure treatment, may be incorporated into a massage treatment making for individually designed treatments that meet the specific needs of the clients.

Angel advice

More and more clients are becoming increasingly sophisticated in their needs and choice of treatments. To be commercial, a masseur/masseuse needs to introduce innovative ways in which to meet these needs whilst enhancing but never compromising standards.

Additions

The introduction of mechanical treatments is common for use on the arms as part of a full body massage:

- Gyratory – hand-held or free-standing gyratory machines are particularly useful if a client prefers a firmer massage. The different heads and varying speeds can be applied to simulate the massage movements ensuring additional pressure. This may be particularly useful for the upper arms.

- Vacuum suction – used specifically to aid the removal of static lymph from congested areas of the body and to stimulate lymphatic drainage. This is particularly useful in areas where there is an excess of fatty tissue which often contributes to sluggish circulation e.g. upper arms. Movements would be directed to the axillary lymph nodes in the armpit.

Tip

Electronic muscle stimulation (EMS) and micro current treatments are popular for tightening the muscles of the upper arm.

Post-treatment procedures

The arms and hands, like all parts of the body, benefit from a variety of post-treatment methods including:

- Individual heat treatments – paraffin wax treatments may be used post-massage as well as pre-massage. Pre-massage eases joints and encourages absorption of massage medium. Post-treatment continues the work of the massage leaving the area luxuriating in warmth and comfort.

- Masks – are particularly beneficial to the hands, the skin of which is often under physical attack through everyday tasks such as washing and cleaning etc. Soothing gel masks, nourishing cream masks and specially mixed clay masks may all be used to treat specific skin types and problems.

- Self-tan – the arms and hands in particular are difficult areas to apply self-tanning products effectively and so the application of such products post-massage is a useful addition to the massage treatment.

Tip

The application of self-tanning products post massage is useful for the client as it ensures even application. For the masseur/masseuse it is a commercial way of attracting more business.

Self-help

The arms and hands are parts of the body under constant pressure and as such need access to care and attention. Whilst a massage treatment offers such care and attention, it may also be necessary for a client to practice self-help techniques for themselves at home. Regular use of self-help techniques soon becomes habit and provides a means to enhancing the general well-being of the whole of the body as well as the parts.

Nutrition

Research has shown that a person's diet can affect the condition of bones generally. As conditions such as arthritis commonly affect the arms and hands thought should be given to:

- Foods to be avoided – including excessive amounts of protein, alcohol and caffeine which are believed to prevent calcium from being stored in the bones. Saturated fats and refined foods should also be avoided.
- Recommended foods – including those high in magnesium and vitamin D as both these minerals encourage the uptake and utilisation of calcium.

Ageing

The skin, bones, joints and muscles of the arms and hands show the effects of ageing in the following ways:

- Skin – irregular areas of pigmentation develop known as age spots. These are more commonly found on the hands.
- Bones – brittleness occurs in ageing bones as hormone levels change. This is particularly common in menopausal women who may develop osteoporosis.
- Joints – the many joints of the arms and hands suffer greatly by gradually stiffening through age, often developing the condition arthritis.
- Muscles – muscle strength and endurance is soon lost through lack of use resulting in weak and loose muscle tone.

It is important to be aware of the things one can do to help delay the ageing process as well as accept the things we cannot change.

Rest

The build-up of tension and restriction or loss of mobility commonly found in the arms and hands is greatly improved by rest. Allowing the muscles time to relax completely between activity will help to prevent the repetitive strain injury associated with many professions. Whilst resting it is important to ensure that the body is kept warm and free from draughts. Tension and mobility in the arms and hands will be aggravated if the limbs are cold. Warms baths provide an ideal way to encourage a restful state. The addition of oils, music and candles adds to the relaxation

Fascinating Fact

Arthritis is a common condition that can affect the joints of the whole body leading to pain and decreased mobility. Arthritis is brought on through the ageing process and physical 'wear and tear' as well as injury.

process which in turn aids sleep. This has a knock-on effect on the whole of the body as well as the parts.

Exercise

A balance between rest and activity results in healthy arms and hands with simple exercises being of benefit in reducing the build-up of tension and aiding flexibility, strength and coordination including:

- Arm shakes – remove the tension out of the entire arm by gently shaking it.
- Shoulder rolls – circle the shoulders forwards and backwards to warm and ease the joints and increase flexibility.
- Wrist circling – circle the wrists in both directions to warm and ease the joints and increase flexibility.
- Finger/thumb rotation – circle the fingers and thumbs in both directions to warm and ease the joints and increase flexibility.
- Weight-bearing exercises – any exercise that incorporates the use of weight will increase muscle strength e.g. *press-ups* using the body weight; or *arm curls* using a dumb bell.

Tip

Increasing the weight used to exercise with will increase muscle *strength*. Increasing the amount of times the weight is lifted will increase muscle *endurance*.

Angel advice

Weight-bearing exercises encourage the bones to store more calcium, helping guard against osteoporosis.

- Playing the piano – playing any musical instrument will help to stimulate neuromuscular pathways and increase brain to hand coordination.

Awareness

Learning to identify the sources of stress in our lives creates a level of awareness that forms the basis for all self-help. It may be necessary for the masseur/masseuse to confirm the effects of such stress in their clients and as a result make suggestions for self-help activities. These suggestions should always be *realistic, justifiable* and within the *scope* of the client:

- Realistic suggestions are more likely to be taken seriously by the client e.g. encouraging a person who drinks only tea and coffee to drink only water is unrealistic. It is much more realistic to suggest a gradual introduction of water together with a gradual decrease of tea/coffee etc.

- Justifiable suggestions ensure that a client understands the reasons why e.g. drinking more water helps to flush away toxins and keeps the body hydrated. Tea and coffee are diuretics which have the opposite effect on the body.

- Suggestions that are within the client's scope are much more attractive than those that are not e.g. visiting the gym three times a week may prove too expensive, too time-consuming, too embarrassing and just too hard, but walking to work three times a week or taking the stairs instead of the lift may be more achievable.

Angel advice

It is important to ensure that as a masseur/masseuse we 'practice what we preach'. Clients will find it difficult to follow our self-help suggestions if it is clear that we are not aware of our own personal stresses and do not bother to apply the principles to our own lives!

Special care

The arms and hands provide the means for receiving and giving special care and as such should not be underestimated. It is as important for human beings to receive special care as it is to give it and touch provides the most primary form of care. Touch, being the most natural form of comfort, can 'soothe like a balm'. The art of touch ensures feelings are passed from one person to another, often without the need for words. It connects us to the world around us helping to instil and maintain self-worth. It is therefore of vital importance to the well-being of each and every person to have some form of special care in their lives. For many people, personal relationships meet their needs for special care. For others it may be their relationship with a special pet. For others still, they may find that having a massage provides a form of special care that helps to enhance the way they feel about themselves e.g. if someone else is prepared to touch them then they must be worthy. In much the same way, a masseur/masseuse can also gain an element of self-worth from the art of giving massage.

Angel advice

The art of touch is the science of love.

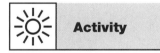

Activity

Practice the suggested order of work on a partner who is also studying massage so that you can continue to give each other feedback on your performance.

Task

Think about the reasons why a person's profession is likely to affect the condition of their hands e.g. hairdresser, doctor, mechanic, secretary etc. Use this knowledge to form a basis for the aftercare advice you give to individual clients.

Knowledge review

1   Name the bone that forms the upper arm.

2   Names the bones of the forearm.

3   How many bones make up the wrist and what are they collectively known as?

4   Where are the biceps and triceps muscles located?

5   How many bones form the hand and what are they called?

6   How many bones make up each finger and thumb and what are they called?

7   Which muscle works with the biceps to flex the elbow?

8   What type of joint enables the forearm and hand to supinate and pronate and where is it formed?

9   Where is the hypothenar eminence located?

10   Which plexus contains the nerves which affect the arms and hands?

11   Where is the olecranon process found?

12   What is the name given to the lymph nodes located in the crook of the elbow?

13   Which area of the arms and hands is more prone to loose saggy skin?

14   Which common condition is associated with inflammation of the joints, pain and decreased mobility?

15   What do the initials RSI stand for?

16   What does vitamin D encourage within the bones?

17   Why are warts a contraindication to arm and hand massage?

18   Why are tapotement/percussion movements generally avoided on the forearm and hand?

19   Which individual heat treatment aids joint mobility?

20   What may be carried out prior to massage to ensure that the massage medium is readily absorbed into the skin?

11

The buttocks, legs and feet

The legs and feet form the lower limbs with the buttocks forming the posterior surface at the top of the backs of the legs. Although the buttocks are not strictly part of the lower limbs, they are generally treated with the legs. This is largely due to the fact that clients may feel embarrassed, vulnerable and exposed if they are treated in isolation. As part of a leg massage, the buttocks may be treated individually, in part or in their entirety depending on the needs of the client.

Anatomy and physiology of the buttocks, legs and feet

The buttocks form the base of the posterior trunk extending to form the hips from which the legs extend. The legs extend to form the lower limbs including the thigh (upper leg), calf (back of the lower leg), shin (front of the lower leg), ankle, feet and toes.

Bones and joints of the buttocks, legs and feet

The buttocks, legs and feet form part of the appendicular skeleton and consist of:

The pelvic girdle:

- Sacrum and coccyx forming the base of the spine and the middle of the pelvic girdle.
- Coxae forming the protruding hip bones attaching to the sacrum and coccyx by fibrous (fixed) joints. Each coxa is made up of three fused flat bones:
  - Ilium
  - Pubis
  - Ischium.

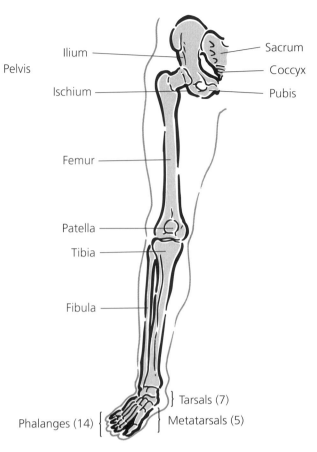

Ilium

Pelvis

Ischium

Sacrum

Coccyx

Pubis

Femur

Patella

Tibia

Fibula

Tarsals (7)

Phalanges (14)

Metatarsals (5)

Bones of the lower limbs

The legs:

● Femur – long bone that forms the upper leg or thigh.

The large joint between the coxa and femur bones is a ball and socket allowing a full range of movement.

● Tibia and fibula bones – long bones that make up the lower leg or shin at the front and calf at the back.
● Patella bone – a sesemoid bone forming the kneecap.

!

Remember

Sesemoid bones are small bones located within tendons and tendons attach muscles to bones.

The joint between the femur and tibia is a hinge allowing the knee to bend and straighten.

The ankle is made up of seven short bones including:

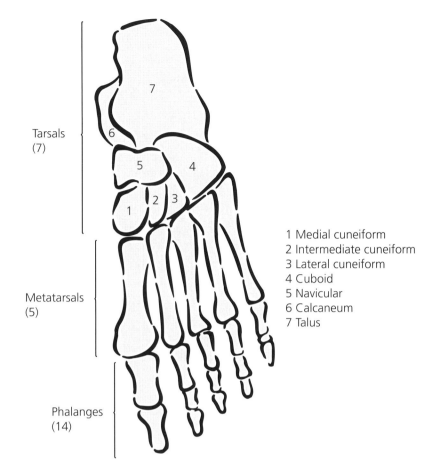

Tarsals
(7)

Metatarsals
(5)

Phalanges
(14)

1 Medial cuneiform
2 Intermediate cuneiform
3 Lateral cuneiform
4 Cuboid
5 Navicular
6 Calcaneum
7 Talus

Bones of the feet

- Calcaneum
- Talus
- Cuboid
- Navicular
- Medial cuneiform
- Intermediate cuneiform
- Lateral cuneiform.

The joint at the ankle between the tibia, fibula and the tarsals is an ellipsoid allowing the foot to bend upwards (dorsi flexion), stretch downwards (plantar flexion), turn in (inversion) and turn out (eversion).

The feet and toes are made up of:

- Metatarsal bones – five miniature long bones forming the length of the foot.
- Phalange bones – fourteen miniature long bones, three to each small toe and two to the big toe.

There are plane joints between the individual tarsal bones as well as between the tarsals and the metatarsals; these allow slight gliding movements only. Between the metatarsals and phalanges there are condyloid joints and between the individual phalange bones there are hinge joints.

Muscles of the buttocks, legs and feet

The muscles of the buttocks and outer thigh include the **iliopsoas, gluteal group** and the **tensor fascia lata**:

- **Iliopsoas**
  - Position – extends from the 12th thoracic to the femur bone.
  - Action – flexes the trunk towards the leg as in sitting up from a lying down position.
- **Gluteal muscle group** – there are three gluteal muscles:
- **Gluteus maximus** – largest most superficial muscle of the group
  - Position – forms the bulk of the buttock region extending from the sacrum to the femur.

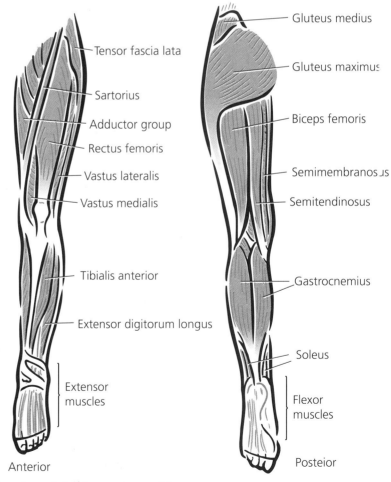

Muscles of the buttocks and legs

- Action – extends the trunk away from the leg as in standing from a bent position and extends the femur as in standing from a sitting position.
- **Gluteus medius**
  - Position – the outer thigh extending from the upper portion of the ilium to the femur.
  - Action – contributes to hip movements e.g. abduction and rotation.
- **Gluteus minimus**
  - Position – the outer thigh extending from the lower portion of the ilium to the femur.
  - Action – contributes to hip movements e.g. abduction and rotation.
- **Tensor fascia lata**
  - Position – upper, outer thigh extending from the front of the ilium to the femur.
  - Action – contributes to hip movements e.g. abduction and rotation.

Tip

The tensor fascia lata and gluteal medius and minimus are collectively known as the *abductor* muscle group due to their combined action of moving the leg away from the mid line of the body.

The muscles of the inner thigh include the **adductor muscle group** and the **gracilis**:

- **Adductor muscle group** – group of four muscles forming the inner thigh: the **adductor brevis**, **adductor longus**, **adductor magnus** and the **pectineus**.
  - Position – collectively this muscle group form the inner thigh extending from the pubis to the femur.
  - Action – adducts the thigh drawing the leg in towards the mid line.
- **Gracilis**
  - Position – inner thigh extending from the pubis to the tibia at the knee.
  - Action – adducts the thigh and flexes the knee.

The muscles of the front of the thigh include the **quadriceps group** and the **sartorius**:

- **Quadriceps muscle group** – there are four quadriceps muscles forming the front of the thigh: the **rectus femoris**, **vastus medialis**, **vastus lateralis** and the **vastus intermedius.**
  - Position – collectively this muscle group forms the front of the thigh extending from the top of the femur to the knee.
  - Action – contribute to hip movements and the extension of the knee keeping it straight when weight bearing.
- **Sartorius**
  - Position – extends from the outer hip to the inner aspect of the knee.
  - Action – contributes to hip movements and flexing of the knee.

The muscles of the back of the thigh include the **hamstring group**:

- **Hamstring muscle group** – there are three hamstring muscles forming the back of the thigh: the **biceps femoris**, **semimembranosus** and the **semitendinosus**.
  - Position – collectively this muscle group form the back of the thigh extending from the ischeum to the knee.
  - Action – extend the hip and flex the knee.

Muscles of the back of the lower leg and foot include the **gastrocnemius**, **soleus**, **flexor hallucis longus** and **flexor digitorum longus**:

- **Gastrocnemius**
  - Position – forms the calf extending from the base of the femur at the back of the knee to the tarsal bones at the ankle.
  - Action – flexes the knee and plantar flexes the foot.
- **Soleus**
  - Position – conjoins with the gastrocnemius muscle to form the lower calf and the Achilles tendon at the ankle.
  - Action – plantar flexes the foot.
- **Flexor hallucis longus**
  - Position – extends from the back of the fibula bone to the phalange bones of the big toe.
  - Action – flexes the big toe.
- **Flexor digitorum longus**
  - Position – extends from the back of the tibia bone to the phalange bones of the four small toes.
  - Action – flexes the small toes.

Muscles of the front of the lower leg and foot include the **tibialis anterior**, **extensor hallucis longus** and **extensor digitorum longus**:

- **Tibialis anterior**
  - Position – forms the shin extending from the top of the tibia bone at the knee to the first metatarsal bone.
  - Action – dorsi flexes the foot pulling it upwards.
- **Extensor hallicus longus**
  - Position – extends from the middle of the front of the fibula bone to the phalange bones of the big toe.
  - Action – extends the big toe.
- **Extensor digitorum longus**
  - Position – extends from the top of the outside of the tibia bone at the knee to the four phalange bones of the four small toes.
  - Action – extends the toes.

Tip

It is possible to massage the calf whilst the client is lying in a supine position by getting them to bend their knee resting their foot flat on the couch.

Some clients may prefer not to have their buttocks massaged in which case the massage routine ends at the top of the leg.

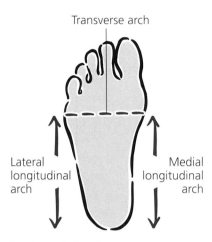

Arches of the feet

Tip

Abductor and adductor muscles form the inner and outer aspects of the lower leg and foot allowing the foot to move from side to side i.e. invert and evert.

The formation of the bones and the muscles of the feet create arches. There are three arches that distribute the weight of the body between the ball and the heel when the body is standing, walking or running:

1. Medial longitudinal arch – running along the inside length of the foot.
2. Lateral longitudinal arch – running along the outside length of the foot.
3. Transverse arch – running across the width of the foot.

Blood and lymphatic vessels

Oxygenated blood is circulated to the buttocks, legs and feet from the heart via the descending aorta which branches out to form the iliac, femoral, popliteal and anterior tibial arteries.

Deoxygenated blood is circulated from the buttocks, legs and feet via the anterior tibial, popliteal, femoral and iliac veins before draining into the inferior vena cava and finally the heart.

Lymphatic capillaries drain waste in the form of lymph from the cells for filtering in the nodes:

- Popliteal nodes – situated behind the knee.
- Inguinal nodes – situated in the groin.

The remaining lymph is circulated to the thoracic duct which drains into the subclavian veins (see Chapter 5 for details).

Nerves

The lumbar and sacral plexuses contain nerves which branch out to supply the skin and muscles of the lower limbs.

- Lumbar plexus – contains the first three lumbar nerves and part of the fourth which branch out to supply the skin and muscles of part of the lower legs.
- Sacral plexus – contains part of the fourth lumbar nerve, the fifth lumbar nerve and the first four sacral nerves which branch out to supply the skin and muscles of the pelvis, the buttocks and part of the lower limbs.

Remember

The sciatic nerve is the longest nerve of the body and extends from the sacral plexus down the lower limbs. It is responsible for the pain associated with the condition sciatica. The nerve supply becomes impeded by excess pressure or damage and pain is experienced in the hips and buttocks down through the knee to the ankle.

Associated organs

There are no specific organs associated with the legs and feet as all of the organs of the body are located within the trunk and head.

The bones and muscles of the buttocks add to the protection of the lower abdominal organs including those of digestion, excretion and reproduction.

Considerations

In order to ascertain the suitability for massage treatment of the buttocks, legs and feet, preferred choice of massage medium and contraindications it is necessary to consider the following:

Skin type and condition

The condition of the skin of the buttocks, legs and feet varies considerably. The skin of the **buttocks and legs** often experiences the following problems:

- Dryness – the skin of the buttocks and thighs of women often suffers with poor circulation caused by hormone fluctuations associated with puberty, menstruation and menopause. This affects cellular function and the renewal of skin cells contributing to skin condition. In addition, the skin of the shin is often excessively dry due to its extreme thinness where it covers the bones. Oil, cream/emulsions are the preferred choice of massage medium for this skin type.

- Superfluous hair – excessive hair growth on the lower limbs is common in people of Latin and Indian extraction and also occurs in females of all extractions during puberty, pregnancy and menopause due to hormone imbalance. The hair growth will often follow a typical male pattern becoming thicker and denser on the legs and bikini line. Powder may be the preferred choice of massage medium.

- Stretch marks are sometimes present on the skin of the buttocks and thighs. These occur when the skin has been overstretched due to excessive and/or rapid weight gain and/or pregnancy. The skin forms in distinct lines (transverse and longitudinal) that appear shiny and discoloured due to loss of elasticity in the dermis layer of the skin.

- Fatty deposits – excess fat from our diet is automatically deposited on the hips and thighs (amongst other areas) of women. This is a genetic factor that ensures that the lower part of the trunk and surrounding area is well protected for childbearing. Men tend to store excessive fat on their abdomens. The way in which the fat cells are positioned also differs between men and women. In men, the fat cells lie horizontally creating a smooth effect to the overlying skin. Conversely, in women, the fat cells point straight up into the skin contributing to the unevenness associated with cellulite. Massage can help to break down fatty tissue making it easier to lose as part of a calorie controlled diet.

- Cellulite – is a skin problem resulting in the characteristic 'orange peel' effect commonly found on the buttocks and legs of women. It is associated with poor circulation which in turn leads to a build up of toxins, reduced breakdown of fatty tissue and eventually cellulite. Cellulite ranges from being soft and barely visible to being hard, lumpy, cold and tender to touch. The harder the cellulite, the more difficult it is to treat. Massage can stimulate the circulation to the affected area helping to reduce the build-up of toxins.

- Bruising – the buttocks and legs are common sites for bruising, especially in women. This is largely due to the health of the circulation in the area. Areas of poor circulation tend to bruise more easily. Injury to the area results in blood leaking out from damaged blood vessels which then seeps into the surrounding body tissue. Bruising is often blue, purple or black depending on the severity of the damage and fades to green and yellow over time.

- Telangiectasis – abnormal dilation of the capillaries or terminal arteries producing blotchy red spots especially on the thighs. May be caused by the pressure associated with pregnancy, obesity and the stimulation associated with the overuse of sun beds etc.

- Varicose veins – valves in the veins that prevent back flow of blood become damaged and defective causing impeded blood flow. This results in swollen, twisted and painful veins. A common site for varicose veins is the legs, particularly the calves.

The skin of the **feet** often experiences the following problems including:

- Hard and cracked skin – commonly found on the heel. Regular exfoliation and massage with a nourishing cream help to keep it under control.

- Athlete's foot – technically known as *tinea pedis*. A form of ring worm resulting from a fungal infection. It affects the soles of the feet and in between the toes and is characterised by itchy, soggy skin which flakes and peels.

- Blister – a swelling caused by an accumulation of clear fluid under the skin. Commonly caused by injury to the skin, heat, irritant substances and friction.

- Callus – thickening of the skin over a bone caused by abnormal pressure or friction.

- Chilblains – painful, red, blue or purple areas of skin resulting from poor circulation.

- Corn – consists of a central core surrounded by thick layers of skin following repeated friction to an area.

Remember

Bruising is a contraindication that restricts the massage treatment.

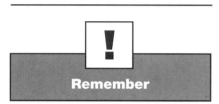

Remember

Tattoos are popular on all parts of the body, including the lower limbs, and the skin may only be massaged if completely healed.

- Ingrowing nails – technically known as onychocryptosis. Nails grow into the surrounding skin which is then prone to infection. Commonly affects the big toe.
- Warts/veruccas – small, solid growths with a hard and often painful central core caused by a viral infection. Commonly found on the soles of the feet.

Muscle tone and condition

The muscles of the buttocks, legs and feet are responsible for keeping the body in an upright position and contribute to the actions associated with walking, running, jumping etc.

- *Good muscle tone* may be experienced when the muscles are fit and healthy and are firm to touch.
- *Poor muscle tone* may be experienced when the muscles are not worked enough resulting in 'flabby', loose muscles that feel flaccid to touch.

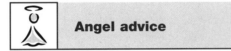

Angel advice

Good muscle tone results in firm muscles and good body shape. Poor muscle tone results in drooping muscles and loss of body contours!

- Muscle *fatigue* may be experienced when muscles are overworked. A chemical reaction takes place within the muscle forming lactic acid which contributes to the resulting aching muscles.

Fascinating Fact

Wearing high heeled shoes forces the muscles of the front and back of the lower leg out of line, resulting in aching calves. The gastrocnemius of the calf is forced to contract tightly whilst the tibialis anterior muscle of the shin is extended. In addition the balls of the feet ache due to the shift in body weight.

Joint mobility

The main joints of the lower limbs are freely moveable synovial joints and include:

- Hip joint – ball and socket
- Knee joint – hinge joint
- Ankle joint – ellipsoid joint.

All of these joints are major weight-bearing joints which means that they come under a lot of pressure just keeping the body in an upright position. The subsequent movements associated with these weight-bearing joints puts additional pressure on the synovial cavities and has a knock-on effect on the hyaline cartilage, which may start to suffer from wear and tear. This results in pain and loss of mobility and joint replacements are increasingly common in the lower limbs especially hips and knees.

Angel advice

A balance between rest and activity is the goal to achieving healthy joints. Lack of use results in loss of use as does overuse!

Stress

Stress may be categorised as being:

- Physical – stress which affects the well-being of the whole body through excessive pressure being placed on the systems e.g. muscle fatigue, obesity etc.
- Psychological – stress which affects the well-being of the whole body through emotional trauma e.g. grief, anxiety, fear, anger etc.

Stress may be real – deadlines for work etc., or imagined – fear of what might happen etc., but whatever form it takes it has the potential to create a seriously debilitating effect on a person as a whole, often resulting in illness and disease. Massage may be seen as a counteracting force that is able to banish the negative effects of this 'unsafe stress' and reinforce the positive effects of 'safe stress' i.e. that which enables the body to perform its various functions throughout life efficiently and effectively.

Contraindications

It is always necessary to conduct a full consultation checking for general contraindications. Specific contraindication considerations relating to the buttocks, legs and feet include:

- Undiagnosed pain and swelling – DO NOT TREAT, refer to GP for advice.
- Infectious disorders e.g. severe athlete's foot and veruccas. DO NOT TREAT – a verucca may be covered with a plaster and the area avoided.
- Circulatory disorders e.g. varicose veins and telangiectasis. DO NOT TREAT if the condition is painful – massage will aggravate the condition.

Tip

Poor circulation results in puffiness and swelling (oedema) in localised areas, e.g. the thighs, around the knees and ankles, and is often associated with the lead up to menstruation. This can be treated effectively with gentle draining movements towards the nearest lymph nodes: popliteal behind the knee and inguinal in the groin.

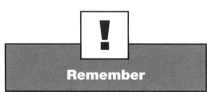

Remember

It is always better to apply caution when checking for contraindications.

Suggested order of work – the front of the legs and feet

The massage to the front of the legs commences with a simple **hold** as the hands are gently placed onto the tops of the feet, and the application of a suitable massage medium with non-directional effleurage movements to the whole of the limb.

The massage continues with:

1 **Directional effleurage**
   - Placing one hand above the other stroke (a) up the front of the limb with pressure, starting at the top of the foot. Reduce the pressure over the knee, increasing it as you work up to the top of the thigh. Separate the hands and (b) stroke down to the toes on either side of the limb without pressure. Take one hand over and one hand under the foot to finish. Repeat 3–6 times.

2 **Directional effleurage to the thigh**
   - Start just above the knee and continue to effleurage from the knee to the top of the leg only. Repeat 3–6 times.

3 **Petrissage to the thigh**
   - Alternate palmar kneading – place one hand on the inner thigh and the other on the outer thigh and work up from just above the knee to the top of the leg.
   - Alternate-handed picking up – both hands used alternately to pick up the tissue in three rows along the inner thigh, top of the thigh and outer thigh.
   - Wringing – across the length of the thigh from the knee to the top of the leg.
   - Rolling – along the length of both sides of the thigh from knee to the top of the leg.

4 **Tapotement/percussion to the thigh**
   - A combination of hacking, cupping, pounding and beating may be used dependent on the amount of fatty tissue present.

5 **Vibration to the thigh**
   - Shaking – may be performed by supporting the thigh with one hand and shaking the muscle groups (adductors, abductors and quadriceps) in turn with the other hand.

6 **Directional effleurage to the thigh**
   - Starting just above the knee apply effleurage with the pressure directed to the top of the leg.

7 **Petrissage to the knee**
   - Thumb kneading – small circles around the knee being careful not to apply firm pressure over the patella.

8 **Directional effleurage to the lower leg**
   - Effleurage from the ankle to the knee with gentle pressure over the shin. Repeat 3–6 times.

Tip

Picking up, wringing and rolling are more effective over areas of fatty tissue. Care must be taken when there is little fatty tissue to avoid discomfort.

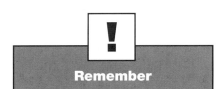

Remember

Tapotement/percussion movements need to be linked with effleurage to re-establish relaxation.

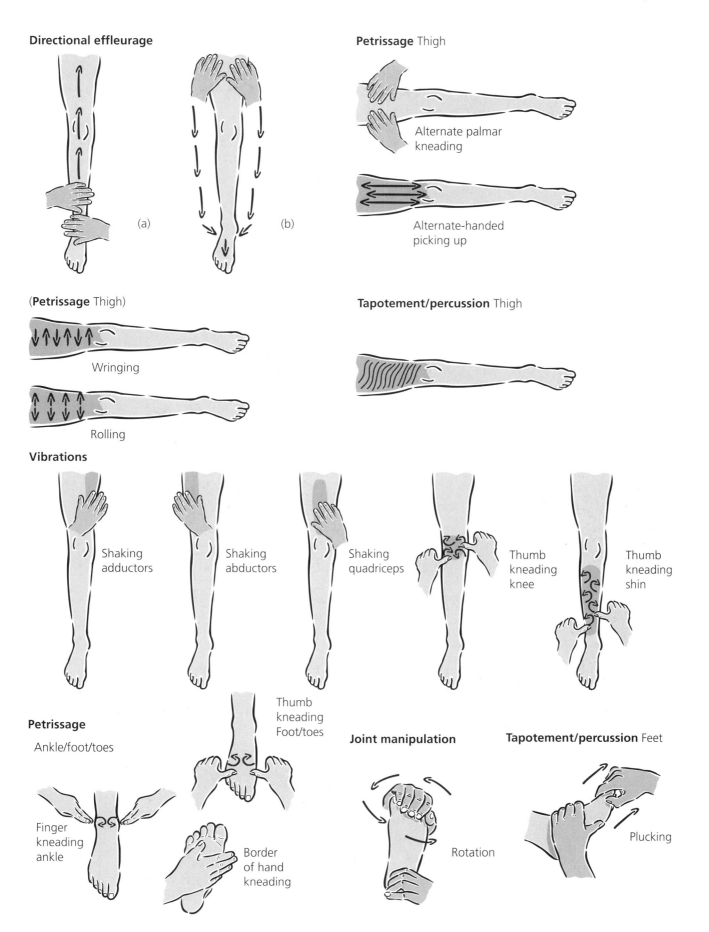

Directional effleurage

(a)

(b)

Petrissage Thigh

Alternate palmar kneading

Alternate-handed picking up

(Petrissage Thigh)

Wringing

Rolling

Tapotement/percussion Thigh

Vibrations

Shaking adductors

Shaking abductors

Shaking quadriceps

Thumb kneading knee

Thumb kneading shin

Thumb kneading Foot/toes

Petrissage

Ankle/foot/toes

Finger kneading ankle

Border of hand kneading

Joint manipulation

Rotation

Tapotement/percussion Feet

Plucking

Remember

The skin of the shin is very thin with little underlying tissue. The tibialis anterior muscle lies to the lateral aspect of the shin and it is only this area that is massaged so as to avoid discomfort.

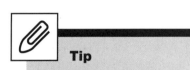

Tip

The protrusion on either side of the ankle joint is known as a *malleolus* and should be avoided so as not to cause discomfort.

9 **Petrissage to the lower leg**
- Thumb kneading – small circles to the lateral (outside) portion of the shin from ankle to knee.

10 **Petrissage to the ankle, foot and toes**
- Finger kneading – using both hands, one on each side of the ankle, apply small circles around the ankle.
- Thumb kneading – with both hands to the top of the foot and toes.
- Border of the hand kneading – support the foot at the toes with one hand. With the thenar eminence of the thumb border apply circular pressure to the medial longitudinal arch.

11 **Joint manipulation to the ankle and toes**
- Lift and support the lower leg with one hand, use the other to gently rotate the foot at the ankle first one way and then the other.
- Each toe may also be rotated in both directions.

12 **Tapotement/percussion to the feet**
- Flicking, plucking/snatching and/or whipping may be performed to stimulate the feet and toes.

13 **Directional effleurage to whole limb**
- Complete the routine with directional effleurage with both hands starting at the foot stroking with pressure up to the top of the leg (reducing pressure over the knee). Separate hands stroking back down to the feet along the outside edges of the legs taking one hand under and one hand over the foot to finish.

Suggested order of work – the buttocks, legs and feet

Massage to the back of the leg and buttocks commences with a **hold** as the hands are gently placed on the bottom of the calf by the ankle and the application of non-directional effleurage movements to introduce the practitioner's hands and the preferred massage medium.

The massage continues with:

1 **Directional effleurage to the whole area**
   - Starting at the heel place one hand above the other and (a) stroke with upwards pressure towards the knee. Reduce the pressure over the back of the knee, increasing pressure as you work up to the top of the thigh. Take the outside hand only up and over the buttock leaving the inside hand at the top of the leg. Separate the hands and (b) stroke down to the heel on either side of the limb without pressure taking the hands over the sole of the foot to the back of the toes. Repeat 3–6 times.

2 **Directional effleurage to the buttock and thigh**
   - Start just above the back of the knee and continue to effleurage the thigh and buttock only. Repeat 3–6 times.

3 **Petrissage to the buttock and thigh**
   - Alternate palmar kneading – place one hand on the inner thigh and the other on the outer thigh; work up from just above the back of the knee to the top of the leg.
   - Single-handed or reinforced palmar kneading – can be performed with the outside hand up and over the buttock. Reinforced palmar kneading offers greater depth of pressure if necessary.
   - Alternate-handed picking up – both hands used alternately to pick up the tissue in three rows along the inner thigh, top of the thigh and outer thigh extending up to include the outside and top of the buttock.
   - Wringing – across the length of the thigh from the knee to the top of the leg. Smaller movements can be applied to the outside edge of the buttock.
   - Rolling – along the length of both sides of the thigh from knee to the top of the leg extending over the outside of the buttock.

4 **Tapotement/percussion to the buttock and thigh**
   - A combination of hacking, cupping, pounding and beating may be used depending on the amount of fatty tissue present.

5 **Vibration to the buttock and thigh**
   - Shaking – may be performed by supporting the thigh with one hand and shaking the muscles groups (adductors, abductors and hamstrings) in turn with the other hand.

Tip

Some clients may prefer to have just their legs massaged and tapotement/percussion movements used on the buttocks over a towel. Adaptations to the massage routine should be made to suit individual client needs.

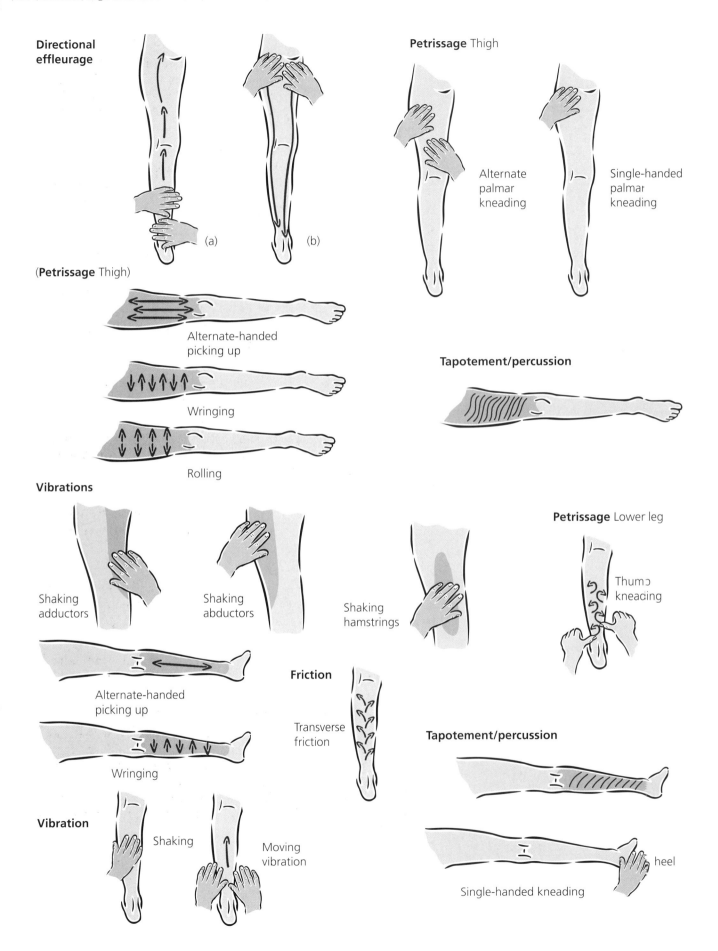

Directional effleurage

(a)   (b)

(**Petrissage** Thigh)

Alternate-handed picking up

Wringing

Rolling

Vibrations

Shaking adductors

Shaking abductors

Alternate-handed picking up

Wringing

Vibration

Shaking   Moving vibration

Petrissage Thigh

Alternate palmar kneading

Single-handed palmar kneading

Tapotement/percussion

Petrissage Lower leg

Thumb kneading

Shaking hamstrings

Friction

Transverse friction

Tapotement/percussion

heel

Single-handed kneading

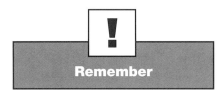

Remember

The popliteal lymph nodes are situated behind the knee and are irritated by excessive pressure.

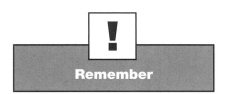

Remember

Picking up and wringing can only be performed if there is adequate fatty tissue.

Angel advice

The skin of the heel of the foot is often dry and cracked. Single-handed kneading provides the means to work maximum product into the area, helping to relieve the symptoms.

6 **Directional effleurage to the buttock and thigh**
- Starting just above the back of the knee apply effleurage with the pressure directed to the top of the leg with both hands and then up and over the buttock with the outside hand. Slide down the sides of the limb to the knee. Repeat 3–6 times.

7 **Directional effleurage to the lower leg**
- Effleurage with both hands as before from heel to just below the back of the knee with upward pressure. Separate hands and stroke down without pressure along the sides of the lower leg. Repeat 3–6 times.

8 **Petrissage to the lower leg**
- Thumb kneading – small circles up the centre of the calf from heel to just below the back of the knee.
- Alternate-handed picking up – both hands used alternately to pick up the tissue along the length of the calf.
- Wringing – across the length of the calf from heel to just below the back of the knee.

9 **Friction to the lower leg**
- Transverse friction – may be performed across the gastrocnemius muscle if there is a lot of tension.

10 **Tapotement/percussion to the lower leg**
- A combination of hacking, cupping, pounding and beating may be used if there is a lot of muscle bulk. Alternatively, plucking/snatching may be used.

11 **Vibration to the lower leg**
- Shaking – may be performed to the gastrocnemius muscle.
- Moving vibration – may be performed running up the calf from heel to knee.

12 **Directional effleurage to the lower leg**
- Stroke with pressure from heel to just below the back of the knee as before. Stroke down the outside of the lower leg. Repeat 3–6 times.

13 **Petrissage to the heel**
- Single-handed kneading – support the foot with one hand and apply single-handed kneading to the heel with the other hand.

14 **Directional effleurage to the whole area**
- Complete the routine with both hands starting at the heel of the foot stroking with pressure up to the top of the leg (reducing the pressure over the back of the knee) with both hands and over the outside of the buttock with one hand. Stroke both hands back down along the outside edges of the buttock and leg taking the hands over the sole of the foot to finish.

Treatment tracker

BUTTOCKS, LEGS AND FEET

The front and the back of the lower limbs are massaged during a full body massage, with the fronts of the legs normally massaged first.

- Massage to the front of the legs includes the feet, shins, knees, sides and front of the thighs – treatment time approximately 5 minutes each leg.

Massage to the back of the legs is usually performed after massage to the front of the legs when the client has turned over.

- Massage to the back of the legs includes the heels, calves, sides and back of the thighs and buttocks – treatment time approximately 5 minutes each leg.

The feet and lower legs may be massaged as part of a pedicure treatment – total treatment time 60–75 minutes including consultation. Massage to the feet and lower legs approximately 10 mins.

Preparation

- Conduct a full consultation.
- Check general and specific contraindications.
- Agree the treatment and preferred massage medium with the client.
- Removal of lower body clothing down to underwear for massage to the legs and buttocks. It is enough to remove shoes and socks/tights and roll up trousers or skirt/dress for massage during a pedicure.
- Skin cleansing with an appropriate cleanser paying particular attention to the feet.
- Exfoliation may be carried out with emphasis on the hard skin of the feet.

Position

As part of a full body massage:
- When massaging the front of the legs the client lies flat or semi-reclined in a supine position on the couch.
- When massaging the back of the legs and buttocks, the client usually lies in a prone position on the couch.

As part of a pedicure:
- The client sits in a chair with their feet resting on the pedicurist's lap, or
- The client lies in a supine position on a reclining couch.

The masseur is positioned on the appropriate side of the couch as part of a full body massage or at the foot of the client for a pedicure.

Client care

Considerations for client comfort when treating the legs and buttocks include:

- A pillow to support the head and back of the neck.
- Rolled up towels or pillows may be used to support the back of the knees and ankles if required.
- A blanket, duvet or towels may be used to ensure modesty and warmth.
- It is good practice to place a towel in between the legs. This ensures client modesty and also prevents massage to the upper, inner thigh area. This area is known as the *femoral triangle* and should be avoided due to its extreme sensitivity.
- Ensure modesty is maintained as the client turns over by the use of towels.
- Clients should be reminded that they may move as and when they feel they need to.

Babies/children – stroking effleurage and gentle petrissage movements may be applied bearing in mind the tickly nature of the feet. Firmer movements applied to the feet have the effect of being extremely soothing and calming and offer an ideal way of inducing relaxation in the young.

Elderly – massage to the lower limbs is of benefit when movement is restricted through stiffness of joints. Care should be taken to avoid excess pressure and never to force movement in a joint.

Male – muscle structure is traditionally stronger, firmer and bulkier in males demanding firmer massage with greater depth of pressure. The area is generally indicated to increased tapotement/percussion movements.

Female – the formation of cellulite requires adaptation of massage movements in this area. Massage should start with gentle pressure as cellulite is often tender to touch, with pressure increasing gradually but never exceeding a client's tolerance. Check body language and ask client for confirmation.

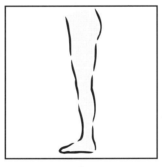

Lymphatic drainage – drainage movements are of special benefit in treating oedema associated with the lower legs and cellulite commonly found on the upper legs and buttocks. Movements should be directed to:
- Lower legs – popliteal lymph nodes behind the knee.
- Upper legs and buttocks – inguinal lymph nodes in the groin.

Posture – poor posture associated with the lower limbs results in muscle fatigue, often leading to postural faults. Care should be taken to ensure correct posture is maintained:
- Pelvis centred.
- Soft knees – not locked.
- Feet facing forward.
- Always bend knees directly over feet.
- Avoid excessive wear of overly high shoes.

- Remove excess massage medium if necessary.
- Move onto next procedure if part of a pedicure.
- Apply post-treatment procedures e.g. masks, self tan etc.
- Cover the foot and leg to ensure warmth and comfort.
- Move onto next leg; turn the client over to treat the backs or next area of the body in a full body massage.

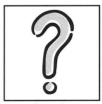

Adaptations

Special emphasis

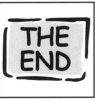

Completion

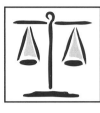

Holistic harmony

The buttocks, legs and feet are areas of the body that come under great amounts of pressure on a daily basis, yet we barely give them a thought except to moan about their size and shape! It is worth spending a few moments reminding ourselves of their uses and the amount of care they duly deserve. Making sure the limbs are well looked after will not only ensure their well-being is maintained but also that of the rest of the body.

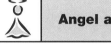

Angel advice

Think how awful you feel when your feet hurt – the pain somehow affects every part of your being making you feel physically and emotionally 'pained'!

Holistic harmony provides the basis for caring for a part that in turn has a knock-on effect on the whole enhancing the effects of massage.

Pre-treatment procedures

As the lower limbs form such a large and useful part of the body, they benefit from a variety of types of care and preparatory treatments are especially beneficial in getting the area ready for massage. Pre-treatment procedures include:

Tip

Cleansing of the feet with antiseptic wipes or spray is necessary as a means to check for contraindications and to ensure the area is odour free!

- Exercise – sluggish circulation is common in the lower limbs due in part to sedentary lifestyles. Exercise as a pre-massage treatment prepares both the body and the mind for massage.

- Cleansing – just like the back, the lower limbs benefit from the directional spray of water from a power shower helping to stimulate and invigorate in preparation for massage.

- Heat treatments – communal and/or individual heat treatments may be used pre-massage to relax muscles especially after vigorous exercise.

- Exfoliation – dry, sluggish skin is often associated with the lower limbs and can benefit greatly from the use of body scrubs and loofahs. Surface tissue will be desquamated and deeper tissue will be stimulated.

- Body brushing – dry or wet brushing can be applied over the skin of the buttocks and thighs in particular to aid circulation and improve skin texture and tone. Care should be taken to avoid damage from harsh bristles.

- Body wraps – a popular way of helping to reduce excess fluid as part of a weight reduction programme. Specific products may be applied prior to the wrap to encourage

Tip

Wax depilation – the semi-permanent removal of hair – is a popular treatment prior to massage. The massage must be carried out with a specific after-wax lotion to prevent skin irritation.

absorption or alternatively the bandages used to wrap around the body are soaked in the product. Popular products used for body wraps include the ingredients seaweed, caffeine, eucalyptus and camphor all of which have a stimulating, detoxifying and purifying effect on the body.

Angel advice

Caffeine stimulates the circulation and increases metabolism. However, this does not mean that increasing the amounts of cups of coffee consumed in a day is going to be of benefit due to the associated side-effects e.g. sleeplessness, headaches etc.

Additions

Mechanical massage treatments offer an additional method of massage which can help to penetrate the tissue effectively. This is of special benefit when there is an excess of fatty tissue present and/or increased muscle bulk. The fatty tissue is often of varying degrees of hardness associated with the formation of cellulite and the large muscle groups when toned become hard and firm to touch. Both conditions may call for increased massage pressure which may be applied more efficiently with the use of mechanical machines including:

- Gyratory – hand-held or free-standing gyratory machines that simulate all of the manual massage movements with the use of different applicator heads and varying speeds provide access to a firm, stimulating massage that may be preferable in some cases to manual massage.

- Vacuum suction – may be included at the close of a buttock, leg and foot massage to aid lymphatic drainage helping to drain the toxins from the area to the nearest lymph nodes e.g. popliteal lymph nodes behind the knee and inguinal lymph nodes in the groin. This has the benefit of improving a sluggish circulation commonly associated with cellulite as well as aid in the removal of toxins from overworked muscles.

Tip

Electronic muscle stimulating (EMS) machines, micro current lifting machines and galvanic machines are commonly used in addition to mechanical and manual massage. EMS aids muscle fitness, micro current improves nerve activity in the muscle and galvanic treatment stimulates the fat cells and surrounding circulation, having an effect on the condition of cellulite. All of these contribute to the overall appearance of the buttocks and legs.

Post-treatment procedures

Post-treatment procedures offer the client a means of enhancing the massage treatment further and may include:

- Masks – a pre-prepared mask e.g. gel or cream may be applied to enhance the action of the massage and accompanying massage medium. For example, if an anti-cellulite oil has been used, a mask could be applied post-treatment to encourage further absorption and to continue the action of the specific ingredients.
- Self-tan – the legs are always a popular area for tanning with the shins being an area of the body most difficult to tan effectively naturally. The application of self-tanning products by the masseur/masseuse helps to ensure an even application as well as offering an additional relaxing service.
- Spritz – removal of excess massage medium may be effectively achieved with a spray of cologne leaving the skin grease free and fresh prior to getting dressed.
- Pedicure – massage of the foot and lower leg often accompanies a pedicure as does a variety of pre-massage procedures e.g. cleansing, exfoliation, heat treatments etc. Regular care of the feet should be recommended and as feet are a difficult area of the body to self-treat, pedicures provide a popular service in the general upkeep of the feet, helping in the prevention of problems and the maintenance of healthy feet.

Remember

A pedicure generally incorporates the treatment of the feet and lower legs with the emphasis on the appearance of the feet and nails.

Self-help

The lower limbs present major problems in the quest for a better body image, with many clients seeking unrealistic expectations from a massage treatment e.g. believing that one treatment will help them to lose weight, eliminate their cellulite etc. In order to maintain body well-being, realistic goals should be set often with the help of the masseuse/masseuse, and then regularly checked and updated. Self-help forms the basis for future maintenance and provides the relevant and regular care needed.

Nutrition

Cellulite is known to be aggravated by certain foods including:

- **Saturated fats** – are found in meat and dairy products and cause the fat cells in the body to be immobile contributing greatly to the formation of the orange peel effect associated with cellulite.
- **Refined foods** – white sugar, white bread, cakes made with white flour etc. do not provide the body with the roughage needed to clear the system of waste.

Fascinating Fact

Fat cells produce the hormone oestrogen which is known to contribute to the formation of cellulite. Being overweight therefore increases the production of oestrogen and the predisposition towards cellulite.

Certain foods have been found to be particularly good at eliminating cellulite including:

- **Water** – although not strictly a food, water is a nutrient and is also found in many foods. Water helps to flush the systems of waste.
- **Fruit and vegetables** – contain roughage vital for its role in the elimination of waste. Some fruits and vegetable also contain pectin which helps to strengthen the immune and detoxification systems of the body.

Ageing

As the body starts to age, its structure (anatomy) and functions (physiology) begin to deteriorate. The structure of the tissue changes and their functions slow down. The specific effects of the ageing process on the buttocks and legs and feet may be experienced in the form of:

- Dropped body contours – the buttocks gradually lose their firmness and start to drop. A previously rounded shape to the buttocks will gradually start to become flatter until there is little definition left at all.
- Restless leg syndrome – a condition which affects one in twelve people. It is characterised by irritating, non-painful sensation in the legs (especially thighs) that gives an overwhelming urge to move the legs. It is more of a problem in the middle-aged and elderly although it can also occur in the young where it is misdiagnosed as 'growing pains'.
- Muscle cramp – muscles go into spasm and refuse to relax. Cramp can last from a few seconds up to fifteen minutes and can recur. Muscle cramp often affects the lower limbs and tends to get worse with age. It is also associated with dehydration, muscle fatigue and low levels of fitness.
- Weight gain – often accompanies ageing as metabolism slows down. It is important to reassess food intake in order to balance daily input with energy output to avoid excessive weight gain and resulting problems.

Leading a balanced life contributes to delaying the effects of ageing as well as helping an individual come to terms with some of the inevitable changes that occur as part of the natural process of ageing.

Rest

It is important to rest the lower limbs in much the same way as it is important to rest the upper limbs. Tension that builds up in the buttocks, legs and feet will manifest itself in the rest of the body, having a knock-on effect on organs and systems. However, we often associate resting the lower limbs with curling up on the sofa, forgetting to observe our general posture when doing so. Getting up from 'curling up on the sofa' is often accompanied by stiffness, pins and needles, numbness and pain as our bodies and in particular our lower limbs have been twisted into unnatural positions:

- Curling legs under us will result in aching joints as the pressure of the weight of the body causes strain.
- Crossing legs and feet over one another impedes blood and nerve flow.
- Twisting the body places strain on the spine and contributes to postural figure faults.

Thought should therefore be given to resting positions to avoid such physical stresses and strains.

Exercise

The large muscle groups of the buttocks and legs are responsible for moving the body from a to b. As such, it is easy to keep these muscles active just by walking around! However, the muscle groups of the inner (adductors) and outer thigh (abductors), although contributing to the movements associated with walking, become slack very easily. Added to which, these are both prime sites for the accumulation of fatty tissue and cellulite. Strengthening exercises are therefore beneficial to keep the muscle groups fit and the fatty tissue away including:

Strengthening exercise for the adductor (inner thigh) muscle group:

1 Lying on the floor face up (supine) with the knees bent.
2 Place a pillow between the knees and press the knees together.

Strengthening exercise for the abductor (outer thigh) muscle group:

1 Lying on the floor face up (supine) with the legs straight and the feet inside the legs of a chair.
2 Push both legs outwards against the legs of the chair holding for the count of ten.

General exercise such as swimming, racket sports, team sports and even yoga and pilates are beneficial in maintaining fitness levels and avoiding the onset of cellulite and 'middle-age spread'!

Awareness

One of the main causes for concern relating to the lower limbs is the formation of *cellulite*.

Fascinating Fact

What most women refer to as cellulite, the medical profession will define as:

- Status protrusis cutis – cellulite that is only apparent when the skin is pinched together
- Derma-panniculosis deformans – cellulite that is visible with the naked eye.

The development of cellulite tends to become apparent in women from around the time of puberty with the production of oestrogen associated with the ovaries. Oestrogen has the following effects on the body:

- Encourages the body to store fat on the buttocks and thighs as part of the process for the preparation of childbearing.
- Contributes to the retention of water in the body.

As a result of the effects of oestrogen on the body, circulation is affected in the following ways:

- Blood flow to the area is reduced making the part feel cool to the touch.
- Lymph flow is sluggish reducing the effective removal of waste and toxins from the area, making the part feel puffy to touch.

There are four phases associated with the formation of cellulite:

1   Slight dimpling of the skin's surface – barely visible.
2   Dimpling and skin depressions that are visible.
3   Severe dimpling and larger skin depressions that feel hard to touch.
4   A combination of hard and soft lumps and skin depressions that may feel tender to touch.

As cellulite worsens the area often feels tender to touch as the hard lumps sometimes compress the nerve endings in the skin.

Angel advice

Surgery is increasingly popular in the treatment of cellulite, including liposuction whereby excessive fat is effectively removed from the problem areas. Post-surgery, care must be taken to ensure the fat and resulting cellulite does not return!

Having an awareness of the factors relating to this condition is the key to understanding. For the masseur/masseuse it means that the massage treatment can be adapted to suit the specific needs of each client ensuring the best possible treatment and aftercare advice. For the client, an increased awareness of the factors affecting their body helps to promote greater self responsibility as people realise that they have the means to help themselves and make a difference to the way in which their body works.

Special care

The lower limbs have a supportive role in maintaining the body and as such need special care in return.

Tip

Sciatica is a painful condition affecting the lower limbs. The sciatic nerve is the largest nerve of the body extending from the sacral vertebrae down to the feet. If the nerve supply becomes impeded by excess pressure and/or damage, pain is experienced in the buttocks extending down the legs through the knee to the ankle.

Fascinating Fact

Nicotine has the effect of narrowing blood vessels, impeding blood flow.

The weight of the body inflicts pressure on the buttocks, legs and feet causing problems to many of the body systems including:

- Skeletal system – pressure on the joints of the hips, knees and ankles affects ease of movement.
- Muscular system – pressure from poor posture affects muscle tone contributing to muscle fatigue.
- Nervous system – pressure can impede nerve responses resulting in the pain, pins and needles and/or numbness.
- Circulatory systems – lymphatic and venous blood flow depend on movement of skeletal muscles as well as valves to prevent back flow. Lack of movement and increased pressure can cause defective valves and subsequent problems including swelling in the tissues (oedema) and the development of varicose veins.

Any special care taken to avoid such conditions will benefit the whole body as a result:

- A balanced diet ensuring that nothing is consumed in excess and that food intake matches energy output. This will ensure additional pressure on the systems is avoided.
- Regular exercise ensuring that the whole body takes part in some form of energetic movement for at least twenty minutes three times per week will help to safeguard the systems.
- Maintaining a lifestyle that has a balanced level of stress i.e. high levels of stress are counteracted by high levels of support and low levels of constraints.

Activity

Practice the suggested order of work on a variety of willing clients. Notice the differing shapes, sizes and condition of skin and muscle tone. Learn to adapt your massage to suit the needs of the client by checking how the massage feels. Note the changes that occur to the area during the massage and monitor how those changes affect the body post-treatment. Continue to experience massage for yourself.

Task

Design a cellulite fact sheet to give to your clients explaining what it is, what aggravates it and how massage helps.

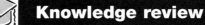

Knowledge review

1   Name the bones that make up the legs.

2   How many tarsal bones form the ankle?

3   Where are the hamstrings located?

4   Name the muscle group of the inner thigh.

5   Name the muscle group that forms the front of the thigh.

6   Name the muscle group that forms the buttocks.

7   Where is the tibialis anterior muscle located?

8   Name the large muscle that forms the calf.

9   What type of joint is the hip joint?

10   What type of joint is the knee joint?

11   What forms the arches of the feet?

12   Name the lymph nodes in the groin and behind the knees.

13   Which is the longest nerve of the body?

14   What may occur if the skin has been overstretched through rapid
     weight gain and/or pregnancy?

15   What is the condition that results in an 'orange peel' effect to the skin?

16   Why is a verucca contraindicated to massage?

17   What are varicose veins the result of?

18   What effect does body brushing have on the circulation?

19   What do the initials EMS stand for?

20   Which foods contain saturated fats?

12

The abdomen

The abdomen is a sensitive area of the body both physically and psychologically and many clients prefer not to have this particular area of their body massaged. However, it can be a problem area in terms of excessive weight gain, stretch marks and lack of muscle tone, all of which are particularly associated with the endomorph body type. Massage can help to tone the muscles by stimulating circulation, improve skin texture by encouraging the absorption of nourishing products and aid in weight loss if accompanied by a reduced calorie diet.

Anatomy and physiology of the abdomen

The abdomen extends from the thorax to the pelvis and incorporates many of the organs of the body associated with the digestive and genito-urinary systems.

Bones and joints

The abdominal region lies below the thorax at the front (anterior) of the body and has no protective bones forming a covering. At the back and sides, it is supported by the lumbar, sacral and coccyx regions of the spine together with the pelvic girdle.

Muscles of the abdomen

- **Rectus abdominus** – longitudinal muscle of the abdomen
  - Position – extends from the 5th, 6th and 7th ribs down to the pubic crest (centre of the pelvic girdle).
  - Action – compresses the abdomen and works with the erector spinae muscles of the back to maintain posture.

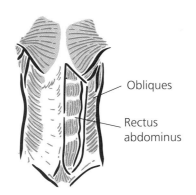

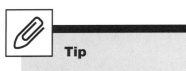

Muscles of the abdomen

> **Tip**
>
> The rectus abdominus muscle contributes to the 'six pack' effect!

- **Obliques** – internal and external muscles forming the waist
  - Position – **internal** – extends from the lower four ribs to the iliac crest of the pelvic girdle; **external** – extends from the lower border of the 8th ribs to the ilium bone of the pelvic girdle.
  - Action – lateral flexion (side bends) and rotation (side twists) of the trunk.

Blood and lymphatic vessels

The abdominal region is associated with portal circulation which involves the flow of blood between the heart and the digestive organs; the stomach, intestines, liver etc. Inguinal lymph nodes in the groin and iliac lymph nodes in the abdomen collect lymph from the abdominal region.

Nerves

The coccygeal plexus contains the peripheral nerves which branch out to supply the muscles and skin of the abdominal region. The autonomic nerves of the thoracic region of the spine supply the abdominal organs. The autonomic nerves are associated with *peristalsis* – the involuntary movement responsible for moving food along the digestive tract, urine through the ureter and urethra tubes, ova along the fallopian tubes and sperm along the vas deferens.

Associated organs and glands

The organs of the digestive and genito-urinary systems are situated within the abdominal cavity.

The digestive and associated organs include:

- Stomach – lies under the diaphragm on the left side of the body.
- Small and large intestines – situated below the stomach.
- Liver – lies under the diaphragm on the right side of the body.
- Gall bladder – located under the liver.
- Pancreas – lies under the stomach on the left side of the body.

The genito-urinary organs include:

- Kidneys – situated either side of the spine at waistline.
- Bladder – located in the lower abdominal cavity.
- Ureter tubes – leading from the kidneys to the bladder.
- Ovaries, fallopian tubes and uterus (female) – situated in the lower abdominal cavity.
- Vas deferens and prostate gland (male) – situated in the lower abdominal cavity.

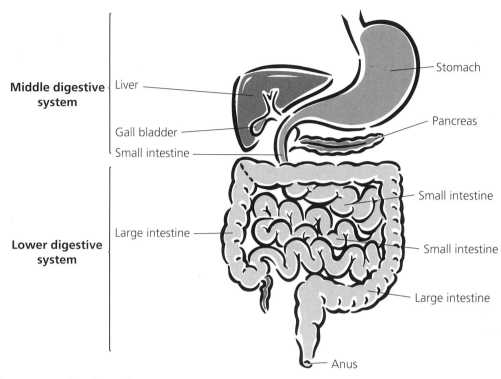

Middle digestive system
- Liver
- Gall bladder
- Small intestine

Stomach
Pancreas

Lower digestive system
- Large intestine

Small intestine
Small intestine
Large intestine
Anus

Abdominal organs – the digestive system

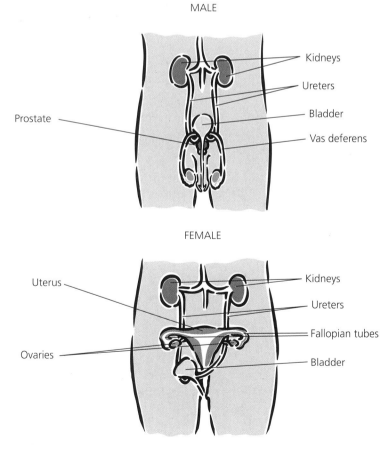

MALE

Prostate

Kidneys
Ureters
Bladder
Vas deferens

FEMALE

Uterus
Ovaries

Kidneys
Ureters
Fallopian tubes
Bladder

Abdominal organs – the male and female genito-urinary organs

Considerations

In order to offer a safe and effective massage treatment it is necessary to consider the following with reference to the abdomen:

Skin type and conditions

Skin of the abdomen varies from person to person with the following common considerations:

- Stretch marks are often present on the skin of the abdomen. These occur when the skin has been overstretched due to excessive and/or rapid weight gain and/or pregnancy. The skin forms in distinct lines (transverse and longitudinal) that appear shiny and discoloured due to loss of elasticity in the dermis layer of the skin. Massage creams/emulsions oils and gels are indicated for use.

- Excess adipose tissue – fat cells stored in the hypodermis under the skin. Whilst this offers protection to the abdominal organs it also contributes to the characteristic pot belly often present in males and the rolls of fat that many women complain about. Firm massage helps to break down fatty tissue.

- A line of hair is often present on males and females growing from the sternum (breast plate) and extending down to the pubic area. This is thought to be protective in nature, often appearing in females during pregnancy.

- Tattoos and piercings are popular on the skin of the abdomen and care must be taken to ensure that in both cases the skin is completely healed prior to the massage treatment. Ideally, any piercings should be removed prior to abdominal massage. However, many clients are unwilling to remove them for fear of skin closure and therefore care must be taken to avoid the pierced area so as not to pull the skin during massage.

- The skin of the abdomen has many sensory nerve endings which when touched can induce a ticklish feeling. Any form of touch to this area of the body should therefore be positive to avoid tickling.

Muscle tone and condition

The rectus abdominus muscle contributes to the desirable flat tummy in females and the six pack effect in males. The obliques are responsible for maintaining a toned waist. However, muscle tone in this area of the body is often poor. The weight gained in obesity and pregnancy is very much associated with poor muscle tone and poor posture. The excess abdominal weight pulls the abdomen forward causing an exaggerated arch in the lower back (lumbar region). This often contributes to the postural figure fault lordosis, resulting in protruding abdomen and buttocks.

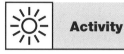 **Activity**

Pinch the flesh around your abdomen. Men should be able to pinch an inch and no more and women should be able to pinch one and half inches and no more!

Joint mobility

The joint between the sacral and coccyx regions of the spine and the pelvis of the pelvic girdle is gliding. This allows a certain amount of movement between the bones during pregnancy.

Stress

One of the first areas of the body to be affected by stress is the digestive system. When we are faced with stressful situations the body goes into the alarm phase of the general adaptation syndrome (GAS). Adrenalin rushes into the bloodstream which has the effect of shutting down the digestive system by diverting blood away from the digestive organs and directing it to the muscles. Indigestion, stomach cramps, bloatedness etc. are many of the symptoms associated with stress and the digestive system. Often digestion becomes sluggish and constipation occurs. Massage can aid sluggish digestion if performed over the large intestine taking care to direct the movements in the natural direction of the elimination of waste through the system. Knowledge of the system and its structures will ensure safe delivery of massage. Massage can also help to relax the body generally, which indirectly stimulates digestion.

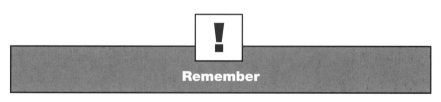

!

Remember

Digestion takes place much more effectively when the body is relaxed.

Contraindications

It is always necessary to conduct a full consultation prior to massaging any part of the body, and information relating to the organs in the abdominal region is an important factor in deciding whether or not a client is contraindicated to treatment.

Specific contraindications include:

- Undiagnosed abdominal pain – DO NOT TREAT, refer to GP for advice.
- First trimester of pregnancy – DO NOT TREAT, due to the possibility of miscarriage.
- Later stages of pregnancy DO NOT TREAT, due to the possibility of bringing on labour. .
- Just prior to and during menstruation – massage to the abdomen can stimulate blood loss and cause discomfort. TREAT WITH CARE with client guidance. Remember some clients will gain comfort from a gentle massage whilst others will not want to be touched.
- Recent scar tissue – surgical operations are common in the abdominal area due to there being good access to many of the internal organs. Operations such as appendectomy, hysterectomy, caesarean etc. all leave scars that must be allowed to heal prior to a massage treatment taking place. DO NOT TREAT, seek medical advice.
- An excessively empty or full stomach are both contraindications to massage. Massaging over the abdomen when the stomach is full will hinder digestion, causing discomfort and possible nausea. Conversely, massaging over the abdomen when the stomach is empty will have a stimulating effect causing the person to feel even hungrier and maybe a little nauseous. The best time to have a massage is approximately two to three hours after a meal when the person is neither full nor hungry.
- Under the influence of alcohol and/or non-prescription drugs is a contraindication to all forms of massage but in particular abdominal massage. Massage has a stimulating effect on the digestive system which in turn will speed up the absorption and resulting side effects of the drink/drugs.

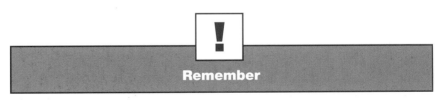

Remember

If massage to the area is likely to make a condition worse – DO NOT TREAT.

Remember

Ask your client if they need to visit the toilet prior to having a massage treatment as massage to the abdomen will put pressure on the bladder and stimulate the elimination of waste through the digestive system!

Treatment tracker

ABDOMEN

The abdomen is rarely massaged in isolation being more commonly treated as part of a full body massage.

As such, massage to the abdomen usually follows that of the legs and precedes massage to the upper body prior to the client turning over.

Treatment time – 5–10 minutes.

Preparation

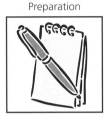

- Conduct a full consultation.
- Check general and specific contraindications.
- Agree the treatment and preferred massage medium with the client.
- Removal of clothing down to underwear for massage to the abdomen.
- Skin may be cleansed with an appropriate cleanser.
- Exfoliation may be carried out.

Position

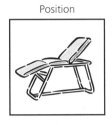

Client – the usual position for receiving massage to the abdomen is lying supine on a flat couch.

Masseur/masseuse – standing to either side of the couch. Most practitioners have a preferred side of the couch that they like to work from. It is usually the left side for right-handed practitioners and the right side for left-handed practitioners. It is important to feel comfortable and to ultimately get used to working on either side of the couch.

Client care

Considerations for client comfort when lying in this position include:

- A pillow to support the head.
- An extra pillow may be needed under the back in cases of postural problems.
- Rolled up towels may be placed under the knees and ankles for support if needed.
- Towels are used to cover the upper and lower parts of the client leaving just the abdomen exposed.
- Clients should be reminded that they may move as and when they feel they need to.

Babies/children – stroking effleurage movements may be performed over the entire length of the abdomen incorporating the chest as well. Gentle petrissage movements may be used around the colon helping to prevent colic, wind and constipation.

Elderly – gentle movements that do not overly stimulate the underlying organs are indicated for this area; take care with position and comfort of the client throughout the treatment.

Male – the abdomen is traditionally an area for males to store excess adipose tissue, so massage may be firm and stimulating to help to soften the fat cells so they may be more easily used up as energy as part of a calorie reduced diet. A combination of tapotement/percussion movements may be incorporated for added stimulation.

Female – care must be taken during pregnancy to avoid overstimulation and the risk of miscarriage in the first trimester and the onset of labour in the final trimester. Gentle massage may be indicated, especially as part of a self-help programme to help avoid the formation of stretch marks and to contribute to the natural bonding between mother and baby. Consideration should be given to client preference prior to and during menstruation to avoid embarrassment, discomfort and excessive stimulation.

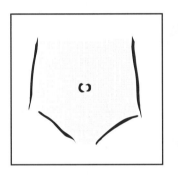

Lymphatic drainage – a build-up of localised toxins may be drained towards the inguinal lymph nodes in the groin.

Posture – a protruding abdomen is a sign of poor posture resulting in poor muscle control. Correct posture associated with this area of the body involves keeping the pelvis centred which in turn encourages the abdomen to be naturally held in. This has the long-term effect of strengthening the general muscle tone. Pelvic floor exercises are particularly beneficial for the external and internal muscles of this area of the body, especially in females.

- Remove excess massage medium if necessary.
- Apply post-treatment procedures e.g. masks, self tan etc.
- Cover the area with a towel, blanket etc. to ensure warmth and comfort.
- Move onto the next area of the body in a full body massage.

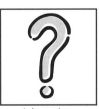

Adaptations

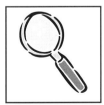

Special emphasis

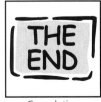

Completion

Suggested order of work – the abdomen

The abdominal massage treatment commences with a simple hold as the practitioner's hands are gently placed onto the centre of the abdomen making a client aware of the fact that it may feel cold. The massage continues with:

1 **Directional effleurage**
   - Both hands together – start at the centre of the abdomen either side of the navel. Stroke in a diamond shape (a) upwards towards the thorax, (b) outwards towards the waist and (c) inwards towards the pubis. Repeat 3–6 times.

2 **Petrissage**
   - Alternate-handed picking up – both hands used alternately to pick up the flesh in two or three rows along the length of the waist and abdomen working both sides of the navel.
   - Wringing – across the length of both sides of the waist in turn. This may be followed by criss-cross wringing over the entire area.
   - Rolling – along the length of both sides of the waist in turn.
   - Kneading to the colon – using flat-handed, finger or ulna border kneading, start at the illeoceacal valve work up the ascending colon, across the transverse colon and down the descending colon.

3 **Tapotement/percussion**
   - Hacking, cupping, beating and pounding may be used with extreme care *only* if there is adequate fatty tissue to allow the movements to take place without causing any discomfort.

4 **Effleurage**
   - Directional – in a diamond shape as performed at the start of the routine.

5 **Holding** – ending the treatment with a gentle hold before lifting off.

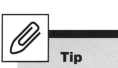

Tip

Kneading to the colon stimulates peristalsis (involuntary muscular action associated with digestion) aiding constipation. It is of great importance that this massage is carried out *only* if needed, with care to ensure the correct direction is followed and without causing discomfort.

Tip

Butterfly movements are likely to feel ticklish so are best avoided on the abdomen.

Tip

It is not generally necessary to perform friction, vibration or joint manipulation movements to the abdomen as the muscle tone is generally normal to poor and there are no specific joints to work on.

Directional effleurage

Petrissage

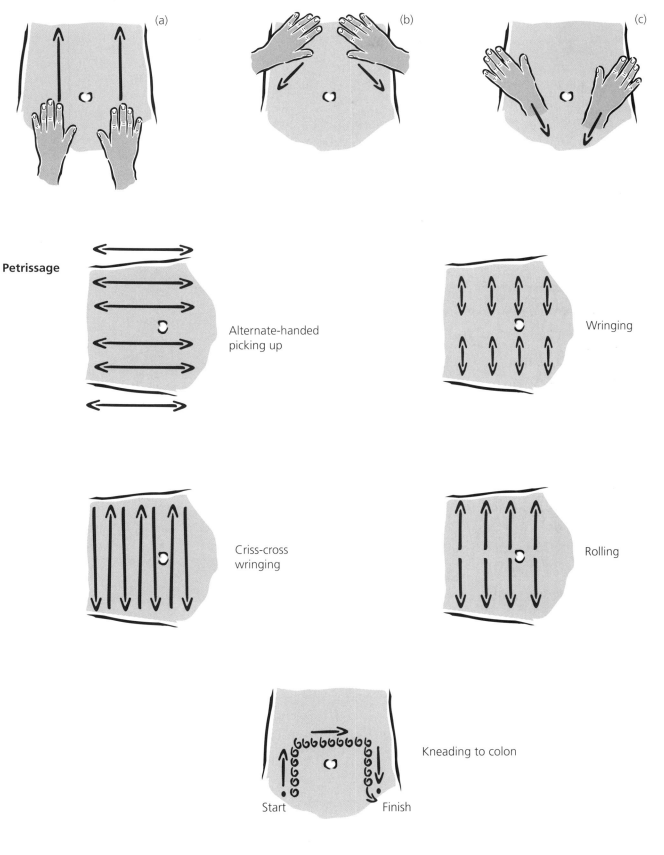

(a)

(b)

(c)

Alternate-handed
picking up

Wringing

Criss-cross
wringing

Rolling

Kneading to colon

Start   Finish

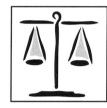

Holistic harmony

The abdomen is an often-neglected area of the body and one the internal functioning of which is very much taken for granted. As such it is useful to consider the procedures that may be followed to ensure that this area is better cared for. Care to the abdominal area of the body results in care of the rest of the body as functions such as digestion and absorption of nutrients and the elimination of waste become more efficient.

Therefore thought should be given to:

Pre-treatment procedures

It is quite usual for clients to seek massage treatment to the abdomen as a means of losing weight. They are often under the misconception that massage will eliminate fatty tissue. Massage will certainly stimulate the area and contribute to other pre-treatment procedures including:

- Exercise and diet – using up more calories in exertion than are consumed by eating will allow the body to use up some of its energy store in the form of fatty tissue. Specific exercises targeted to work the abdominal muscles will strengthen and tone producing a more flattering body image.
- Body wraps – can be used to encourage absorption of products that have a direct effect on the fatty tissue and surrounding circulation. Heat may also be applied which stimulates sweating and the removal of excess fluid which may be a contributory factor in the quest for weight loss.
- Exfoliation – body scrubs used on the surface of the skin can improve texture and tone and encourage greater absorption of massage mediums, improving the general appearance.

Tip

Electronic muscle stimulating (EMS) treatments are popular on the abdomen and have the effect of tightening and toning the muscles. Micro current treatments are also increasingly popular and have the effect of re-educating and toning muscles that have become slack over time.

Additions

Mechanical massage treatments may be used in addition to the manual massage including:

- Gyratory – hand-held or free-standing gyratory machines have the benefit of stimulating fatty tissue as well as the circulation. This is particularly beneficial if there is excess fatty tissue as different applicator heads and speeds can be used depending on the amount of tissue present.
- Vacuum suction – used specifically to aid lymphatic drainage which is of direct benefit to areas of the body associated with excess fatty tissue. Movements should be directed towards the inguinal lymph nodes in the groin.

Post-treatment procedures

It is rare to treat the abdomen in isolation – it is usually treated as part of a full body massage treatment, in which case the treatment would continue with massage to other areas of the body. However, post-treatment procedures relating to other areas of the body can still apply to the abdomen if required e.g. masks, spritzing, self-tanning etc.

Self-help

Many clients feel too embarrassed to have another person massage their abdomen; providing information on self-help procedures as part of a full body massage treatment ensures that a person has the knowledge to perform relevant home care to aid their specific problem. Specific advice relating to the abdomen includes:

Nutrition

The abdomen is an area where excess fat is often stored. To avoid this, care should be given to maintaining a healthy, balanced diet. Thought should be given to matching input with output i.e. the intake of calories should be enough to allow the body to function efficiently. *More* calories than are needed result in weight *gain* and *less* calories result in weight *loss*. It is therefore important to have an awareness of the *vital nutrients* and the role they play in the maintenance of the body as a whole. In addition it is equally important to have an awareness of the *anti-nutrients* i.e. those substances that hinder the beneficial nutrients from being absorbed and used by the body.

Vital nutrients include:

- Carbohydrates for energy.
- Proteins for growth and repair.
- Fats for energy store.
- Minerals and vitamins for cell functions.
- Water for hydration.

Anti-nutrients include:

- Alcohol, cigarettes, synthetic chemicals, pesticides and antibiotics.

Anti-nutrients produce *free radicals*. Free radicals are the toxic by-product of energy metabolism which causes damage and destruction to the cells of the body. Antioxidants fight against free radical damage and include vitamins A, C, E and the minerals selenium and zinc. Main food sources include fruit and vegetables.

Fascinating Fact

There also exists substances known as *super antioxidants*. These substances are oligomeric proanthocyanidins (OPCs) and include extracts of pine bark and grape seed.

Ageing

As skin and muscles age, they often become thinner, looser and less effective in their functions. In many cases this fact is worsened by the effects of overexposure to the ultra violet rays from the sun as well as excessive use of sunbeds. The abdominal area is an area that is kept covered most of the year and is often subjected to intense exposure over a short period of time e.g. two week holiday. As a result burning is often experienced on the delicate skin of the abdomen which heightens the possible risks of skin cancer. The use of sun screens and after-sun products are essential for this area of the body.

Rest

The organs of the abdominal area respond well to rest e.g.

- Digestion is more effective if the body rests after eating, when large amounts of blood are required. Blood is diverted to other systems of the body during periods of activity.
- The production of urine is reduced during sleep enabling the body to utilise water over a period of time.

Exercise

Muscle strengthening exercises for the abdomen and waist are of benefit to body image as well as helping to rectify postural figure faults e.g. lordosis.

- Lying on the floor face up with bent knees, press the small of the back into the floor, tilting the pelvis backwards and pulling the abdomen in. Hold and release. Breathe out as you hold and in as you release.
- Lying on the floor face up with bent knees, press the small of the back into the floor tucking the head down onto the chest and lifting the head and shoulders slightly. Lift and release. Breathe out on the lift and in on the release.
- Lying on the floor face up with bent knees, place hands behind head and twist to touch one knee with the opposite elbow. Repeat on the other side. Breathe out with the twist.
- Standing with feet hip distance apart, maintain correct posture. Taking the arm down the corresponding leg, stretch down to the side. Repeat on the other side, breathing out on the stretch.

The first two exercises help to strengthen the lower back and abdomen and will help to achieve a flat tummy.

The latter two exercises target the oblique muscles, helping to develop a toned waist.

Angel advice

Fertility problems are often associated with lack of rest through stress. Taking time out to allow the body as a whole to rest will have a positive effect on the associated organs.

Awareness

Having an awareness of the underlying organs and body systems associated with the abdominal region of the body will help to provide a suitable, safe and effective massage treatment.

In addition, having an awareness of the problems associated with these organs and systems will help to provide vital aftercare advice.

Common digestive problems include:

- Indigestion – pain (heartburn) associated with eating certain foods which are more difficult to digest. It is also associated with overeating, hunger and stress.
- Constipation – infrequent passing of waste from the anus resulting in dry, hard faeces as much of the water is absorbed, making it increasingly difficult to pass.
- Diarrhoea – abnormally frequent elimination of faeces during a peristaltic 'rush' resulting in dehydration and weakness as too much fluid and too many nutrients are lost from the body too quickly.
- Irritable bowel syndrome (IBS) – a condition commonly associated with high stress factors. Symptoms include alternate bouts of constipation and diarrhoea.
- Coeliac disease – an intolerance of gluten (a protein found in wheat).
- Crohn's disease/ileitis – an inflammation of the latter section of the small intestine (ileum).
- Ulcers – a break in the surface of any part of the alimentary canal caused by the overproduction of acid in the gastric and intestinal juices.

Common genito-urinary problems include:

- Cystitis – inflammation of the bladder resulting in a frequent urge to pass urine with subsequently small quantities of urine being passed often accompanied by stinging and pain in the lower abdomen.
- Endometriosis – cells from the uterus form in the fallopian tubes or ovaries, causing pain especially during menstruation.
- Kidney stones – formed by an excess of salts in the blood. These salts crystallise in the urine and can cause obstruction to the flow of urine resulting in extreme pain.
- Pre-menstrual tension (PMT) – physical and psychological tension leading up to menstruation caused by an imbalance in hormones in the ovaries.
- Prostatitis – inflammation of the prostate gland.

Angel advice

Deep breathing exercises may be carried out at the beginning and/or end of the massage treatment and practice encouraged on a regular basis to aid against the effects of stress.

Special care

Many factors contribute to the care of the abdominal region of the body, including:

- **Breathing** – efficient breathing using the diaphragm, intercostals and abdominal muscles gently massages the internal organs, aiding their action.
- **Posture** – good posture allows the organs to sit comfortably within the body. Bad posture forces organs to compress against each other putting added pressure on them.

Angel advice

Posture checks may be carried out as part of the consultation and massage treatment with self-help exercises given for posture correction and maintenance.

- **Self massage** – gentle massage movements over the abdomen can soothe the pains associated with poor digestion and elimination as well as those that often accompany menstruation. Massaging a nourishing product into the skin of the abdomen may help to avoid stretch marks and improve those that have already developed. Self massage during pregnancy is a way of communicating with the foetus as well as encouraging a person to become more in tune with their own bodies.

Activity

Practice the suggested order of work with a partner who is also studying massage to ascertain the correct execution of movements and depth of pressure. Continue to practice on male and female clients observing the differences in skin and muscle tone.

Task

Think about how you would go about contacting a client's GP in the event of a contraindication preventing massage treatment from taking place e.g. undiagnosed abdominal pain. Write a sample letter to a GP paying particular attention to professionalism and client confidentiality. Always get permission from the client prior to any contact with their GP.

Knowledge review

1   Which areas of the spine support the abdomen?

2   What is the name given to the muscle that runs along the length of the abdomen?

3   What are the names of the muscles associated with the formation of the waist?

4   Which abdominal muscles are worked when doing sit-ups?

5   Which abdominal muscles are worked when doing side bends?

6   What is portal circulation associated with?

7   What is peristalsis?

8   Name the organs associated with the digestive system.

9   What are stretch marks?

10 Which figure fault results in a protruding abdomen and buttocks?

11 Why is massage contraindicated in the latter stages of pregnancy?

12 Which massage movements start and finish an abdominal massage treatment?

13 When are tapotement/percussion movements used as part of an abdominal massage treatment?

14 Give three examples of anti-nutrients.

15 What are antioxidants?

16 What are the main food sources of antioxidants?

17 What do the initials IBS stand for?

18 Which common disorder is associated with the frequent urge to pass urine often accompanied by pain?

19 What effect does deep breathing have on the organs associated with the abdominal region?

20 How does good posture contribute to the well-being of the abdominal organs?

The upper body

13

The upper body consists of the chest, shoulders, face, ears and scalp, constituting the areas of the body commonly treated as part of a traditional facial. If treating a male client the chest and abdomen may be treated as one large area. If treating a female, however, the breasts are usually kept covered leaving the abdomen as a separate treatment.

Tip

The *décolletage* refers to the neck, shoulders and upper chest and is a term commonly used to describe this area when treated as part of a facial.

Anatomy and physiology of the upper body

The upper body contains many anatomical structures which contribute to maintaining an upright posture. In addition many of the major organs are located in the upper body contributing to the vital functions associated with respiration, sensitivity and movement.

Bones and joints of the upper body

The chest and head form part of the axial skeleton and include:

Thorax

The thorax is made up of flat bones forming the chest.

- 12 thoracic vertebrae of the spine to which 12 pairs of ribs attach.

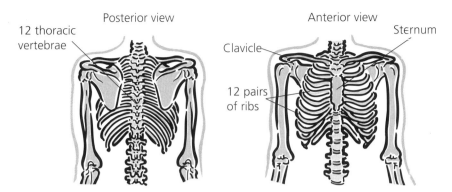

Bones of the thorax

There are plane joints between the ribs and the vertebrae allowing a slight gliding movement which enables the chest to expand during breathing.

- Seven of the ribs (true ribs) attach to the sternum or breast plate at the front of the chest.
- The next three pairs of ribs attach to the ribs above them and are called false ribs.
- The final two pairs of ribs do not attach at the front and are known as floating ribs.

Skull

The skull is made up of bones forming the cranium (head) and face most of which are flat or irregular in shape with fixed joints or sutures.

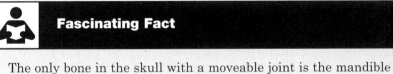

Fascinating Fact

The only bone in the skull with a moveable joint is the mandible which forms the lower jaw.

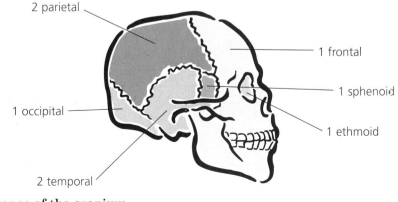

Bones of the cranium

The cranium is made up of eight bones:

- 1 frontal bone forms the forehead and contains two sinuses, one above each eye.

Remember

Sinuses are air spaces in the bones which connect to the nasal passageways. They are lined with epithelial tissue containing goblet cells that secrete mucus. The sinuses are prone to blocking, easily becoming infected as part of the symptoms associated with the common cold.

- 2 parietal bones form the crown of the skull.
- 1 occipital bone forms the base of the skull and contains the opening (occipital cavity) for the spinal cord.
- 2 temporal bones form the temples at the sides of the skull.
- 1 ethmoid bone forms part of the nasal cavity and contains many small sinuses at the sides of each eye.
- 1 sphenoid bone forms the eye socket and contains two sinuses, one either side of the nose.

The face is made up of 14 bones:

- 2 zygomatic bones form the cheeks.
- 2 maxillae bones fuse together to form the upper jaw containing the sockets for the upper teeth as well as the largest pair of sinuses.
- 1 mandible bone forms the lower jaw containing the sockets for the lower teeth. It forms an ellipsoid joint with the temporal bone on each side of the face allowing the jaw to move up and down and side to side as in chewing and talking.
- 2 nasal bones form the bridge of the nose.

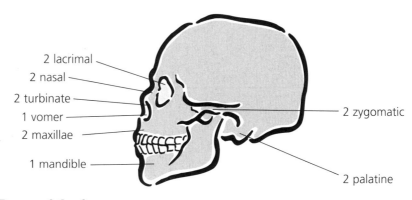

Bones of the face

- 2 palatine bones form the floor and wall of the nose and roof of the mouth.
- 2 turbinate bones form the sides of the nose.
- 1 vomer bone forms the top of the nose.
- 2 lacrimal bones form the eye sockets containing the opening for the tear duct.

Muscles of the upper body

Muscles of the chest and neck include:

- **Platysma/depressor anguli oris**
  - Position – a broad muscle group covering the front of the neck extending from the chest and shoulders to the mandible bone of the lower jaw.
  - Action – draws the jaw and lower lip downwards as in sadness and contributes to the **necklace lines** on the neck.
- **Sterno cleido mastoid**
  - Position – extends from the sternum and clavicle bones at the sides of neck to behind the ear.
  - Action – the muscles work together to bring the head **forward** and in opposition to move the head from **side to side**.
- **Pectoralis – major and minor**
  - Position – covering the chest area; the **pectoralis major** extends from the clavicle and sternum to the humerus at the shoulder joint and the **pectoralis minor** extends from the outer surface of the 3rd, 4th and 5th pair of ribs to the scapula.
  - Action – together the pectoral muscles contribute to the shoulder movements involved with **throwing** and **climbing** and the elevation of the ribs in forced inspiration.

Muscles of respiration (breathing) include:

- **Diaphragm**
  - Position – large dome-shaped muscle separating the thorax from the abdomen.
  - Action – flattens on contraction to increase the area to allow the lungs to fill with air as we **breathe in**. Returns to normal shape as we **breathe out**.
- **Intercostals** – internal and external
  - Position – situated in between the ribs forming the shape of the thorax.
  - Action – the intercostals work together to increase the space in the thorax (external intercostals) when **breathing in** and to depress the ribs (internal intercostals) when **breathing out**, **coughing** and **blowing**.

Anterior view

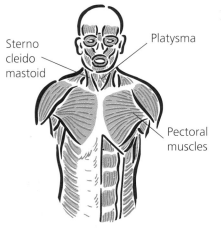

Sterno cleido mastoid

Platysma

Pectoral muscles

Muscles of the neck and chest

!

Remember

The *trapezius* muscle forms the upper back and part of the shoulders together with the *deltoid* muscles.

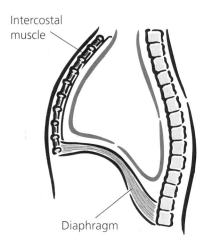

Intercostal muscle

Diaphragm

Muscles of respiration

Fascinating Fact

Many of the small facial muscles attach to one another or to the facial skin itself, pulling the face a specific way as they contract, forming the facial expressions.

Muscles of facial expression

● **Occipito-frontalis**

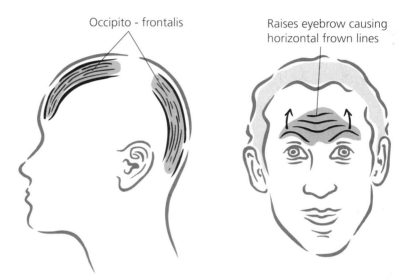

Occipito - frontalis

Raises eyebrow causing horizontal frown lines

Occipito-frontalis

- Position – covering the occipital bone at the base of the cranium and the frontal bone at the front of the cranium forming the forehead.
- Action – raises the eyebrows in **surprise** and is responsible for **horizontal frown lines**.

● **Corrugator supercilli**

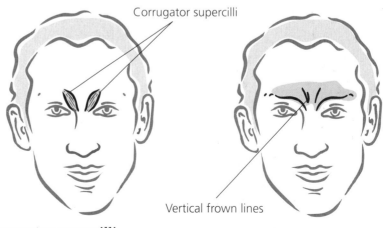

Corrugator supercilli

Vertical frown lines

Corrugator supercilli

   – Position – situated between the eyebrows.
   – Action – draws the eyebrows together creating a
     vertical frown line.

- **Orbicularis occuli**

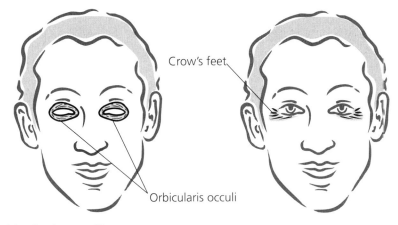

Orbicularis occuli

   – Position – a circular muscle surrounding the eye.
   – Action – closes the eye and contributes to the fine lines
     that first appear when you close your eyes tightly,
     developing into **crow's feet** over time.

- **Zygomaticus**

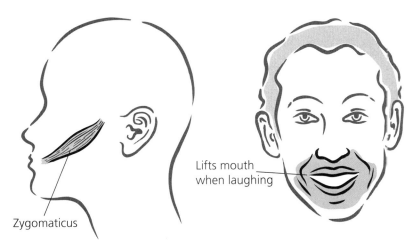

Zygomaticus

   – Position – covers the zygomatic bones and is attached to
     the muscles of the mouth.
   – Action – lifts the mouth and the cheeks as we **laugh**.

● **Risorius**

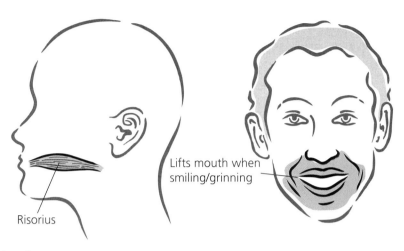

Lifts mouth when smiling/grinning

Risorius

Risorius

– Position – situated in the lower cheek area and is attached to the corners of the mouth.
Action – lifts the mouth in a **smile** extending to a **grin**.

● **Nasalis**

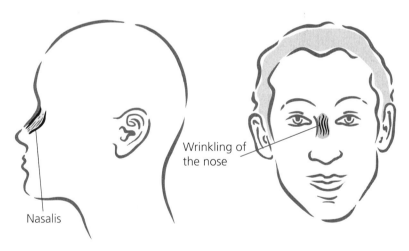

Wrinkling of the nose

Nasalis

Nasalis

– Position – covers the front of the nose.
– Action – causes **wrinkling** of the nose when the muscle is compressed.

● **Procerus**

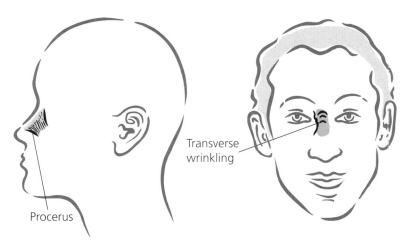

Procerus

- Position – covers the bridge of nose.
- Action – draws the eyebrows downwards puckering up the skin of the top of the nose into **transverse wrinkles**.

● **Orbicularis oris**

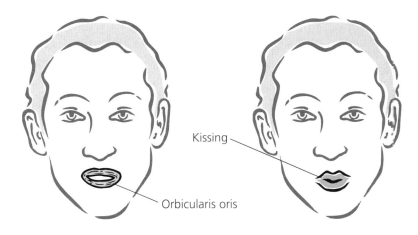

Orbicularis oris

- Position – a circular muscle surrounding the mouth forming its shape during use.
  Action – puckers and compresses the mouth as in **kissing**.

● **Triangularis**

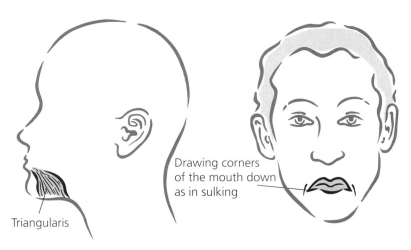

Drawing corners
of the mouth down
as in sulking

Triangularis

Triangularis

    — Position – extends along the side of chin.

    — Action – draws the angles of the mouth down as in **sulking**.

● **Mentalis**

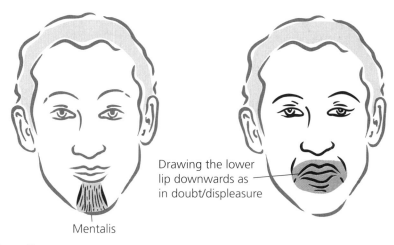

Drawing the lower
lip downwards as
in doubt/displeasure

Mentalis

Mentalis

    — Position – situated at the top of chin.

    — Action – raises the lower lip as in **doubt** or **displeasure** causing the chin to wrinkle.

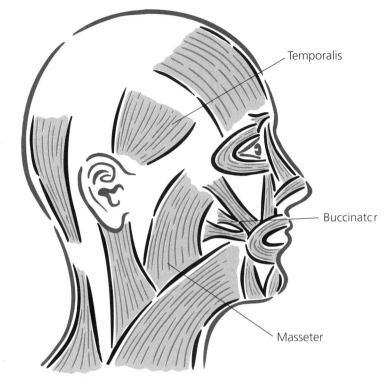

Temporalis

Buccinator

Masseter

Muscles of mastication

Muscles of mastication (chewing) include:

- **Temporalis**
  - Position – situated at the side of the head extending from the temporal bone to the mandible bone.
  - Action – lifts the mandible closing the jaw and draws it back when **chewing**.
- **Masseter**
  - Position – situated in the cheek extending from the zygomatic to the mandible bones.
  - Action – raises the mandible and is responsible for closing the jaw and **clenching** the teeth.
- **Buccinator**
  - Position – situated between the upper and lower jaw.
  - Action – draws the cheeks together as we **chew**.

Fascinating Fact

Grinding the teeth, a common stress-related disorder, is responsible for 'jaw ache'!

Blood and lymphatic vessels

Oxygenated blood is circulated to the upper body from the heart via the ascending aorta which branches out to form the subclavian and carotid arteries.

Deoxygenated blood is circulated from the upper body via the anterior jugular and subclavian veins before draining into the superior vena cava and finally the heart.

Lymphatic capillaries drain waste in the form of lymph from the cells for filtering in the nodes:

- Auricular nodes – situated behind the ear.
- Buccal nodes – situated in the cheek.
- Submandibular nodes – situated under the jaw.
- Occipital nodes – situated in the base of the skull.
- Cervical nodes – situated in the neck.

The remaining lymph is circulated to the thoracic duct from the left side of the head, neck and chest and to the right lymphatic duct from the right side of the head, neck and chest before draining into the subclavian veins (see Chapter 5 for details).

Nerves

There are twelve pairs of cranial nerves which radiate from the central nervous system (brain and spinal cord) to all areas of the face and neck:

1 **Olfactory** nerves – associated with our sense of smell.
2 **Optic** nerves – associated with our sense of sight.
3 **Oculomotor** nerves – associated with the movement of the eyes and eyelids.
4 **Trochlear** nerves – assist with the movement of the eyes.
5 **Trigeminal** nerves – associated with activity in the eyes and the jaw.
6 **Abducent** nerves – help with eye movements.
7 **Facial** nerves – associated with the taste buds, the salivary glands, the tear ducts and facial expressions.
8 **Vestibulocochlear** nerves – help with our sense of balance and hearing.
9 **Glossopharyngeal** nerves – associated with the tongue and the pharynx and help to control swallowing.
10 **Vagus** nerves – associated with speech and swallowing as well as being associated with the heart and the smooth muscles of the thorax and abdomen.
11 **Accessory** nerves – associated with the neck and back.
12 **Hypoglossal** nerves – associated with speaking, chewing and swallowing.

The cervical plexus contains the first four cervical nerves which branch out to supply the skin and muscles of the neck, shoulder and chest.

Fascinating Fact

The phrenic nerve stimulates the contraction of the diaphragm during respiration and is contained within the cervical plexus.

Associated organs

The brain is the main organ associated with the central nervous system and is situated in the skull, protected by the overlying bones, muscles and skin. Additional organs include the sensory organs:

- Eyes – associated with the sensory function of sight.
- Ears – associated with the sensory function of hearing and balance.
- Nose – associated with the sense of smell.
- Tongue – associated with the sense of taste.

The main organs associated with circulation and respiration are situated within the chest (thorax) and include:

- Heart – located slightly towards the left side of the upper body. The heart is about the size of the owner's fist. It is a hollow muscular organ that acts like a pump circulating blood around the body.
- Lungs – two balloon-like structures situated either side of the heart. The left lung is slightly smaller than the right because of the position of the heart. They are responsible for the action of breathing air in and out of the body during respiration.

As the ear is often included as an area for massage it is important to have a working knowledge of its associated anatomy and physiology.

The ears are attached to the head by muscles and tendons with the earflap or pinna forming the external portion. The pinna consists of a lower section or earlobe and an upper section or helix. The

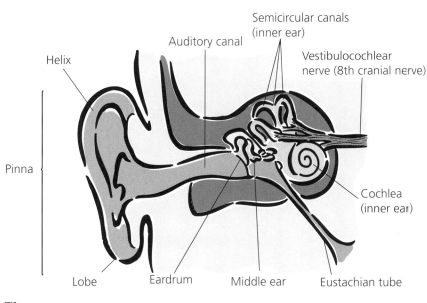

The ear

earlobe is composed of fibrous and adipose tissue with a rich blood supply and the helix is composed of elastic cartilage with a poor blood supply.

The auditory canal forms a tube leading into the ear from the pinna. It is lined with fine hairs and glands which are responsible for forming cerumen (earwax). The auditory canal leads on to the ear drum, middle and inner ear:

- The eardrum is cone-shaped and lined with mucous membrane.
- The middle ear is an irregular shaped cavity which contains the Eustachian tube linking the ears with the nasopharynx.
- The inner ear consists of fluid filled canals, the cochlea and the vestibulocochlear nerve linking the ears to the brain.

The functions of the ear include those associated with **hearing**, **balance** and **pressure**:

- Hearing – sound waves are picked up by the pinna and directed into the auditory canal to the eardrum where they pass through the middle ear to the inner ear, are picked up by the cochlea and transmitted to the brain by the nerve for interpretation.
- Balance – the ears detect changes in the position of the head and send messages via the nerve to the brain. The messages are interpreted and the skeletal muscles are instructed to maintain posture and thus balance.
- Pressure – pressure in the body is equalised by the Eustachian tube which opens when we yawn and/or swallow. This is often experienced as a 'popping' sensation in the ears.

Fascinating Fact

The word cochlea takes its origins from the Greek word *kokhlias* which can be translated as 'spiral in the form of snail-shell'. This translation gives rise to the popular saying 'a word in your shell-like'!

Considerations

In order to ascertain the suitability for massage of the upper body as well as be able to adapt the treatment to meet the needs of the different areas it is necessary to consider many factors including skin types and skin conditions.

Skin types

The skin of the face and upper body may be classified into the following skin types:

- **Normal skin** – ideal skin type commonly associated with children when the skin is balanced in texture and tone.
- **Oily skin** – puberty marks the age when the sebaceous glands of the body become more active often producing

excessive amounts of sebum (natural oil). This is common on the face, chest and back. The skin appears sallow, uneven and feels greasy to the touch.

- **Dry skin** – ageing skin has a tendency to dryness as sebaceous activity slows down. Less sebum is produced reducing the effectiveness of the protective acid mantle. The skin becomes dull, lifeless and uneven in texture and tone.

- **Dehydrated skin** – is associated with a general lack of moisture in the body which has a knock-on effect on the surface of the skin. The skin appears dull, uneven and superficial wrinkles will be more apparent.

- **Sensitive skin** – fine, pale skin tends to be more prone to sensitivity than darker, thicker skin types. The blood capillary network is close to the surface and is more readily and easily stimulated leading to surface redness. This may be caused by the use of overly harsh products, exposure to extreme temperatures and allergies as well as stress and emotions e.g. skin flushing and blushing etc.

- **Combination skin** – any combination of the former skin types constitutes a combination skin. The most common combination is an oily centre panel i.e. forehead, nose and chin and normal/dry/sensitive cheeks and neck.

- **Mature skin** – skin that is suffering with the effects of ageing. This may be premature and due to external forces e.g. excessive sunbathing and/or use of sunbeds, stress, illness, misuse etc. as well as the natural passing of time. As the skin ages its processes slow down and it begins to lose its protective functions.

Skin conditions

The skin of the upper body may exhibit some of the following conditions:

- **Freckles** – small areas of pigmented skin. Commonly associated with fair and red-headed people. Freckles darken when exposed to the sun.

- **Papules** – small raised areas of unbroken skin. Solid and painful to touch often developing into a pustule.

- **Pustules** – often referred to as a 'whitehead', spot or pimple. Raised, pus-filled area of skin often developing from a papule.

- **Comedones** – also known as 'blackheads'. The opening of a pore becomes blocked with excess dried sebum, dead skin cells, sweat and dirt etc. oxidising to form a blackened plug.

Acne is an inflammatory condition characterised by the formation of an eruption of papules, pustules and comedones. Acne may be classified as:

Tip

Massage mediums are chosen depending on skin type. Oils, creams/emulsions and gels are commonly used on the upper body and many of them contain active ingredients that have specific actions on the skin e.g. aloe vera which nourishing, camphor which is detoxifying, chamomile which is soothing etc.

Tip

Papules, pustules and comedones are commonly associated with an oily skin type and may be present on the face, neck, back and chest.

Tip

Pre-menstrual acne is a form of cyclical acne that appears shortly before (rarely after) the onset of menstruation.

Tip

Massage can help to disperse milia.

Tip

Sun damage may be seen in thinned skin that has lost its natural elasticity, wrinkles when compressed and appears leathery in texture. This may often be seen first on the décolletage area.

Angel advice

The heart chakra is located in the area of the upper chest, contributing to our feelings of connection with those around us. When we feel unloved and generally disconnected it is a natural reaction to try to protect ourselves by rounding the body inwards. This has the effect of tightening the pectoral muscles.

- **Acne vulgaris** – chronic acne, usually occurring in adolescence, with comedones, papules and pustules on the face, neck and upper parts of the trunk i.e. chest and back.
- **Acne rosacea** – a severe and extensive form of acne incorporating comedones, papules and pustules together with a reddening of the nose and cheeks characterised by the shape of a butterfly caused by the dilation of minute blood capillaries in the skin.
- **Milia** – small, harmless pinhead cysts. Commonly found around the eyes and cheeks on dry skin.
- **Telangiectasis** – abnormal dilation of capillaries or terminal arteries producing blotchy red spots. Commonly found on the face and associated with a sensitive skin type.
- **Superfluous hair** – a male pattern hair growth in women often accompanies hormone imbalance. Hair becomes thicker and darker around the upper lip, chin and sides of the face often leading to distress and lack of self-confidence.
- **Wrinkles and dropped contours** – as skin ages it becomes thinner and responds more readily to the pull of gravity contributing to the formation of lines, wrinkles and dropped contours.
- **Stretch marks** – may be present on the skin of the décolletage in women. These occur when the skin has been overstretched due to excessive and/or rapid weight gain and/or pregnancy, generally on the breasts. The skin surrounding the breasts forms in distinct lines (transverse and longitudinal) that appear shiny and discoloured due to loss of elasticity in the dermis layer of the skin.
- **Piercings** – are increasingly popular on the upper body including the nipples, eyebrows, mouth, nose, ears and tongue. Ideally these should be removed prior to the massage treatment. However, if this is not possible, care should be taken to avoid the area to prevent dragging the skin.
- **Scar tissue** – as a result of piercings and surgery e.g. face lifts, breast augmentation etc. may be present.

Muscle tone and condition

The many muscles of the upper body contribute to the functions of this area including:

- **Shoulder and arm movements** – pectoralis muscles often experience tightening and shortening through postural problems such as kyphosis. Hunched and rounded shoulders may accompany feelings of low self-esteem and lack of confidence and contributes to the formation of tight pectoral muscles.
- **Head movements** – platysma and sterno cleido mastoid muscles work together with the trapezius muscle of the upper back. All of these muscles suffer greatly when

posture is out of line because the head is being continuously tilted forward or back.

- **Breathing** – diaphragm and intercostals muscles contract with the inward breath pushing abdominal organs down and the rib cage out to let maximum amounts of air into the body. The muscles relax with the outward breath. Breathing is very soon affected if muscle tone is poor resulting in inefficient and ineffective breathing.

Fascinating Fact

The act of breathing helps to gently massage the internal organs and has the effect of stimulating venous blood and lymphatic flow within the body generally.

- **Jaw movements** – masseter, buccinator and temporalis muscles contribute to the processes of mastication (chewing) and talking and as such also contribute to the grinding of teeth. The masseter muscle in particular can become very tight and sore as a result.

Angel advice

Many people find that they grind their teeth at night without knowing it. This is generally associated with stress and the inability to totally relax.

Fascinating Fact

Dentists are fast realising the beneficial effects that massage and holistic treatments have on the well-being of the teeth. Stress-related grinding of teeth wears them down creating long-term problems. Treatments such as massage relax a person to the extent that they do not grind their teeth anymore!

- **Facial expressions** – many of the facial muscles attach to each other and/or the skin helping to pull the face into the various facial expressions that we associate with feelings of pleasure, despair, surprise, fright, anger etc. Repetitive movements associated with these muscles affect their tone and condition, often leaving the marks of overwork in the form of:
  - horizontal frown lines – occipito-frontalis muscle
  - vertical frown lines – corrugator supercilli muscle

- crow's feet around the eyes – orbicularis occuli muscle
- fine lines around the mouth – orbicularis oris muscle
- jowls – platysma muscle etc.

Joint mobility

Tight muscles result in loss of mobility affecting the overall functioning of the body. As head, neck, shoulder and chest muscles become tired and tight there is a general loss of flexibility and mobility. Movements become strained, painful and restricted. This can have an effect on our psychological well-being, making us feel emotionally strained, pained and restricted! Feelings of frustration, anger, fear, anxiety etc. often accompany a loss of mobility as the body and mind fail to function in harmony.

The opposite may also be seen as being true. If we are feeling frustrated, angry, frightened and anxious we tend to hold our bodies differently resulting in a lack of physical well-being. The saying 'what goes around, comes around' is very apt!

Stress

As we have seen, the upper body is an area that tends to hold onto physical and psychological stress but is also an area of the body that is prone to cause us stress.

Face and body image is very important in today's culture and we very quickly learn the importance of physical appearance. The face in particular provides an insight into a person and first impressions are often founded on appearance and whether or not it conforms to the norm. It is human nature for people to want to 'fit in' and anyone that is different is often seen as being 'abnormal'. As we enter the various physical milestones associated with human development e.g. puberty, menopause etc. the body experiences changes that can cause excessive stress and can in turn be worsened by stress e.g. acne.

Massage treatments to the whole body and/or the parts can help a person feel physically and psychologically better about themselves:

- Physical appearance may be improved as skin types and conditions are recognised and treated through massage and appropriate use of skin care products.
- Psychological well-being may be improved through recognition and subsequent treatment making a person feel 'normal'.

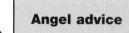

Angel advice

Be aware and accept the fact that things which at first appear 'out of the norm' are in fact quite normal!

Remember

Good functioning relies on good muscle tone just as poor functioning results from poor muscle tone.

Contraindications

It is important to conduct a full consultation prior to any form of massage treatment to check for general contraindications. Specific contraindications to massage of the upper body include:

- Undiagnosed pain and swelling in the area. DO NOT TREAT, refer to GP for advice.
- Recent scar tissue. DO NOT TREAT until completely healed. Obtain medical advice if necessary.
- Migraines – massage is likely to make a person suffering with a migraine feel worse before they feel better. They are advised to rest in a darkened room until the migraine has completely gone.

Tip

Mild tension headaches are not a contraindication to massage. In fact massage may help to disperse the toxins in the muscles that are contributing to the pain.

Infectious disorders are common on the face and the following conditions are classified as contraindications:

- Infected acne – the condition is aggravated by a bacterial infection.
- Herpes simplex – a viral infection commonly known as a cold sore. The mouth is the most common site.
- Conjunctivitis – inflammation of the conjunctiva which covers the whites of the eyes and the inner surface of the eyelids. The eyes become red and/or sticky.
- Stye – a boil-like infection of the glands at the root of the eyelashes.

It is important never to diagnose a medical condition. It is however necessary to recognise a condition that could be made worse by massage and/or one that could cause cross-infection. In any situation, the area should not be treated until it is completely cleared of all infection.

Tip

An area of the body that is painful, raised, inflamed, red and/or contains a pus formation is considered a contraindication to massage.

Treatment tracker

UPPER BODY

The upper body involves massage treatment to the décolletage, face and neck, ears and scalp and may be massaged in their entirety or as:

- Décolletage as part of a full body massage – treatment time approx. 5 minutes.
- Face, neck and décolletage as part of a facial – 20 minute massage as part of an hour facial including consultation.
- Ears and/or face and neck as part of thermal auricular therapy – massage time approx. 5–20 minutes as part of a 45–60 minute treatment including consultation.

There are many variations of treatment combinations and timings for massage to the upper body and the emphasis should be on adapting to meet the needs of the individual client and treatment plan.

Preparation	Position	Client care
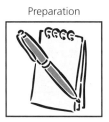	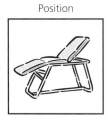	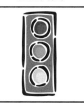

Preparation

- Conduct a full consultation.
- Check general and specific contraindications.
- Agree the treatment and preferred massage medium with the client.
- Removal of lower body clothing down to underwear for massage to the entire upper body.
- Ensure hair is secured away from the face.
- Removal of jewellery e.g. necklaces and dangling ear rings etc.
- Skin cleansing with an appropriate cleanser paying particular attention to the face and neck.
- Exfoliation may be carried out with emphasis on the face and neck and décolletage.

Position

Client – the client usually lies flat or semi-reclined on the couch in a supine position.

Masseur/masseuse – is usually positioned at the head of the couch behind the client, although they may work from the side when working the décolletage. If working for any length of time at the head of a couch the practitioner may be seated for additional comfort.

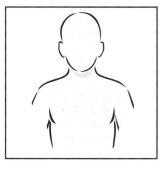

Client care

Considerations for client comfort when lying in this position include:

- A pillow to support the head and neck.
- Additional pillows to support the spine in cases of postural figure faults.
- Rolled up towels to support the back of the knees and ankles if necessary.
- A blanket, duvet and/or towels may be used to ensure modesty and warmth.
- Clients should be reminded that they can move as and when they feel they need to.

Babies/children – the chest may be massaged as part of the abdomen thus covering the whole of the front of the torso at one time. Stroking effleurage and gentle petrissage movements are ideal over the face, ears and scalp providing comfort as well as soothing body and mind, inducing relaxation and often sleep. The neck is often omitted due to its extreme sensitivity.

Elderly – gentler depth of pressure is usually indicated in the area of the upper body with the emphasis on the superficial absorption of product and the deeper stimulation of the circulation. Extra care should be taken to ensure client comfort when in a supine position to avoid excessive joint stiffness.

Male – when treating the upper body on men, it is possible to extend the massage to the chest area to include the abdomen as well. Depth of pressure should be adapted to suit the muscle bulk and amount of adipose tissue which not only varies from person to person but also over different areas of the upper body.

Female – the décolletage area is usually treated in isolation as part of a full body massage or as part of a facial and the breasts are covered with a towel. However, many product companies are introducing breast treatments in which case, the massage can be adapted to suit the needs of the client/treatment plan.

Lymphatic drainage – tightness associated with tension in the muscles and puffiness associated with blocked sinuses and congested skin can be successfully aided with drainage movements. Movements should be directed to:

- Décolletage – axillary lymph nodes under the arms.
- Neck – deep and superficial cervical lymph nodes.
- Face – buccal and submandibular lymph nodes in the cheek and jaw.
- Ears – parotid and auricular lymph nodes in front and behind the ears.
- Scalp – occipital lymph nodes at the base of the skull.

Posture – poor posture associated with the upper body often results in poor breathing techniques. Rounding the shoulders down and forwards is a common postural figure fault associated with physical and mental stress resulting in limited space in the chest. The lungs are then unable to extend to receive a maximum capacity of air which has a knock-on effect on the rest of the body. Attention should be paid to keeping:

- Shoulders centred
- Head held with the chin parallel to the floor.

- Remove excess massage medium if necessary.
- If oils have been used in the hair they may be left to soak in further or shampooed out.
- Apply post-treatment procedures e.g. masks, self tan etc.
- Apply remedial products in the form of moisturisers paying particular attention to the eyes and neck.

Adaptations	Special emphasis	Completion
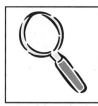		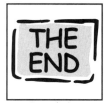

Suggested order of work – the décolletage

Tip

The massage to the décolletage as described is performed with the practitioner positioned at the head of the couch behind the client's head for ease of access. The movements may be adapted for working at the side of the client.

The décolletage includes the upper chest and shoulders.

The massage to the décolletage commences with a simple **hold** as the hands are gently placed on the chest and the application of a suitable massage medium with non-directional effleurage movements. This allows the introduction of the practitioner's hands as well as the product, both of which may be cool to start.

The massage continues with:

1 **Directional effleurage**
   - Both hands start at (a) the top or base of the neck and work down to the start of the breasts and (b) out to the arms with pressure and then (c) over and under the shoulders and up the back of the neck without pressure. Repeat 3–6 times.

2 **Petrissage**
   - Finger kneading – using the fingers of both hands to make small circles over the chest from sternum to underarms, over the shoulders and up the back of the neck.
   - Thumb kneading – thumbs of both hands may be used to apply small circles to the back of the shoulders.
   - Knuckling – over the chest working into the pectoral muscles.

3 **Friction**
   - Circular friction – using the thumbs, may be applied to areas of tension found on the back of the shoulders and up the back of the neck.

4 **Tapotement/percussion**
   - Butterfly – may be performed over the décolletage and neck.

5 **Joint manipulation**
   - Stretching – using the fingers of both hands placed in the occiput (base of the occipital bone at the top of the back of the neck) gently pull the head towards you.
   - Rocking – placing the palmar surface of the hands over each shoulder and gently press alternate shoulders in a rocking motion. Complete the movement with a gentle press with both hands.

6 **Directional effleurage**
   - Complete the routine with effleurage directed from the neck to the start of the breasts, out to the arms, over and under the shoulders and up the back of the neck. Repeat 3–6 times.

Directional effleurage

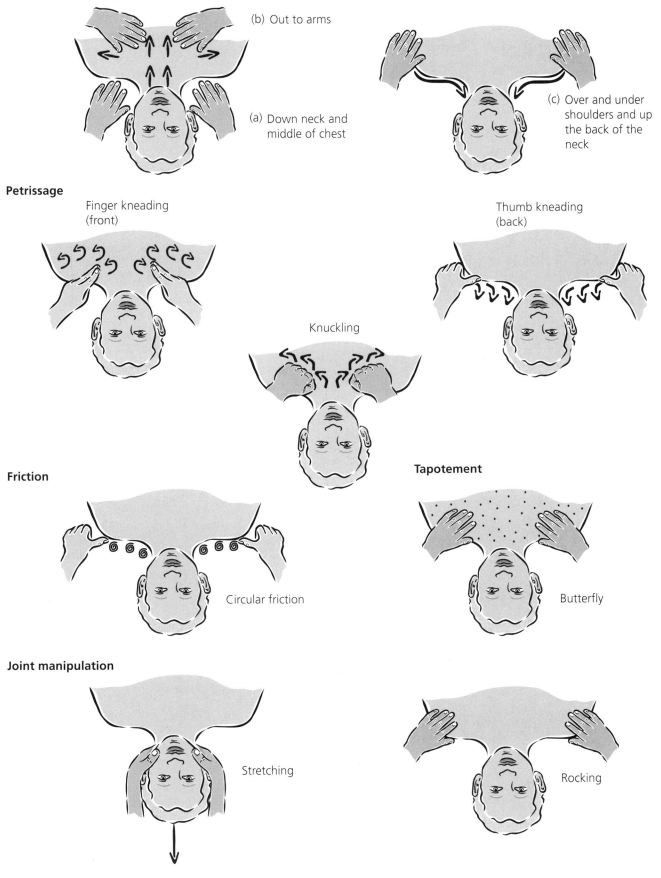

(b) Out to arms

(a) Down neck and middle of chest

(c) Over and under shoulders and up the back of the neck

Petrissage

Finger kneading (front)

Thumb kneading (back)

Knuckling

Friction

Circular friction

Tapotement

Butterfly

Joint manipulation

Stretching

Rocking

Suggested order of work – the face and neck

The face and neck may be treated in isolation and/or with the décolletage, scalp or ears.

The massage commences with a simple **hold.** This is usually performed at the temples with one hand at either side. This ensures that the client is aware that the treatment is about to start. Non-directional effleurage may be used to apply the massage medium of choice to the whole area being careful to avoid the eyes, mouth and nostrils.

The massage continues with:

1 **Directional effleurage**
   - Using both hands alternately to work with upward pressure (a) up the front of the neck, (b) around the chin, (c) up each cheek, (d) around and over the nose and (e) up and across the forehead.
   - Both hands may be used alternately with increased pressure at the centre forehead and both sides. Repeat 3–6 times.

2 **Petrissage**
   - Kneading – finger and/or thumb kneading may be used with both hands (a) up the neck, (b) around the chin, (c) around the mouth, (d) up each cheek, (e) around the nose, (f) around the eyes (g) along the forehead.
   - Picking up – using the thumb and forefinger of both hands pick up and squeeze the tissue (a) along the eyebrows, (b) along the jaw line.
   - Rolling – using the middle two fingers of both hands, the tissue of the cheeks can be rolled in three horizontal rows (a) along the jaw line, (b) from the corner of the mouth to the ear and (c) from the sides of the nose to the temples.

3 **Friction**
   - Circular friction – using the fingers/thumbs may be used to work around the nose.
   - Transverse friction – using two fingers from one hand and one from the other in a scissor like action across the forehead.

4 **Tapotement/percussion**
   - Butterfly – gentle tapping movements may be used all over the face and neck.

5 **Vibration**
   - Static vibration – may be applied with the fingers of each hand to the zygomatic bones (cheek).

6. **Directional effleurage**
   - Using both hands alternately to work with upward pressure (a) up the front of the neck, (b) around the chin, (c) up each cheek, (d) around and over the nose and (e) across the forehead.

Tip

When working around the eyes it is advisable to use the ring finger as it applies the least amount of pressure on this delicate area.

Directional effleurage

Up the neck	Around the chin	Up the cheeks	Around the nose	Across the forehead

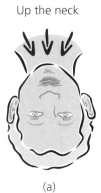
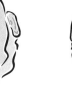
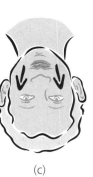
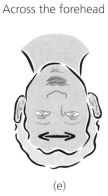

(a)   (b)   (c)   (d)   (e)

Kneading

Up the neck	Around the chin	Around the mouth	Up the cheeks	Around the nose

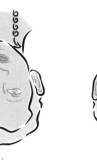
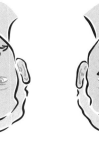
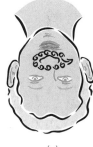

(a)   (b)   (c)   (d)   (e)

Around the eyes   Along the forehead

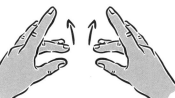

(f)   (g)

Rolling
(a) Along jawline
(b) From corner of mouth to ear
(c) From nose to temple

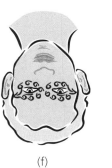

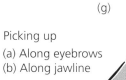
Picking up
(a) Along eyebrows
(b) Along jawline

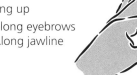

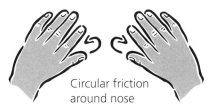
Circular friction
around nose

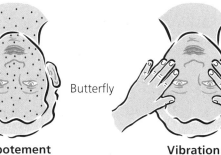

Static vibration

Butterfly

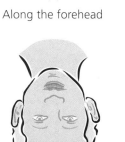

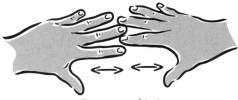
Transverse friction
across forehead

Tapotement   **Vibration**   **Friction**

Suggested order of work – the ears

Ears are often a forgotten area of the body in terms of massage. The ears form a miniature representation of the whole body and are often treated as part of a reflexology treatment and/or self treatment. They respond well to massage and may be massaged as part of a facial and/or scalp treatment.

Massage to the ears starts with a simple **hold** to introduce the practitioner's hands. Non-directional effleurage may be used to introduce a massage medium if required. The massage continues with:

1   **Directional effleurage**
    - Using both hands gently stroke the ears with downward pressure from helix to lobe and up the back of the ear without pressure. Repeat 3–6 times.

2   **Petrissage**
    - Kneading – using the thumb and index finger of both hands apply small alternate kneading movements along the pinna of each ear.
    - Picking up – using the thumb and index finger of both hands apply small picking up movements along the pinna of each ear.

3   **Friction**
    - Circular friction – using index finger or thumbs of both hands apply small circles to areas of tension along the pinna of the ear and surrounding area.

4   **Tapotement/percussion**
    - Flicking – using the index finger and thumbs of each hand gently flick the pinna.

5   **Joint manipulation**
    - Stretching – holding the ears between the index fingers and thumbs of each hand gently pull the ear out from the head. Work all along the pinna with gentle stretching pulls

6   **Direction effleurage**
    - Using both hands gently stroke down the front of the ear with pressure and up the back of ear without pressure. Repeat 3–6 times.

Directional effleurage

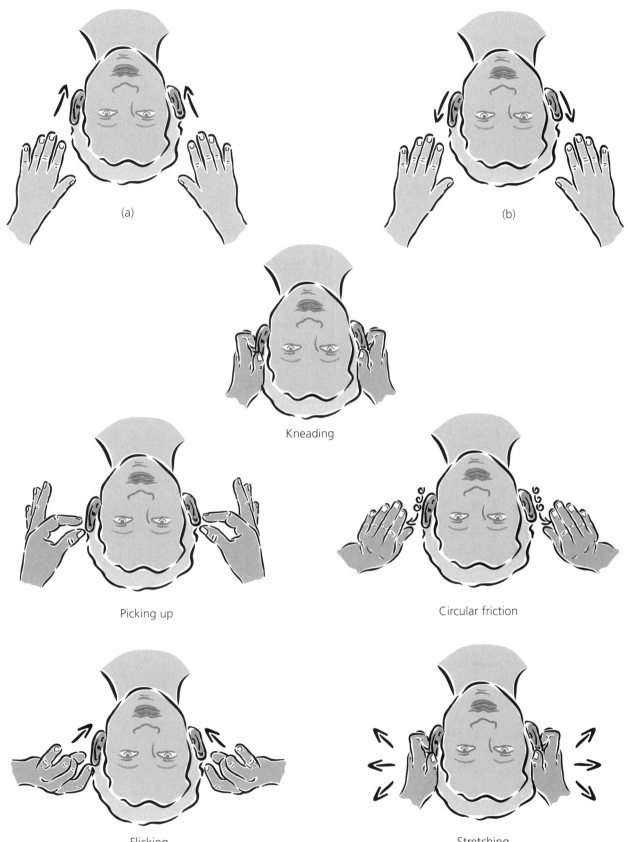

(a)

(b)

Kneading

Picking up

Circular friction

Flicking

Stretching

Suggested order of work – the scalp

Tip

Specific hair conditioners and oils may be used to massage the scalp as an alternative to other massage mediums.

Tip

It is not always necessary to lift the client's head whilst applying scalp massage in this position. It may be more comfortable to avoid the area resting on the pillow and work around it and/or gently ease your fingers beneath the head taking the full weight of the head as you do so.

A scalp massage is an ideal accompaniment for facial massage and may be applied with or without the use of a massage medium.

A scalp massage commences with a simple **hold** with both hands at the temples (as for facial massage) as a means of introduction. Non-directional effleurage may be used to introduce the massage medium if required, stroking it through the hair as well as onto the scalp.

The scalp massage continues with:

1 **Directional effleurage**
   - Using both hands to gently stroke over the scalp and through the hair. Hands are used alternately with the pressure applied down the lengths of the hair. Repeat 6–12 times.

2 **Petrissage**
   - Kneading – pads of the fingers and thumbs of both hands may be used to apply small kneading movements over the entire scalp. The movements may be superficial, e.g. skimming over the surface tissue, and/or deep e.g. moving the underlying tissue from the bone.
   - Border of the hand kneading – using the hypothenar eminence of the little finger side of the hand at the temples.

3 **Friction**
   - Circular friction – using the pads of the fingers and/or thumbs to apply firm circles to specific areas of tension e.g. along the hairline.

4 **Tapotement/percussion**
   - Butterfly – gentle tapping over the entire scalp.
   - Plucking – gentle plucking of the hair over the entire scalp.
   - Hacking – gentle hacking over the entire scalp.

5 **Vibration**
   - Shaking – using the fingers of both hands through the hair to gently shake or 'ruffle' the hair from the scalp.

6 **Joint manipulation**
   - Stretching – placing the fingers of both hands in the occiput apply a gentle pull towards you.

7 **Directional effleurage**
   - Complete the treatment using both hands to gently stroke over the scalp and through the hair. Hands are used alternately with the pressure applied down the length of the hair. Repeat 6–12 times.

Directional effleurage

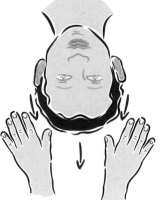

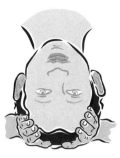

Kneading

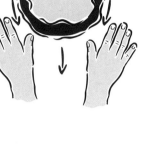

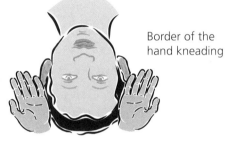

Border of the hand kneading

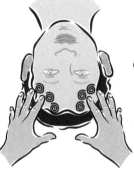

Circular friction

Tapotement/percussion

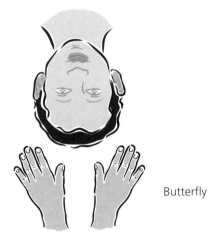

Butterfly

Plucking

Hacking

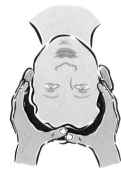

Shaking

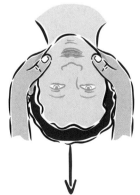

Stretching

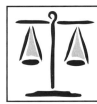

Holistic harmony

The upper body and most especially the face is often the area of the body responsible for creating the all important first impressions. We are judged by our appearance, the formation and symmetry of our features, our facial expressions, eye contact and speech. Personal confidence and levels of self-esteem are also often measured in these terms. If we feel good about how we look and the impression we create our confidence levels improve, as does social interaction. If, however, we feel bad about such things our self-esteem is affected and personal interaction is often avoided.

A person's sense of worth is very much reflected in their appearance. A strong sense of self-worth will be demonstrated in a person's desire to take care of themselves and their appearance. The opposite is true of those people suffering a lack of self-worth.

Massage may be seen as a useful tool in increasing a person's sense of self-worth through the art of touch. This can have a knock-on effect on how a person subsequently cares for themselves post-treatment. Therefore effective pre- and post-treatment advice is vital in providing a service that has the potential to be life enhancing and even life changing.

Pre-treatment procedures

Massage of the upper body is traditionally carried out as part of a facial and as such many preparatory treatments may be applied, including:

- Cleansing – it is important to remove all traces of make-up from the skin prior to massage. Specialist products may be used for cleansing dependent on skin type and skin problems.
- Toning – it is important that the skin is grease free prior to massage and the use of a toner removes any traces of grease left on the skin from the cleansing process. A grease free skin will absorb the massage products more effectively.
- Exfoliation – dead skin cells tend to congest the skin, especially if there is an excess of sebum. In addition, make-up can become clogged resulting in an uneven texture. Gentle exfoliation removes the dead skin cells, excess sebum and clogged make-up leaving the skin smooth and even.
- Steaming – the use of facial steamers can gently warm the skin, softening the surface cells and encouraging impurities to the surface. Warm flannel mitts may be applied as an alternative ensuring that the temperature is not too great.

Although these pre-treatments are considered to be part of a facial, there is no reason why they cannot be included in a body massage.

Additions

Mechanical massage treatments may be used in addition to and/or
to complement the manual massage including:

- Audio sonic vibrator – may be used pre- or post-manual
  massage to relieve tension in the muscles. It is particularly
  effective on the shoulders but may be used on the face,
  neck and chest with good results.
- Brush cleanse – may also be used pre- or post-manual
  massage. Pre-massage treatment works to deep cleanse the
  skin preparing it for massage. Post-massage treatment
  works to encourage further absorption of the massage
  medium.
- Vacuum suction – is generally used as an alternative to
  manual massage to aid lymphatic drainage. This is
  particularly useful for congested, problematic skin, aiding
  in the removal of static lymph which is often a contributory
  factor. Movements are directed to the auricular, buccal and
  submandibular lymph nodes of the face, the cervical lymph
  nodes of the neck and the supraclavicular and/or axillary
  lymph nodes of the upper chest and underarms.

Post-treatment procedures

As with all areas indicated for massage, post-treatment procedures
are beneficial. They not only provide an additional service but also
ensure the most effective treatment and offer that little bit extra in
terms of treatment enhancements that may make the difference
between a client coming to you for treatment rather than the
practitioner down the road!

- Masks – traditional facial treatments will always include
  the application of a mask which may be in the form of a
  pre-mixed, specially prepared or thermal mask. The choice
  of mask is dependent on the skin type and skin problems.
  Face masks are multipurpose and may be used to soothe,
  nourish, purify, warm, cool or even exfoliate the skin.
- Self-tanning – another popular post-treatment procedure
  for the upper body that ensures an even application of

product without streaking as well as a safer option to obtaining a much sought after tan.

Remedial treatments in the form of moisturisers/nourishers that hydrate and protect the skin of the face, eyes, neck and décolletage including:

- Gels – provide a means to protect and moisturise the skin. Face, neck and eye gels are a good choice for the remedial treatment of the skin of the 14–30 age group. Gels have a cooling and tightening effect on the surface tissue helping to gently moisturise and protect as well as prevent fine lines and wrinkles from becoming ingrained.

- Creams/emulsions – provide the basis for moisturising day and nourishing night products that provide protection to the skin's surface. Day creams are generally thinner in consistency and may be used under make up and/or in isolation with many containing a sun protection factor (SPF). Night creams are thicker in consistency and as such, more nourishing. Specific eye and neck creams are the preferred choice for the fine skin surrounding the eyes as well as that of the neck as ageing begins to become apparent.

- Oils – offer an alternative to creams/emulsions as some people prefer the feel of oil on the skin.

- Serums – concentrated ingredients may be applied to the skin of the face, neck, eyes and décolletage prior to the application of gels, creams/emulsions and/or oils. The active ingredients contained in the serums offers effective remedial action on all types of skin including oily, dry, dehydrated, sensitive and ageing.

Self-help

It is of equal importance to recommend suitable treatments, remedial products and correct application along with additional ways in which a person can learn to help themselves. Taking responsibility for personal well-being encourages a person to actively take more control which in turn creates a more positive outlook.

Nutrition

What we eat greatly affects the condition of the skin and maintaining a balanced diet is the one of the main factors in achieving healthy skin. The skin of the upper body presents the main area of concern for most people, with many finding that psychological problems associated with lack of self-esteem and confidence accompany a problem skin.

Research is constantly discovering the links between certain foodstuffs and skin conditions, for example:

- Acne results from an oversecretion of sebum resulting in papules, pustules and comedones. The skin appears sallow and dull. Fatty foods compound the condition and should be avoided in excess. In addition, a lack of vitamin A in the diet has been found to produce skin congestion. Acne conditions respond well to a low-fat, low-sugar diet that is high in fruit and vegetables. Drinking plenty of water is a prerequisite for improved skin.

- Eczema and dermatitis are common skin conditions characterised by a dry, itchy, inflamed skin. Any area of the body may be affected with common sites being on the upper body. They can be triggered by allergies, stress and food. Coffee has been found to be a common trigger. Eating oily fish and fruit containing vitamin C is believed to significantly improve both conditions.

- Herpes simplex is a virus that causes cold sores commonly found on the mouth. Research has shown that salt and mucus-forming dairy products can contribute to an outbreak. Conversely, a diet high in protein has been found to safeguard against an attack as proteins are needed by the body to make antibodies.

Fascinating Fact

Eczema and dermatitis are often associated with allergies to wheat or dairy products.

Ageing

One of the main concerns relating to the upper body for both men and women is the signs associated with the passing of time and the effects of the ageing process. The skin and underlying fatty tissue, muscles and bones are all affected by this process with the resulting gradual deterioration of structure and slowing down of functions. Whilst massage treatment and self-help techniques can significantly slow down the ageing process it can in no way put a stop to it. An increasing number of people, both men and women, are seeking medical intervention in their quest to stay young. Popular medical procedures include:

- Chemical peels – acid solutions are applied to the skin to remove blemishes, sun damage and the effects of ageing.

- Botox injections – a series of injections of *botulinium toxin* are administered to the lines around the eyes, between the eyebrows and on the forehead which have the effect of paralysing the muscles and nerves.

- Lip augmentation – *collagen* or *hyalurionic* gel are injected to temporarily plump up the lip line. A more permanent alternative is to have tissue extracted from a person's own tendons in the wrist or mouth which is then threaded into the lip line. Both procedures have the effect of ridding the lip line of the effects of ageing.

- Laser resurfacing – a laser is passed over the skin burning the surface tissue to create a smoother effect.

- Face lift (rhytidectomy) – an incision is made usually at the back of the ear from the hair line to the lobe. The skin of the face is then pulled back, excess skin is removed and the tightened skin sewn back into its new position. Brow lifts and eye lifts (blepharoplasty) are also popular procedures.

Rest

Sleep is vital for regeneration of the body as a whole and the effects of sleep are clearly visible in the condition of the skin. Sleep is a period of rest for both the body and mind. Whilst asleep the body is in a state of partial unconsciousness allowing the 'recharging of batteries' to take place. This has the effect of ensuring cellular replenishment and regeneration can take place.

Mental and physical weariness soon manifests itself in the condition of the body as a whole, and in turn that of the upper body and most especially the face often resulting in:

- Greater definition of expression lines as muscles become overworked.
- Dropped contours as muscles become fatigued.
- Dull skin colour due to reduced circulation of oxygen and inefficient removal of cellular waste.
- Dry, dehydrated skin caused by lack of adequate replenishment of water and nutrients to the cells.

Long-term sleep deprivation has a knock-on effect on all of the organs and systems of the body, making the body extremely vulnerable. The body becomes less able to perform its vital functions and more prone to illness and disease.

The amount of sleep needed is dependent on age, activity and lifestyle with the average daily amount for an active adult being between seven and eight hours.

Exercise

During the course of the day the facial muscles are used to express our feelings through the formation of facial expressions, and to perform various functions e.g. eating, talking, blinking etc.

The use of the facial muscles is not always balanced as we repeatedly frown whilst working; continuously strain our eyes whilst focusing on the computer screen or talk incessantly whilst cradling the phone to our ear etc. These repetitive actions tire the muscles which in turn become fatigued from constant use and ache from a build-up of the toxin lactic acid.

Gentle facial exercises may be used as a way of helping to relax the muscles and stimulate the circulation, bringing fresh oxygen to the area and helping to eliminate the lactic acid and associated aches and pains.

At the end of the day cleanse over your face to clean away the effects of the day. Whilst doing so try some of the following exercises:

Remember

Muscles continue to work even when energy levels are low. This is associated with the anaerobic energy system whereby lactic acid is produced as a by-product.

1. Gently rub the whole face with your fingertips to loosen the muscles and stimulate the circulation.

2. Lift your eyebrows and open your eyes as widely as possible, helping to stretch the muscles of the upper face. Circle your eyes feeling the tension start to disappear.

3. Open your mouth as wide as possible and move your lips into the shape of the vowels saying them out loud e.g. 'a', 'e', 'i', 'o', 'u'. This will help to stretch the muscles of the lower face. If you exaggerate the movements you will also feel the stretch in the muscles of the neck.

4. Remove the cleanser and tone the skin. Gently pat the skin to invigorate and stimulate. The toner will evaporate leaving the skin feeling refreshed.

5. Apply a moisturiser using gentle massage movements. Start at the neck and work upwards with flowing movements as you feel the skin and underlying muscles become gently restored and rejuvenated.

Activity

Research exercises suitable for the face and neck and devise an exercise plan suitable for client use at home as part of a self-help programme.

Awareness

The quality of the air breathed into the body has a direct effect on the condition of the skin as a whole and of the skin of the face specifically due to the amount of exposure it receives. Toxins from the environment are absorbed into the skin breaking down the acid mantle leaving the skin, and in turn the rest of the body, vulnerable. Nicotine is one of the most harmful toxins that the skin may find itself regularly exposed to:

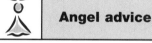

Angel advice

Relaxation time associated with having a massage treatment encourages deep breathing. Ensure that the treatment room is well ventilated and odour free so that a client may benefit from the physical act of better breathing and the physiological intake of clean, fresh air.

- Passive smokers absorb the toxins from the cigarette smoke into the layers of the skin, hair and nails. The toxins, colour and odour are all absorbed affecting their function, colour and odour. In addition, the toxins are absorbed into the blood through respiration and circulated to all of the internal organs and systems of the body affecting their function and well-being.

- Active smokers experience all of the above effects but at more concentrated levels. The direct heat of the smoke adds to the overall aggravation of the body by dehydrating surface cells and the act of smoking encourages fine lines around the mouth the eyes.

Special care

The whole body including its parts requires special care in the form of antioxidants which help to fight against free radical attack.

Free radicals contribute to the condition of the body and are another factor that greatly affects the external appearance of the skin of the upper body. They include pollution, radiation and over-processed foods e.g. fried and toasted. Free radicals cause damage to individual cells because of their effect on the cell's ability to take in nutrients and release waste products.

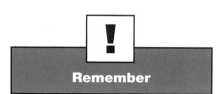

Remember

Free radicals are the toxic by-product of energy metabolism e.g. oxidation.

Antioxidants provide protection against the effects of free radicals. Antioxidants are able to safeguard the body against the effects of oxidation and are present in certain foods including:

- Vitamin A – found predominantly in red/orange/yellow fruits and vegetables.
- Vitamin C – found predominantly in citrus fruits as well as vegetables.
- Vitamin E – found predominantly in 'seed' foods e.g. nuts and nut oils.
- Selenium – a mineral found in abundance in seafood and seeds.
- Zinc – a mineral found in abundance in seafood, most especially oysters.

The body itself is able to produce antioxidants as part of the immune system. However, adding antioxidants to a well balanced diet enhances the body's ability to cope with free radical attack helping to maintain homeostasis and prevent illness, disease and the effects of premature ageing.

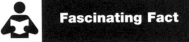

Fascinating Fact

Zinc is also essential for fertility in both women and men and oysters are said to be powerful aphrodisiacs!

Activity

Practice the suggested order of work, adapting the treatment accordingly. Put the whole routine together and practice on as many people as possible of varying sizes and ages in order to gain as much practical experience as possible.

Task

Plan a treatment list to give to clients outlining the variations of massage treatments you can offer. Give information on timing, effects and benefits and price.

Knowledge review

1   How many pairs of ribs make up the rib cage?

2   What are sinuses?

3   What is the name of the bone that forms the base of the skull?

4   What does the mandible bone form?

5   Which muscle separates the thorax and the abdomen?

6   Where is the orbicularis oris located?

7   Which muscle is responsible for lifting the mouth into a smile?

8   Name the muscle that surrounds the eye.

9   Name the lymph nodes situated in the neck.

10   Give the three functions of the ear.

11   What is the outside portion of the ear called?

12   What is the technical term for a blackhead?

13   What is telangiectasis?

14   Name the three muscles associated with mastication.

15   What type of facial lines do the frontalis and corrugator supercilli muscles form?

16   When is scar tissue a contraindication to massage?

17   What is herpes simplex commonly known as?

18   Name the two main types of acne.

19   What do botox injections cause in the muscles and nerves?

20   Which three vitamins are classed as antioxidants?

Part 5
Massage progression

Learning objectives

After reading this part you should be able to:

- Recognise the need for pathways of progression.

- Identify the links between client needs and treatment choice.

- Understand the origins and procedures associated with each treatment.

- Be aware of the links between the East and the West and the old and the new.

- Appreciate your place within the massage industry and the contribution you can make.

In order to look forward to the progression of massage, we need to once again look back through time. Whilst certain parallels have been observed in the development of massage therapies within the Eastern and Western cultures clear divides have also existed.

The progress that we are now experiencing in beauty and holistic treatments takes as its origin the basic art of massage which has been passed through the ages from generation to generation as something vital to all aspects of a person's life and well-being. This is a predominantly Eastern phenomenon which has gained momentum in the Western world since the 1960s and the hippy movement. However, the science of massage which as the development of mechanical massage procedures in the fields of sport and medicine has been a predominantly Western phenomenon has provided an undercurrent for progression albeit sometimes losing sight of the basic art.

The following chapters aim to explore the progress of both the art and science of massage by answering the following questions:

- Where do I go from here?
- How can I advance my massage skills?

The answers to these questions will make reference to the recognised areas of study to which national standards and subsequent qualifications have been defined as being advanced techniques.

These chapters do not offer a definitive guide or even a means to acquiring a qualification in each treatment area. What they do offer, however, is an introduction and a means of understanding the origins and procedures and the unique place they have each established within the realms of massage. The result of which is the ultimate realisation that none of these treatments can be effective without the basic knowledge that is the art and science of massage.

14

Mechanical massage

The use of electrotherapy to simulate the effects of manual massage

The introduction of mechanical massage occurred as a direct result of medical developments in the West largely contributing to the fall in the application of manual massage by physicians. The American brothers Dr George Taylor and Dr Charles Taylor were amongst the early pioneers of mechanical massage in the mid-nineteenth century. They and other physicians of their time invented a whole host of machines designed to administer '**mechanical Swedish massage**' as an aid to a variety of medical conditions including those associated with the nervous, digestive, muscular and skeletal systems.

 Angel advice

It may be said that whilst mechanical massage can be used as a substitute for manual massage it will never totally replace the use of the human hand or indeed be equal to the variations and sensitivity of touch administered by the human hand. Nowadays it is common practice to combine the uses of both mechanical and manual massage.

Many of the original machines developed for the medical profession have been adopted and adapted for the beauty, sports and holistic industries. Their use complements that of manual massage providing the masseur/masseuse with an additional means of massage including:

- Percussion and audio sonic – vibratory massage machines which create a tremulous motion causing rapid movements to and fro.

- Hand-held and free-standing gyratory machines – which create a convolution causing circular movements around a central point.
- Vacuum suction massage machines – which create a vacuum causing a mild suction effect through pressure.

Fascinating Fact

The vibrating chair was an early invention by J. H. Kellog MD in 1883 and variations of this concept are still in use today as salons, spas and health clubs often incorporate updated devices as part of post-treatment relaxation.

Where do I go from here?

Having acquired the fundamental procedures associated with traditional Swedish massage, a natural progression may be to advance these skills to incorporate mechanical massage in order to aid the specific physical problems that individual clients often complain about. This enables a masseur/masseuse to become more commercial and offers the client additional services as well as providing further means of aiding specific and general physical problems. Working with clients on a regular basis using the basic massage techniques often highlights specific problems that may be further aided by the introduction of the advanced skills associated with mechanical massage.

Such problems include:

- Excess fatty deposits associated with weight gain.
- Cellulite, sluggish circulation and fluid retention.
- Muscular tension and associated postural figure faults.

Mechanical massage offers a complementary form of massage that can be adapted to meet the needs of these common problems.

How do I advance my massage skills?

Mechanical massage treatments may be studied alongside Swedish massage, sports massage and/or as part of an electrical and mechanical treatments course for either the face or body which accompanies a traditional beauty therapy qualification (at NVQ level 3 or equivalent) or as part of the rising trend in spa treatments.

Angel advice

Many clients feel embarrassed by the thought of manual massage, preferring to be treated with a less personal form of treatment i.e. mechanical machine.

Tip

If studying mechanical treatments as part of an electrical treatments course additional training is offered in the use of **electrical muscle stimulation (EMS)**, **galvanic**, **high frequency** and **micro current** treatments for the body and/or face.

Vibratory massage machines

Percussion vibrator

- **Use** – portable hand-held machine for use primarily on the face, neck and shoulder area.
- **Effects** – 'tapping' the skin simulating traditional **tapotement** massage movements.
- **Products** – may be used with or without a massage medium.
- **Variations** – different applicator heads may be used. The rate of tapping is in the region of 100 taps per second and the intensity of each tap may be altered enabling the practitioner to vary the depth and length of treatment to suit the needs of the client i.e. 5–15 minutes.

Tip

It can be difficult to maintain manual tapotement movements for any length of time so the introduction of the percussion machine is a useful aid.

- **Benefits** – stimulates circulation to the skeleton/muscular and integumentary systems improving muscle and skin tone.
- **Precautions** – avoid overuse.

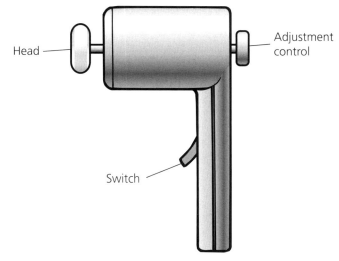

Percussion vibrator

Audio sonic vibrator

- **Use** – portable hand-held machine used primarily on the face, neck and shoulders but may also be used on any localised areas of tension.
- **Effects** – an electromagnet produces sound waves which create a compression and decompression of the tissue when applied to the skin's surface. The vibrations penetrate the tissue having a stimulating effect on the deep tissue and a gentler effect on the surface tissue.

Fascinating Fact

Audio refers to *sound* and **sonic** refers to the production of *soundwaves*. The audio sonic machine therefore produces a vibration that can be both *heard* (humming) and *felt*.

- **Products** – may be used with or without a massage medium.
- **Variations** – the machine may be applied directly onto the surface of the skin for a deep effect or alternatively applied over the practitioner's hand for more surface stimulation. Flat or rounded applicator heads may be used for different areas.
- **Benefits** – stimulates deep tissue easing tension in the muscles and joints. Has a gently stimulating effect on the surface tissue.
- **Precautions** – avoid bony areas and overuse.

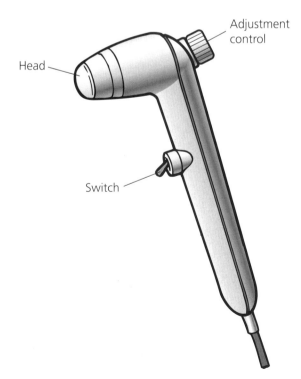

Audio sonic vibrator

Gyratory massage machines

Brush cleanse

- **Use** – motorised hand-held applicator for use primarily on the face, décolletage and upper back.
- **Effects** – a choice of applicator attachments are used that are able to rotate in a clockwise or anti-clockwise direction. This has the effect of deep cleansing, aiding desquamation and encouraging the absorption of nourishing products into the skin.
- **Products** – cleansers, massage creams/emulsions, oils and gels may be used depending on the treatment plan.
- **Variations** – speed, direction of rotation, length of treatment and applicators may be altered for use on

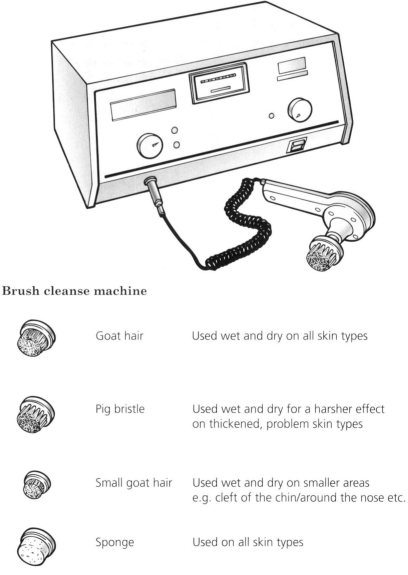

Brush cleanse machine

	Goat hair	Used wet and dry on all skin types
	Pig bristle	Used wet and dry for a harsher effect on thickened, problem skin types
	Small goat hair	Used wet and dry on smaller areas e.g. cleft of the chin/around the nose etc.
	Sponge	Used on all skin types

Brush cleanse applicators

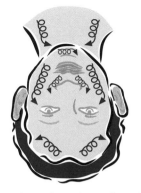

Upwards on the neck

Upwards on the face

Around the nose and chin

Across the forehead

Direction of application – brush cleanse

different areas and skin types depending on the treatment plan. Brush and sponge applicator heads may be used wet for a gentler effect and/or dry for a harsher effect.

- **Benefits** – provides an alternative method of skin care for nervous clients. It is also particularly beneficial for male clients and all clients with a congested and oily skin type. Brush cleanse may also be used on the back.

- **Precautions** – avoid use on excessively loose skin and do not overuse on any skin type.

Hand-held and free-standing gyratory machines

- **Use** – heavyweight machines that are primarily used on the bulky areas of the body including the legs, buttocks etc.

- **Effects** – a rotary electric motor turns a crank which creates gyratory movements which simulate effleurage, petrissage, friction and tapotement/percussion massage movements.

- **Products** – powder is traditionally used for the application of gyratory machines to the body although creams/emulsion and oils may also be used.

- **Variations** – in order to simulate the variations of effleurage, petrissage, friction and tapotement/percussion massage, different applicator heads may be used with varying speeds and length of treatment time.

Tip

Some practitioners advocate the use of protective disposable covers for the applicator attachments which are changed for each client. Thorough cleansing and sanitising of the attachments is essential after each use if this practice is not adhered to.

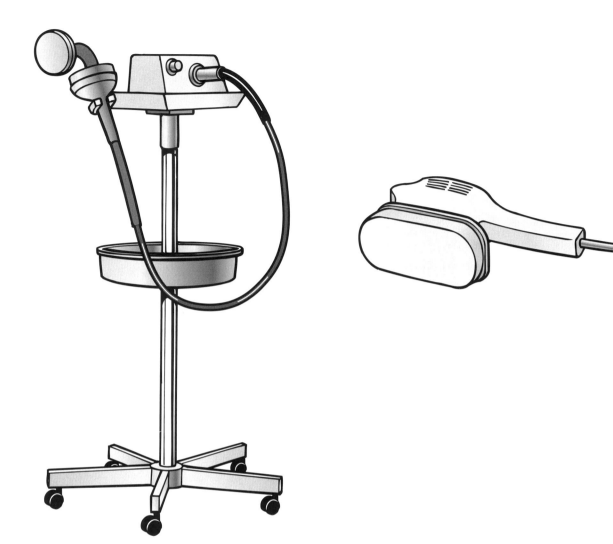

Hand-held and free-standing gyratory machines

🖇️ **Tip**

Gyratory massage is ideally combined with manual massage to enhance the effects. The amount of manual massage may vary depending on the needs of the client.

Name of attachment	Illustration	Use and effect
'Eggbox' applicator		used on bulky muscular areas and fatty tissue such as the gluteals and the thighs
'Spiky' applicator		used generally over the body to stimulate the nerve endings
Smooth applicator		used for effleurage and petrissage effects

Applicators for hand-held machine

Name of attachment	Illustration	Use and effect
Round smooth rubber applicator	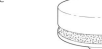	client who has sensitive skin which may be irritated by sponge; used for effleurage and petrissage effects
Round smooth water massage head		warm or cold water creates a stimulating/invigorating or relaxing effect; used for effleurage and petrissage effects
Round sponge applicator		used on the trunk to induce relaxation at the start and end of massage of the treatment part used for effleurage effect
Curved sponge applicator		used on the arms and legs to induce relaxation at the start and end of massage of the treatment part; used for effleurage effect
'Eggbox' rubber applicator		used on bulky muscular areas and fatty tissue such as the gluteals and thighs; used for petrissage effect
'Pronged' rubber applicator		used on bulky muscular areas and fatty tissue such as the gluteals and thighs; used for petrissage effect
'Football' rubber applicator		used on loose flabby areas of the skin such as the abdominal walls; also used over the colon to promote peristalsis; used for petrissage effect
'Spiky' rubber applicator		used generally over the body to stimulate the nerve endings and create a rapid hyparemia; improves a dry skin condition by removing surface dead skin cells; used for percussion effect
'Lighthouse' rubber applicator		used to treat tension nodules on the upper trapezius and may be used either side of the spine and around the knee; used for friction effect

Applicators for free-standing machine

- **Benefits** – ideal for use on clients who are nervous and/or dislike excessive manual massage. A strong, firm effect can be achieved increasing the depth of pressure that can be applied manually which is of benefit to spot reduction in cases of localised fatty deposits aiding in the treatment of cellulite.
- **Precautions** – heavy and prolonged use may cause bruising and damage to surface capillaries. Avoid areas of the body that are excessively hairy as the treatment may cause discomfort. Direction of use should always follow venous blood flow and the lymph nodes to aid circulation.

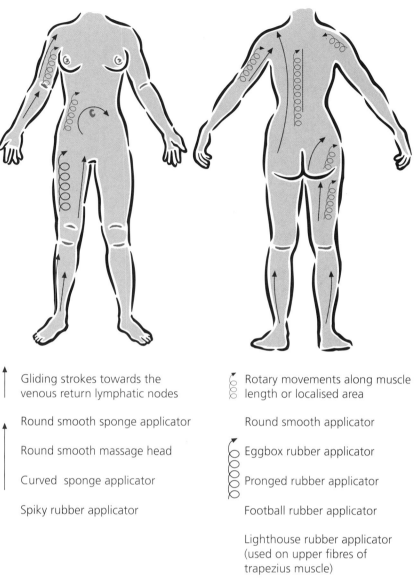

↑ Gliding strokes towards the venous return lymphatic nodes	Rotary movements along muscle length or localised area
Round smooth sponge applicator	Round smooth applicator
Round smooth massage head	Eggbox rubber applicator
Curved sponge applicator	Pronged rubber applicator
Spiky rubber applicator	Football rubber applicator
	Lighthouse rubber applicator (used on upper fibres of trapezius muscle)

Direction of application

Vacuum suction massage machines

Vacuum suction machine

- **Use** – a mechanical treatment incorporating the use of external suction that may be applied to the face and body.
- **Effects** – suction may be continuous, intermittent, static and gliding; all of which have the effect of lifting and releasing the tissue in a simulation of petrissage massage movements.
- **Products** – oils are more commonly used for vacuum suction but creams/emulsions are equally effective in providing the necessary slip.

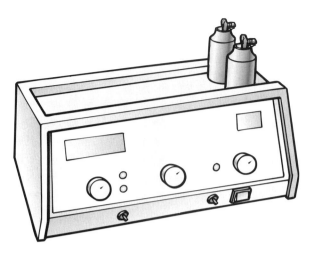

Facial/body vacuum suction machine

- **Variations** – applicators in the form of glass or plastic cups of varying sizes are used for the body and smaller cups and ventouse are used for the face. The type and amount of suction can be varied as can the length of treatment.
- **Benefits** – vacuum suction offers all of the benefits of manual petrissage with the added benefits of being able to treat localised areas of fatty deposits, cellulite and non-medical swelling and puffiness associated with fluid retention extremely effectively.
- **Precautions** – avoid areas of excessively loose and hairy skin. Avoid overuse and excessive amounts of suction which could lead to bruising and damage to surface capillaries.

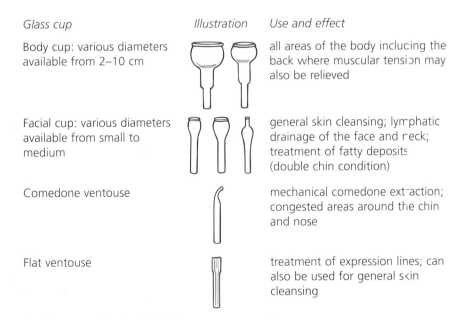

Glass cup	Illustration	Use and effect
Body cup: various diameters available from 2–10 cm		all areas of the body including the back where muscular tension may also be relieved
Facial cup: various diameters available from small to medium		general skin cleansing; lymphatic drainage of the face and neck; treatment of fatty deposits (double chin condition)
Comedone ventouse		mechanical comedone extraction; congested areas around the chin and nose
Flat ventouse		treatment of expression lines; can also be used for general skin cleansing

Applicators for facial/body vacuum suction

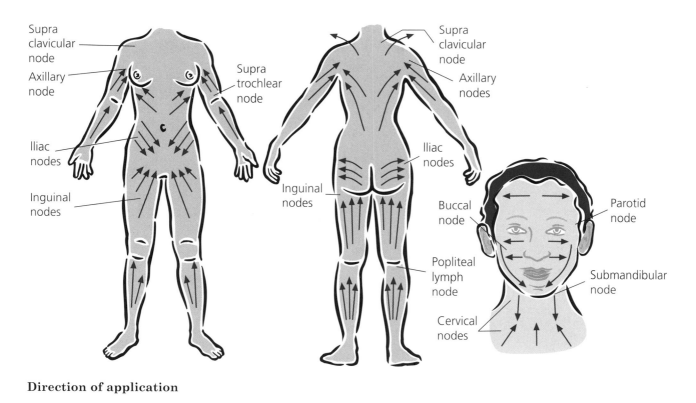

Direction of application

Pre-heat treatments

It is common practice to include the use of pre-heat treatments in association with mechanical massage treatments including:

- **Infra red/radiant heat lamp** – localised application of electromagnetic rays to heat the area in preparation for massage. This has a relaxing effect on the whole body and a soothing effect on the localised surface and deep tissue making the application of massage potentially more effective.

- **Steam** – localised application of wet heat in the form of hand-held and free-standing steamers and/or general application in the form of steam baths and steam rooms. Steam has the effect of raising the body temperature, inducing sweating thus cleansing the body, as well as making the underlying tissue more receptive to manual and/or mechanical massage.

- **Sauna** – general exposure to dry heat within a pine wood cabin that is heated by an electric stove. The humidity is very low but can be increased with the introduction of water which is poured over the stones that are placed on top of the stove. The heat of the sauna which ranges from between 50–120° Centigrade brings about a general rise in body temperature which stimulates circulation, heart rate and cell metabolism. Sweating is induced which has a detoxifying effect on the body. The heat encourages relaxation, surface and deep tissue is warmed, nerve endings are soothed and pain and stiffness relieved making it a useful preparatory treatment for mechanical and/or manual massage.

- **Spa** – baths or pools that incorporate jets of water and air. The jets of water act as a form of water massage exerting pressure on localised areas of the body. The air jets form bubbles which perform gentle massage on the surface of the skin. The temperature of the water may be varied but is generally kept warm in order to induce the benefits associated with the application of heat pre-massage.

- **Heat inducing products e.g. paraffin wax** – localised application of warm liquefied paraffin wax is ideal for easing stiff joints prior to the application of manual or mechanical massage.

All mechanical massage and heat producing/inducing machines and products can only be used on clients when all relevant theoretical and practical training has been undertaken, a recognised qualification achieved and appropriate insurance obtained. Manufacturers' guidelines should also be adhered to at all times to ensure safe and effective treatments that are suitable for the agreed treatment plan.

Activity

Book a mechanical massage at a local salon, health club or college and compare the treatment with that of a purely manual massage treatment. Try to have a full range of mechanical treatments as well as a range of pre-heat treatments to understand the physical, physiological and psychological effects and benefits from a personal point of view.

Task

Use your growing theoretical and practical knowledge to produce an information sheet for your clients and/or employer (if they are unaware of the treatments). Use this exercise as a marketing tool to see if your clients would be interested in you adding such services to your treatment list. This will help to direct you onto the appropriate pathway in terms of possible career progression.

Treatment tracker

MECHANICAL MASSAGE

Tools

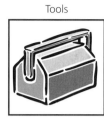

Vibratory massage machines

- Percussion producing superficial 'tapping' movements.
- Audio sonic producing sound waves that compress and decompress the deeper tissue.

Gyratory massage machines

- Hand-held and free-standing heavy weight machines that produce a variety of massage movements ideally suited to the bulky areas of the body.

Vacuum suction massage machines

- Facial vacuum suction aiding skin problems associated with poor circulation e.g. congested oily skin types.
- Body vacuum suction aiding the treatment of fatty deposits and cellulite.

Indications for treatment

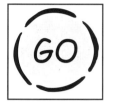

- Excess fatty deposits associated with weight gain. Gyratory and vacuum suction machines are very effective in the 'breaking down' and softening of fatty deposits so they are more easily absorbed as energy as part of a reduced calorie diet.
- Cellulite, sluggish circulation and fluid retention. Vacuum suction and gyratory machines offer a means of stimulating the circulation with the emphasis on lymphatic drainage and detoxification.
- Muscular tension and associated postural figure faults. All mechanical machines aid in the breakdown and removal of tension in the muscles and joints helping to reduce aches and pains and improve joint mobility.

Contraindications

Contraindications to Swedish massage also apply to mechanical massage including:

- Undiagnosed pain or swelling.
- Skin diseases and disorders.
- Broken, inflamed and/or itchy skin.
- Hypersensitive skin i.e. skin that reacts adversely to pressure and stimulation.
- Excessively hairy skin.
- Excessively loose skin.
- Bony areas.
- Varicose veins.

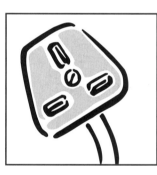

- Preparation of treatment area and checking of machines.
- Conduct a full consultation.
- Agree a treatment plan with the client.
- Removal of appropriate clothing.
- Positioning on couch to ensure comfort of client and practitioner.
- Application of cleansing and/or pre-massage heat treatments as necessary.
- Application of preferred choice of massage medium.
- Application of treatment in combination with manual massage as appropriate.
- Removal of massage medium.
- Treatment of whole body or the part in accordance with treatment plan and commercially accepted timings.

- Erythema – reddening of the area due to surface stimulation.
- Bruising caused by a treatment that is too firm, too lengthy or used incorrectly i.e. wrong applicator attachment and/or wrong setting.
- Damage to surface capillaries due to excess stimulation to the skin.
- Skin drag, irritation and scratching caused by incorrect choice of treatment, contraindicated client and/or excessive use.

- Drink plenty of water to aid the removal of toxins and increase kidney function.
- Exercise routines to complement the effects of the mechanical massage.
- Dietary advice in terms of maintaining healthy eating.
- Home care products including cleansers, exfoliators, toners, moisturisers and remedial products.
- The need for regular treatments depending on the individual treatment plan.

Preparation

Contra actions

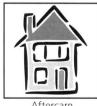

Aftercare

Knowledge review

1   What did the American brothers Dr George and Dr Charles Taylor invent in the 1800s?

2   Which types of mechanical massage machines produce a tremulous motion?

3   Which types of mechanical massage machines produce a convolution?

4   What type of manual massage movement does a percussion machine simulate?

5   Which mechanical massage machine produces sound waves?

6   Do sound waves have a greater stimulating effect on deep or superficial tissue?

7   Which mechanical massage machine may be used for skin cleansing?

8   Which type of mechanical massage machines offers a more heavyweight treatment of bulky areas of the body?

9   Which type of manual massage movements do the vacuum suction machines simulate?

10   What possible contra actions could accompany the excessive and overuse of mechanical massage machines?

11   Which types of heat treatments administer wet heat?

12   Which types of heat treatments administer dry heat?

13   What type of wood is a sauna traditionally made from?

14   Which type of heat treatment is associated with low humidity?

15   What does humidity refer to?

16   Which type of heat treatment incorporates water massage?

17   What effect does heat have upon the circulation?

18   When should heat treatments be used: before or after massage?

19   Give an example of a heat-inducing product.

20   What must be obtained prior to treating clients with mechanical and heat treatments?

Advanced massage

These are massage techniques that offer enhanced effects and benefits to those achieved with the basic techniques associated with traditional Swedish massage. Experience of massage through the centuries has brought about a set of practical techniques that draw from all cultures and beliefs throughout history. The result is a wide range of soft and deep tissue manipulations that provide a natural extension of the basic massage skills. These so-called advanced techniques are still primarily intuitive and instinctive although a detailed knowledge of anatomy and physiology is required in order to perform them with the intelligence needed to be effective. In addition, a working knowledge of the traditional Eastern beliefs associated with the flow of energy which they refer to as being the 'life force' enables greater understanding of the spiritual effects and benefits of advanced massage techniques. The history of massage helps us to appreciate the origins of these techniques, which take their influences from both Western and Eastern developments.

- Western influences developed healing systems of massage based on research associated with physical and psychological science and the subsequent knowledge of anatomy and physiology of the human being. Swedish massage, mechanical massage, sports and remedial massage developed as a direct result of this research.

- Eastern influences developed healing systems of massage based on more spiritual experiences and the idea that each person is linked to everything around them by the flow of energy or life force. Acupressure, acupuncture and shiatsu etc. developed as a direct result of such thinking.

Where do I go from here?

Advanced massage techniques involve the potential for the integration of both Western and Eastern influences to produce a greater involvement in the art and science of massage and therefore require a greater level of commitment between the giver and the receiver at all levels.

- The masseur/masseuse needs to be able to analyse and understand the needs of the client in order to adapt their use of all massage techniques to aid specific problems.
- The client needs to be able to put their total trust in the masseur/masseuse in order gain maximum benefit from the application of appropriate massage techniques for physical, psychological and spiritual benefit i.e. treatment of the whole person – body, mind and spirit.

Advanced massage skills provide a natural route of progression for many masseurs/masseuses who want to be able to extend their basic skills. The progression into advanced techniques may take place during and/or immediately after a Swedish massage course. More often however, a masseur/masseuse needs to gain experience with the basic skills first until they achieve a level of competency and confidence that enables them to work intuitively before extending their skills further.

How do I advance my massage skills?

Many training centres offer qualified masseurs/masseuses one-day or weekend courses in specific advanced techniques which provide an initial insight into the skill with some practical application. This provides a good introduction to the associated advanced skills as well as an ideal means to refresh basic skills as part of ongoing professional development. Alternatively, more detailed training may be undertaken in advanced massage techniques generally as well as in specific areas of study – Shiatsu, Bowen technique, Rolfing and Hellerwork etc.

The general skills associated with advanced massage include:

- **Palpation** – a means to identify changes in the structure of the soft tissue i.e. skin and muscles.
- **Deep tissue work** – a means of understanding and working with the structural layers that make up the body to improve and maintain general function.
- **Relaxation** – the use of Swedish massage and breathing techniques to improve physical, psychological and spiritual well-being at the beginning, during and at the close of a treatment.

Task

Breathing techniques form a large part of activities such as body building, yoga, Tai Chi, dance etc. Research one of these techniques with the emphasis on the effects of breathing on the ability to perform to the optimum level. Think about how this information will help in the application of advanced massage techniques as well as provide clients with effective aftercare advice.

The specific skills associated with advanced massage include:

- **Deep effleurage** – the use of deep stroking movements to help to break down adhesions and stretch and realign muscles.

- **Lymphatic drainage** – the use of massage to simulate the action of the skeletal muscles to provide a pumping action moving the lymph from the cells towards the nodes for filtering.

- **Neuromuscular technique** – the use of pressure applied to local areas of muscular tension, stimulating the release of endorphins which has the effect of suppressing the associated pain and thus releasing tension.

- **Acupressure** – the use of pressure applied to key points on the surface of the skin to stimulate the natural healing mechanisms of the body.

- **Stretching and strengthening** – the use of assisted passive exercises and soft tissue release to rebalance muscles.

- **Balancing** – a means of working with the body's natural life force to encourage homeostasis.

Deep effleurage

Effleurage movements are applied with smaller strokes and deeper pressure. Deep effleurage may be applied both longitudinally and/or transversely.

- Longitudinal deep effleurage aims to stimulate local circulation and stretch muscle fibres helping to realign them.
- Transverse deep effleurage aims to stimulate local circulation and break down adhesions in the muscle fibres.

Deep effleurage may be performed with the palmar surface of the hands, wrists, fists, forearms and elbows, depending on the areas being worked and the amount of pressure indicated.

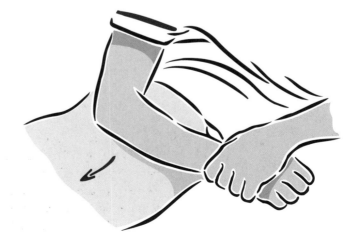

Deep effleurage

Lymphatic drainage

Adaptations of massage techniques specifically to aid lymphatic drainage were developed in France in the 1930s. Until that point it had been well documented that massage increased circulation generally and that directing the pressure of the massage movements towards the heart had a direct effect on both venous blood and flow of lymph. However, massage had not previously been used to create a direct effect on the flow of lymph and the treatment of oedema associated with static lymph and fluid retention in the tissues.

Lymphatic circulation is a one-way system that relies on the movement of the skeletal muscles to stimulate the flow of lymph through the lymphatic vessels. When muscles experience tension and fatigue they not only accumulate more waste but also become less effective in moving the lymph through its vessels. This has the knock-on effect of slowing down the removal of waste and lowering immunity, resulting in fluid retention and swelling (oedema) as well as congestion and problem skin conditions e.g. cellulite, acne etc.

Specific techniques include the application of pressure using the palmar surfaces of the hands in the direction of the lymph nodes to *pump, push, scoop* and *drain.*

- *Pumping* involves the application of intermittent pressure over an area.
- *Pushing* involves circular movements applied with the pressure on the upward curve of the circle.
- *Scooping* involves lifting movements to bulky tissue with the pressure applied to the upward motion.
- *Draining* involves effleurage stroking movements towards the lymph nodes.

Angel advice

Pumping, pushing and *scooping* movements all have the effect of freeing static lymph whilst *draining* movements help to smooth the area, ridding it of congestion.

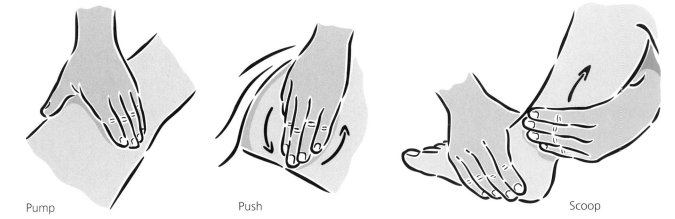

Pump   Push   Scoop

Lymphatic drainage

Neuromuscular technique

Neuromuscular technique works on the basis of the flow of electrical impulses through the nervous system and the principles of dermatomes.

Dermatomes are segmented regions of the body, each of which are supplied with a spinal or cranial nerve as part of the peripheral nervous system linking the body with the central nervous system (spinal cord and brain) and vice versa.

When a muscle has experienced any sort of trauma a natural reflex action increases the tension around the damage as a form of protection against further damage. The muscle may eventually become used to this level of tension and the body begins to view it as being normal. Repetitive strain and postural problems often occur as a result as the muscles find it difficult to return to their former state.

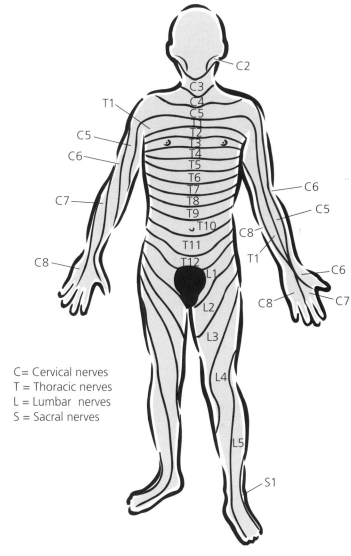

C = Cervical nerves
T = Thoracic nerves
L = Lumbar nerves
S = Sacral nerves

Dermatomes

Tip

Breathing techniques should be encouraged with the use of neuromuscular technique, encouraging the client to take a deep breath in followed by a deep breath out. The application of pressure may be increased with the outward breath when the body experiences greater relaxation.

Neuromuscular technique focuses the application of pressure on the area of tension, which will feel tight and tender to touch. As deep pressure is applied, it will induce pain. The natural reaction of the body is to move away from the pain, but if a client is encouraged to resist this urge and relax into the pain it will gradually ease. In addition to this, endorphins are released which have the effect of suppressing the pain and tension is released. As this occurs it is possible to reverse the reflex action and return muscles to their natural state.

The application of pressure associated with neuromuscular technique should be applied only after the area has been adequately prepared with effleurage, petrissage etc. Pressure may be applied for as little as a few seconds increasing to up to a few minutes.

Neuromuscular technique may be applied with the thumbs, fingers, knuckles and elbows. Thumbs and fingers may be reinforced for greater pressure.

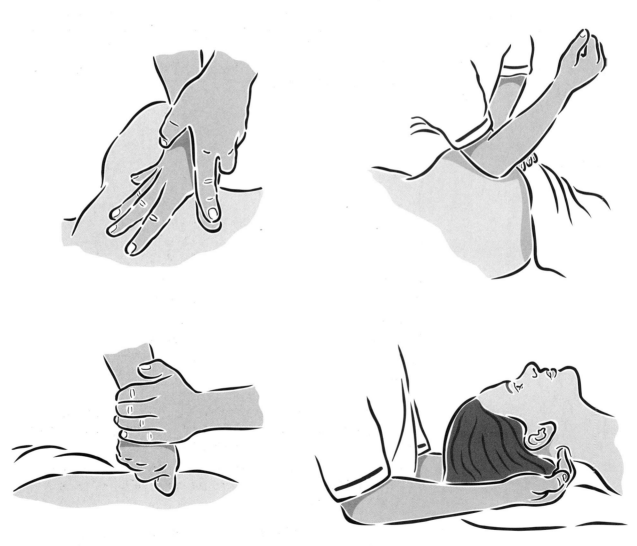

Neuromuscular technique – thumbs, elbows, knuckles and fingers

Acupressure

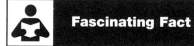

Fascinating Fact

Acupuncture developed from *acupressure* as a means of applying intense and accurate pressure with fine needles to key points of the body. The key points are the same as those used for manual acupressure.

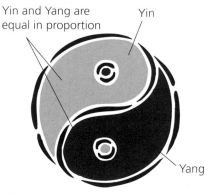

Yin and Yang are equal in proportion

Yin

Yang

Yin and Yang

Acupressure developed from the ancient Chinese art of healing and forms a large part of traditional Chinese medicine. It literally means the application of *intense* and *accurate* pressure. Different styles and interpretations of acupressure have evolved over the years, the most popular being Shiatsu. The Japanese adopted and subsequently adapted the ancient Chinese skills to form their unique version. Shiatsu literally means 'finger pressure' (although, thumbs, knuckles, elbows etc. are also used as the 'fingers') and is often referred to as being 'acupuncture without needles'.

The differences in styles and interpretations of acupressure are largely associated with the application of pressure e.g. Shiatsu involves firm pressure being applied to a point for three to five seconds. Another variation known as Jin Shin advocates the use of gentle pressure held on a point for up to one minute.

All forms of acupressure work on the Yin and Yang principal and associated energy flow. Yin and Yang may be described as being the basis of all life and form the principals on which traditional Chinese medicine is based. They are opposite forces yet are complementary and interdependent and also form a part of one another. Inside Yin there is some Ying and vice versa.

According to traditional Chinese medicine yin and yang form the following characteristics:

Yin	Yang
Water	Fire
Night	Day
Still	Activity
Cold	Heat
Soft	Hard
Slow	Quick
Quiet	Loud
Internal	External
Yielding	Resisting
Female	Male
Psychological	Physical
Front	Back
Lower	Upper

Yin and Yang are opposite energies that form one with Yin providing the calm and Yang providing the stimulation: when the body is in full health they balance perfectly.

The energy they produce is referred to as '**chi**' or 'Qi' by the Chinese and '**ki**' by the Japanese and is classified as being *congenital* and *acquired*:

- Congenital chi – the inherited life force of a person.
- Acquired chi – the air we breathe and the food we eat etc.

Chi is closely linked to the blood. Both blood and chi are vital substances providing the body with nourishment and protection.

Whilst blood flows through vessels in the form of arteries and veins, chi flows through corresponding vessels or channels called *meridians*. Meridians form a connection between the internal organs and the exterior surface of the body. Networks of fine linking channels connect the meridians to one another forming the link between the body systems. There are twelve main meridians and two extra meridians that are divided into six Yin meridians and six Yang meridians, each associated with and taking its name from individual organs or body systems including:

- **Yin meridians** – heart, liver, spleen, lungs, kidney and pericardium (circulation).
- **Yang meridians** – small intestine, gall bladder, stomach, large intestine, bladder and triple heater (temperature regulation).

The two extra meridians are known as *Du* and *Ren*:

- **Du** runs along the posterior midline and governs the Yang meridians. For this reason it is also known as the *governing vessel*.
- **Ren** runs along the anterior midline and monitors, regulates and directs the Yin meridians. It is also known as the *conception vessel*.

The meridians form a continuous network of vessels through which chi flows in a twenty-four hour cycle with two hourly surges during which time one meridian and its associated organs will be stimulated and its opposing meridian and associated organs will be calmed.

The flow of chi may be disturbed and even blocked by the effects of stress and illness resulting in imbalance between Yin and Yang which will cause specific symptoms within the body e.g.

- Symptoms associated with imbalance in the Yang organs include inflammation, heat, redness, pain and swelling etc.
- Symptoms associated with imbalance in the Yin organs include water retention, weight gain, heightened emotions, reduction of movement etc.

Tip

General massage movements applied against this energy flow will produce a calming effect whilst applying massage with the flow will serve to stimulate energy flow.

Fascinating Fact

People who are **Yin** dominant tend to be overweight, pale skinned with a slow metabolism and poor circulation. They are quiet, slow moving and complain of the cold. People who are **Yang** dominant tend to have a build up of muscular tension, have a stimulated complexion, are loud and often aggressive and have a tendency to hyperactivity.

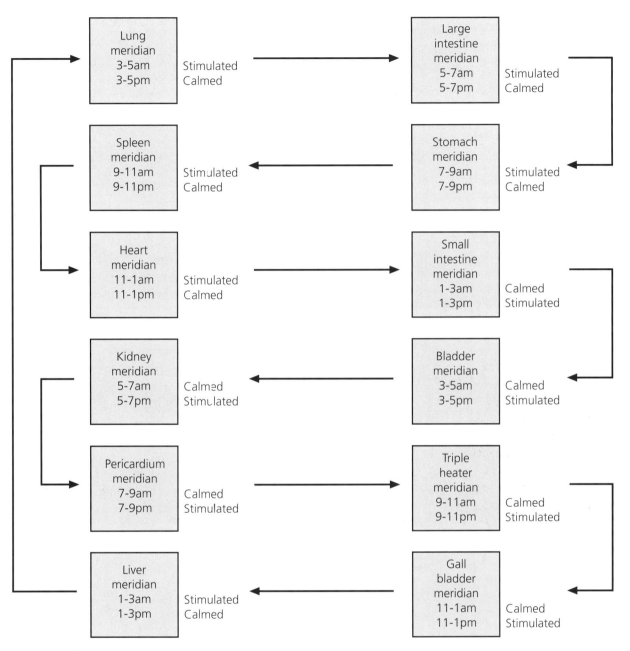

Flow of chi through the meridians

Remember

Pressure applied to the body will also have an affect on the blood circulation.

As a result, Yang organs need calming and Yin organs need stimulating in order to rebalance the body. All forms of acupressure use the application of pressure to key points along the meridians to release blocked energy and restore free flow. This has the effect of activating the body's natural healing mechanisms in order to restore natural homeostasis. Acupressure therefore aims to restore the body to a natural state of balance (homeostasis) by balancing Yin and Yang to ensure free flow of energy.

The key points are believed to be small holes in the meridians and are known as *acupoints* or *potent* points of which there are some 365 located at various points along the meridians. They are found along body landmarks, e.g. eyebrows, hairline etc., within indentations in bones and muscular fibres or knots of tension and may be felt as very slight depressions in the tissue. Sometimes they may be identified simply because they feel 'different' and so require sensitive palpation in order to locate them.

Fascinating Fact

Ayurvedic massage also works on the principal of energy flow (*prana*) and the existence of 107 special pressure points or *marmas*.

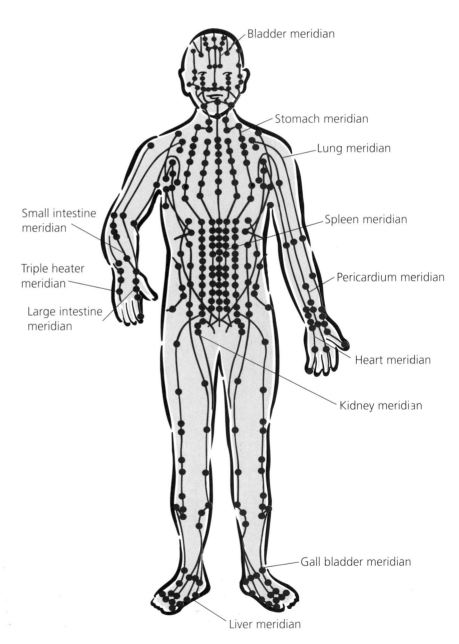

Bladder meridian
Stomach meridian
Lung meridian
Small intestine meridian
Spleen meridian
Triple heater meridian
Pericardium meridian
Large intestine meridian
Heart meridian
Kidney meridian
Gall bladder meridian
Liver meridian

Meridians and acupoints

Acupoints may be further classified as being *local, trigger* and *tonic* points.

- **Local points** – refer to areas where pain or tension is felt when pressure is applied to the point. These points are also known as *ashi* points.
- **Trigger points** – refer to areas which 'trigger' an associated point elsewhere in the body when pressure is applied to the point.
- **Tonic points** – refer to specific areas which stimulate health and well-being when pressure is applied to the point.

The treatment of *local points* may be likened to that which is associated with neuromuscular technique and works on the same principal as the reflex effect.

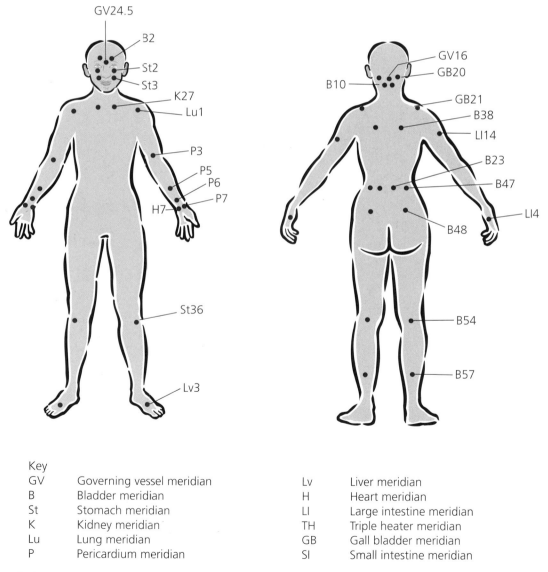

Key			
GV	Governing vessel meridian	Lv	Liver meridian
B	Bladder meridian	H	Heart meridian
St	Stomach meridian	LI	Large intestine meridian
K	Kidney meridian	TH	Triple heater meridian
Lu	Lung meridian	GB	Gall bladder meridian
P	Pericardium meridian	SI	Small intestine meridian

Acupressure points

The treatment of *trigger points* relates specifically to the meridian system and energy flow with the application of pressure focused on key points which in turn trigger an effect in the corresponding organ/body system.

The treatment of *tonic points* relates to specific acupressure points that have been found to strengthen the functions of the associated body systems helping to maintain homeostasis.

Pressure is applied using the thumbs or fingers although knuckles and elbows may also be used. The application of slow pressure creates a deeply relaxing effect whereas pressure applied quickly and intermittently creates a more stimulating effect. Light pressure has a toning effect with deeper pressure producing a sedative effect.

Acupressure points

Each acupoint was originally described by the use of a Chinese character, an identification number relating to the associated meridian, its location described in measurements and/or anatomical position and its associated effects and benefits and cautions for use listed.

The diagram highlights some of the acupoints including:

Third Eye point, **GV 24.5** – directly between the eyebrows – stimulates immune function and calms the spirit.

Drilling bamboo, **B 2** – either side of the eye sockets where the bridge of the nose meets the ridge of the eyebrows — clears the head and sinuses and brightens the eyes.

Four whites, **St 2** – one finger width below the lower ridge of the eye socket in line with the centre of the iris in the indentation of the cheek – clears and relaxes the eyes and face.

Facial beauty, **St 3** – at the base of the zygomatic bone directly below the pupil – clears the sinuses and face.

Elegant mansion, **K 27** – in the hollow below the clavicle bone either side of the sternum – benefits the lungs, throat and kidneys.

Letting go, **Lu 1** – outer part of the chest, three finger widths below the clavicle bones – strengthens the lungs and clears the emotions.

Crooked marsh, **P 3** – on the inside of the arm at the lower end of the elbow in the crease – regulates the heart and balances the emotions.

Intermediary, **P 5** – four finger widths above the centre of the inner wrist crease – balances the internal organs and calms the spirit.

Inner gate, **P 6** – in the centre of the forearm one-and-a-half finger widths from the wrist – balances the internal organs and calms the spirit.

Big mound, **P 7** – in the middle of the inside crease of the wrist – regulates the stomach.

Spirit gate, **H 7** – on the ulna side of the forearm at the crease of the wrist – regulates the heart and strengthens the spirit.

Three mile point, **St 36** – four finger widths below the patella towards the outside of the shin – aids digestion and restores the immune system.

Bigger rushing, **Lv 3** – on top of the foot between the first two metatarsal bones – invigorates, transforms and clears the systems.

Wind mansion, **GV 16** – in the occipital cavity – clears the head and the nose.

Gates of consciousness, **GB 20** – just below the base of the occipital bone in the hollow either side of the spine – alleviates head and neck pain.

Heavenly pillar, **B 10** – half an inch below the occipital either side of the spine – opens the sensory organs and relaxes the body.

Shoulder well, **GB 21** – highest point of the shoulder, one to two inches from the sides of the neck – eases muscular tension.

Vital diaphragm, **B 38** – between the scapulae bones and spine at the level of the heart – calms the emotions and promotes relaxation.

Outer arm bone, **LI 14** – outer surface of the upper arm between the shoulder and the elbow – aids reduction of muscle tension inducing relaxation.

Sea of vitality, **B 23 & B47** – between the second and third lumbar vertebrae, two and four finger widths away from the spine at waist level – strengthens the digestive and genito-urinary organs and stimulates the immune system.

Joining the valley, **LI 4** – in the webbing between the thumb and index finger – clears and balances the digestion system.

Womb and vitals, **B 48** – one to two finger widths on either side of the sacrum – relieves backache.

Commanding middle, **B 54** – in the centre of the back of the knee crease – strengthens the lower back and knees.

Supporting mountain, **B 57** – in the centre of the base of the gastrocnemius muscle – strengthens the lower back and relaxes the legs.

These acupoints offer an introduction and a guide only. Further study is required to locate the remaining acupoints.

Stretching and strengthening

Stretching and strengthening techniques may be classified as:

- Muscle energy techniques (MET)
- Soft tissue release (STR)
- Strain–counter strain (SCS)

Muscle energy techniques

Muscle energy techniques work on imbalance in muscle tone. Neuromuscular problems, i.e. postural faults, result from an imbalance in muscle alignment. Muscles work in pairs or groups to initiate a movement by *reciprocal inhibition*. This involves one muscle (or group) performing the contraction whilst the opposing muscle (or group) relaxes. This is a natural reflex response initiated by the central nervous system. A tight muscle transmits the same message to the central nervous system as a naturally contracting one therefore initiating the reflex response in the opposing muscle. This results in an excessively tight muscle and a corresponding weak muscle.

Muscle energy technique works at stretching the tight muscle (or group) and strengthening the weak muscle (or group).

- Palpation techniques are used to identify areas of tightness.
- The muscle is taken into a passive stretch by moving the associated joint.
- The position is held when a mild stretch is felt.
- To stretch the muscle the client tries to extend the stretch.
- To strengthen the muscle the client tries to resist the stretch.

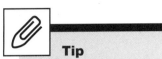

Tip

If a muscle is very tight, it may be too painful to apply massage. If the opposing muscle is contracted the tight muscle will relax and become free to be massaged without undue discomfort.

Soft tissue release

Soft tissue release incorporates stretching to release tension and adhesions within the muscles. It may be used in a sitting or standing position and can be applied through clothes.

- Tension in the muscle is located and the muscle is relaxed and held in a shortened position by moving the associated joint.
- Pressure is applied to the muscle to fix the position.
- Tension is released by stretching the muscle away from the fixed point by moving the joint.

Strain–counter strain

Secondary muscular tension may build up as a result of damage to the muscles. The reflex action of the body causes the muscles surrounding the damage to tighten, acting as a protective function against further damage. This situation also occurs in muscles that are habitually held tight which can have the effect of restricting blood flow and preventing relaxation.

Strain–counter strain techniques work by:

- A passive movement into the direction of the tightness until it is comfortable.
- This position is held for 90 seconds in which time the tension is released from the muscle.
- The muscle is then slowly and passively stretched beyond its previously restricted range.

- This position is held for up to one minute in which time the muscle is able to adapt and the tightness significantly reduced.

Balancing

Balancing involves techniques that have an effect on the energy (chi and blood) that flows through the body linking organs and body systems. This energy also links us with the people around and with the world that surrounds us.

 Angel advice

> A person is not seen as being separate from their surroundings, instead he/she is seen as being a part of it, in relationship with it and influenced by it.

All forms of massage have an effect on energy flow to release, unblock, stimulate and/or calm depending on depth and direction of pressure, speed and adaptation of movements etc. Balancing techniques help to maintain energy free flow by helping to create a more even rhythm and include:

- **Holding** – a gentle placing of hands onto or slightly above an area of the body. Sensitive hands will 'feel' the energy and the position may be held until the energy feels balanced.
- **Breath awareness** – depth of breathing is a natural response to the needs of the body and is controlled by the autonomic nervous system. Stress initiates shallow breathing in order to take in air quickly. Although this is useful in short bursts it is not beneficial in the long term when deeper, slower breathing is needed to counteract the effects of stress. Breath awareness provides a means to enhance the effects of the advanced massage techniques helping to create balance and harmony.
- **Visualisations** – form a means of utilising left brain activity into a mental picture of something that is associated with and/or brings about feelings of pleasure which in turn encourages the deep relaxation needed to allow the body to activate its own healing mechanisms.
- **Affirmations** – form a means of utilising right brain activity with powerful statements that amplify the benefits of the massage. Positive statements of intent, e.g. letting go of emotional strain and tension, have a knock-on effect on physical strain and tension helping to activate the level of relaxation needed for the body to once again activate its own healing mechanisms.

Advance massage techniques require study and practice in order to perfect the skills and fully appreciate the effects and benefits. Advanced massage techniques ultimately become an integral part of every massage treatment without the need to differentiate between styles, interpretations or methods. A masseur/masseuse intuitively alters and adapts their techniques to meet the specific needs of each individual client on each separate occasion.

Activity

Try to experience as many different massage treatments as possible to broaden your knowledge and outlook generally. Look in the Yellow Pages for details of complementary practitioners and when on holiday try to find out about the local massage treatments.

Task

Find out more about the various styles of acupressure by looking on the Internet or at your local library. Make yourself a chart of the acupressure points and practice them on yourself. This will help you to become more familiar with the techniques and ascertain whether or not this is a possible career pathway for you.

Treatment tracker

ADVANCED MASSAGE

Tools

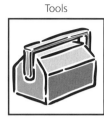

Advanced massage techniques may be performed with the fingers, thumbs, hands knuckles, fists, elbows and forearms in order to apply greater and more specific pressure. Attention should be paid to the care of these 'tools':

- Regular hand and arm exercises.
- Avoid overstraining any one area.
- Try to make use of both hands and arms so as not to overtire one or the other.
- Do not overextend the joints as this will lead to damage.

Remember that your career relies on the health of your 'tools'.

Indications for treatment

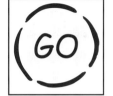

Advanced massage techniques are generally used to aid specific problems associated with:

- Stress – relaxation techniques are used to encourage relaxation.
- Poor circulation – lymphatic drainage movements remove static lymph.
- Muscular imbalance – stretching and strengthening techniques help to rebalance postural muscles.
- Pain – neuromuscular technique and acupressure help to relieve pain and reverse reflex action associated with tight muscles.
- Energy imbalance – acupressure, holding, breath awareness, visualisations and affirmations help to encourage energy free flow.

Advanced massage techniques have the effect of stimulating the body's own healing mechanisms helping to restore homeostasis.

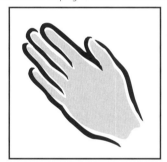

Contraindications

The contraindications that apply to advanced massage are the same as those that apply to all other massage techniques.

Care should be taken to identify contraindications that:

- Restrict treatment – bruising, cuts, abrasions etc.
- Prevent treatment – injury, undiagnosed pain etc.

Special care should be taken in the case of:

- Conditions of the skeletal system e.g. osteoporosis where the use of pressure may be detrimental.
- Circulatory disorders where the skin is prone to bruising.
- Nervous disorders where the skin is particularly sensitive.
- Certain acupoints should be avoided during pregnancy.

- Conduct a full consultation.
- Agree a treatment plan with the client.
- Position of the client and choice of massage medium should be suitable for the proposed treatment and area to be treated.
- Apply Swedish massage movements to prepare the area.
- Apply palpation techniques to identify problem areas.
- Apply specific advanced techniques in combination with Swedish massage as appropriate to the needs of the area.
- Adapt the treatment in terms of choice of massage techniques, depth of pressure, speed of movements etc.

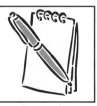

Preparation

Advanced massage techniques may result in the following contra actions (in addition to those associated with Swedish massage) including:

- Muscle soreness as the muscle adapts and begins the healing process.
- Tingling sensation as blood and chi are stimulated.
- Distension or swelling as the healing process is activated.

It is worth noting that if a treatment has no contra actions then it may not have been deep enough or long enough.

It is also worth noting that excessive treatment in terms of depth of pressure and length of treatment may result in fainting as the body shuts itself down.

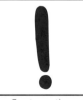

Contra actions

It is important that a person becomes aware of the factors which caused the problem e.g.

- Stress forces a person to hold their body tightly resulting in muscle fatigue.
- Repetitive strain is caused by overuse of body parts resulting in weakness and damage in associated joints, muscles etc.
- Poor posture encourages imbalance in postural muscles.
- Loss of confidence and low self-esteem is accompanied by poor posture.
- Negative thought promotes negative health.

If a person is made aware of the root of the problem they can put in place avoidance techniques which will help to prevent further problems in the future.

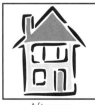

Aftercare

Knowledge review

1   What is palpation?

2   In which directions may deep effleurage be performed?

3   When was lymphatic drainage massage developed in the Western world?

4   What type of pressure is applied during the pumping lymphatic drainage movement?

5   What causes the increased tension around a damaged muscle?

6   What type of pressure is used to apply the neuromuscular technique?

7   What action do endorphins have?

8   Where does acupressure originate from?

9   What is the Japanese form of acupressure known as?

10 Are the following characteristics Yin or Yang – still, cold, soft and female?

11 What is chi?

12 What is acquired chi?

13 What are the channels through which energy flows called?

14 What is the name given to the small holes along the meridians?

15 What do the initials MET stand for?

16 What does soft tissue release help to relieve?

17 What effect does secondary muscle tension have on blood flow?

18 What affect do holding movements have on energy?

19 Which side of the brain is associated with visualisations?

20 Which side of the brain is associated with affirmations?

Sports and remedial massage

This is a combination of Swedish massage and advanced massage techniques in the form of deep tissue massage applied before sport activity to aid performance, between sport activity to enhance performance and/or post-sport activity to aid recovery. All through history, we can find evidence of massage being used to prepare for sporting activities as well as in the treatment of post-sporting problems e.g. the treatment of gladiators and warriors etc. The sports may have changed over the centuries but the need for advanced massage techniques to treat the body pre, during and post sporting activities continues to be necessary for every serious sports person, club or team.

Swedish massage takes its origins from sports culture. Per Ling founded the 'Swedish Movement Cure' in the early nineteenth century. It comprised passive, active and remedial exercise together with massage for both health and well-being. Sport and remedial massage differs from traditional Swedish massage in that it is more specific in its treatment, generally firmer and brisker in its application and performed on clients who are often fitter and healthier than the average client yet suffer greater injuries as a result of their sporting activities. Such clients usually have a greater knowledge and awareness of their own body.

Nowadays as more and more people are partaking in an increasing amount and variety of sporting activities on a professional and amateur basis the need for such massage skills has grown.

Where do I go from here?

Sports and remedial massage provides another possible career pathway for those practitioners qualified in Swedish massage. Sports and remedial massage qualifications provide the means to specialise in an area of massage that is increasingly popular. Sports clubs, leisure centres and health spas are becoming a natural part of today's culture offering ways of increasing physical and mental well-being. The additional use of sport and/or remedial massage enables a practitioner to become more specialised and more adaptable in their use of massage skills. This enables a masseur/masseuse to become more commercial and ultimately more employable and/or more able to offer their services on a freelance basis.

The training and use of sports and remedial massage enhances the basic massage skills providing a challenging and rewarding career route.

How do I advance massage skills?

Having completed a Swedish massage qualification a possible career pathway may lead a practitioner along the sports and leisure route. Various qualifications exist at different levels including:

- **Sports massage** – the treatment of athletes with *massage* pre, post and between sporting activities.
- **Remedial massage** – the treatment of injuries with *massage* pre, post and between sporting activities.
- **Sports therapy** – the treatment of athletes and their associated injuries with *massage* and *exercise* as part of an ongoing training programme.

Sports and remedial massage involves a combination of Swedish massage techniques together with advanced massage techniques and specific remedial skills. Sports therapy takes this a stage further with the added knowledge of exercise for training and remedial treatment.

Sports and remedial massage and sport therapy all involve working with a team of people whose main focus is on the body's ability to perform at the optimum level e.g. athlete, trainer or coach, medical specialist etc. This therefore requires the practitioner to be familiar with the anatomy and physiology of the body, the nature of different sporting activities, common injuries associated with different sports and the psychological and sometimes spiritual factors affecting competitive performance at both amateur and professional levels.

- An amateur sportsperson is likely to have varying levels of interest in their body and the way it performs depending on their sporting commitment.
- A professional sportsperson will have a team of people focusing their attention on all aspects of their performance at all levels at all times.

It is also necessary to have detailed knowledge of how the body reacts to sporting injuries in terms of contra actions, contraindications and indications and frequency of treatment.

Finally, it is of equal importance to be aware of how competing affects a person in terms of success and failure and how the resulting mental attitude affects physical well-being and the possible impact it may have on future performances.

Sports and remedial massage techniques

Swedish massage techniques are frequently used including:

Effleurage

- Superficial stroking may be used to prepare the area and to locate specific problem areas associated with possible strain and injury.
- Deeper stroking may be performed to stimulate local circulation and break down adhesions as well as stretch muscles helping to realign them.

Petrisssage

A combination of kneading, picking up, wringing and rolling are effective in stimulating the circulation to specific bones, muscles and joints. Movements may be reinforced for additional pressure and/or applied with the elbows, clenched fist and/or heel of the hands.

Friction

Circular and/or transverse frictions using thumbs, fingers or elbows may be used with care to break down adhesions and scarring in the muscle fibres.

Tapotement/percussion

A combination of hacking, cupping, pounding and beating effectively stimulates and invigorates the muscles.

Vibrations

- Static and moving vibrations are effective in releasing tension and associated build up of toxins and/or fluid.
- Shaking is useful on sore tight muscles when deeper movements are too painful.

Joint manipulation

Gentle mobilising movements may be performed and/or mobilising exercises used to warm up prior to the event and cool down post event as appropriate.

Remember

Massage itself may be likened to an exercise work out. Effleurage movements prepare the body in terms of warming up. Petrissage and percussion/tapotement movements work the body in terms of improving muscular strength and endurance and effleurage movements offer a way of cooling down the body.

Advanced and specific remedial massage techniques used in sports and remedial massage include:

Lymphatic drainage

Gentle compression and releasing movements using thumbs, fingers and/or hands in pumping, pushing and scooping actions may be used over an area to aid lymphatic drainage. These movements usually accompany superficial and/or deep effleurage movements depending on the area being treated.

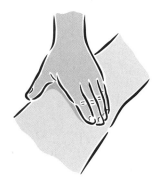

Lymphatic drainage – pump action

Tip

Superficial movements aid drainage of superficial muscles and deeper movements aid in the drainage of deeper muscles.

Neuromuscular technique (NMT)

NMT involves using palpation techniques to feel for underlying muscle stress. General massage techniques are then used to warm and soften the area followed by more palpation techniques to determine the point or points in the muscles where the tissue feels most tense. Pressure is applied using the thumb, fingers, knuckles, heel of hand and/or elbow to just within the client's tolerance levels.

The client may then be asked to take some deep breaths; inhaling through the nose and exhaling through the mouth. The pressure of the movement can be maintained or decreased during inhalation and increased during exhalation as the body relaxes more. This technique is maintained for up to 90 seconds, increasing or decreasing the amount of pressure applied as appropriate.

Tip

If the pressure applied is too great and applied too quickly the muscle will experience a reflex tightening and the client will automatically flinch which will prevent the neuromuscular technique from working.

Tip

A gradual reduction in pain should accompany NMT as endorphins are released and relaxation occurs. If the pain starts to increase, there may be some associated inflammation in which case the technique should be stopped.

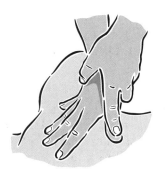

Neuromuscular technique

Muscle energy technique (MET)

MET involves a series of techniques that help to release the strain and tension associated with overworked, tired and imbalanced

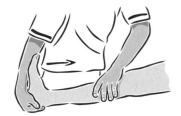

Muscle energy technique

muscles. Palpation techniques are used to identify tightness and/or weakness in the muscles. Assisted stretching movements may then be applied to take the muscles through an extended movement in order to increase elasticity in the muscle. The stretch is held for 5–10 seconds and then extended further and held before being released. Muscle strength is achieved through the application of resistance by the client and held for 5–10 seconds before being released. Breathing deeply will help performance and the stretch or resistance may be increased during the outward breath as the body relaxes.

Soft tissue release (STR)

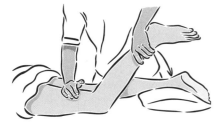

Soft tissue technique

Palpation techniques using static pressure and movement of the underlying tissue to determine the state of the muscle fibres. The muscle is relaxed and held in a shortened position by moving the associated joint. Pressure is applied to the muscle using the thumb, fist, heel or palm of the hand. The joint is then moved so that the muscle is in a stretched position keeping the pressure focused on the same point which may be pulled slightly in the opposite direction. The resulting stretch lengthens the muscle fibres helping to release adhesions.

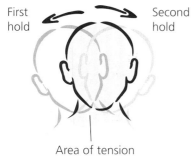

Strain–counter strain

Strain–counter strain (SCS)

SCS may be used when secondary tension builds up around overworked, tired or damaged muscle fibres. The joint is moved in the direction of the tension to shorten the muscle fibres. This has the effect of easing the tension and reducing any pain. The position is held for 90 seconds in which time relaxation occurs in the muscle fibres. The muscle can then be slowly and carefully stretched by moving the associated joint. Again the position is held encouraging the muscle fibres to return to normal.

Connective tissue manipulation (CTM)

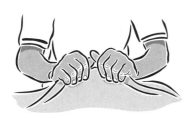

Connective tissue manipulation

CTM may be used to release tension and thickening in the connective tissue that binds the muscle fibres together to form a complete muscle. This technique is applied without the use of a massage medium and is often performed through a towel for extra grip. The skin is gripped above the muscle and a stroke is applied feeling for the underlying tissue. The subcutaneous layer is pulled across the connective tissue of the muscle helping to release tension and adhesions. The skin is released before the next stroke begins. CTM is felt as a scratching sensation in the deeper tissue as friction is produced between the layers.

Sports and remedial massage incorporates the combined use of these massage techniques for the following applications:

Tip

Massage is used between activity in sports such as boxing and wrestling as well as during multiple activity sports e.g. triathlons involving three sports and pentathlons involving five sports.

- **Pre-event massage** – used prior to any sporting activity taking place to prepare the body and mind for the intended sport and to maximise performance.
- **Post-event massage** – used immediately or up to two hours after any sporting activity has taken place to help to return the body back to a normal pre-exercise state.
- **Between-events massage** – used in between activity to help to treat tired, overworked and damaged muscles post-event as well as prepare for further activity.
- **Treatment massage** – corrective massage used in the treatment of sports injuries to encourage more effective and speedier recovery.
- **Training massage** – preventative massage used as part of a training programme to build on strengths and work on weaknesses in order to optimise long-term performance.

Pre-event massage

Pre-event massage occurs before the sporting activity takes place, enhancing the effect of the warm up session. It is used to focus the body and the mind in preparation for the performance of specific physical and mental requirements of a sport. Pre-event massage involves:

Tip

Massage should only be applied pre-event when an athlete is used to massage as part of their training programme. If they are unused to massage treatment, the effects may disturb their natural timing potentially affecting their overall performance.

- The use of a massage medium e.g. oil or cream.
- Massage to the main parts of the body needed for the event.
- Short in duration 5–10 minutes for each area.
- A combination of massage movements e.g. petrissage, tapotement/percussion performed at a brisk rate to stimulate the body into activity.
- Some relaxation movements may be used to help to calm the mind, reduce anxiety and soothe the mental nervous tension associated with competing.

Pre-event massage warms the muscles, stimulates the circulation and energises the mind creating the potential to maximise performance.

Post-event massage

Post-event massage should take place as soon after the event as is practicable to combat the effects on the body. Taking part in most sports results in a certain amount of damage to the muscle which is not always immediately apparent. This is referred to as micro trauma and can result in long term problems if not treated. Post-event treatment can help to identify any micro trauma in the muscles and the massage is then adapted to break down and release the associated tension. Post-event massage involves:

- The use of a massage medium as appropriate to the technique used.
- A combination of massage techniques to relax, stretch and treat the muscles.
- Massage techniques performed at a slower rate in order to work specific areas of muscle fibres.
- Palpation techniques to identify micro trauma.
- Light pressure should be applied at the start of the treatment increasing slowly and rhythmically as relaxation of the muscles is experienced.
- Communication with the client should confirm any pain and discomfort so the treatment can be adapted accordingly.

Post-event massage relaxes the muscles, encouraging them to rest which in turn allows the natural healing mechanisms of the body to become activated. Circulation is stimulated to the area helping to replace toxins with nutrients in order to maximise recovery.

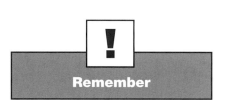

Remember

Pre- and post-event massage do not replace a warm up or a cool down session; they merely enhance their effectiveness.

Between-events massage

Between-events massage occurs when an athlete has a natural break in their sporting activity and should include a combination of both post- and pre-event massage as necessary. This type of sports massage has the potential to prevent excessive damage in tired and overworked muscles, restore efficient muscle use and enhance performance for the next stage of the event.

Treatment massage

Treatment massage is used to correct any problems associated with injury by promoting healing. Immediate action should be taken in the event of a sporting injury and treatment massage is performed post-event only after medical approval has been sought with the emphasis on achieving a complete recovery.

Immediate action involves *rest, ice, compression* and *elevation* – RICE:

- Rest immobilises the area to prevent further injury.
- Ice should be applied to constrict blood flow to the area.

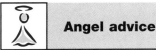

Angel advice

Massage must not be given immediately after injury due to the risk of further damage.

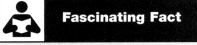

Fascinating Fact

Research has shown that the body recovers from a strenuous workout at a faster rate as a result of having a massage than it does from just resting.

- Compression helps to reduce swelling.
- Elevation aids drainage away from the affected area.

Treatment massage can take place once a medical diagnosis has been made and appropriate post-injury treatment has taken place. In cases of minor injury treatment massage may begin after a minimum of two days. In more severe cases treatment must be postponed until medical approval is given.

In any event, treatment massage begins slowly, tentatively and superficially, gaining in pressure as healing takes place.

Training massage

Training massage is used as a regular treatment to prevent long-term problems and maintain peak condition and thus performance in an athlete. It is similar to post-event massage but the emphasis is on maintenance of the body. Training massage is used to combat the effects of continuous strain on the body as an athlete performs their sport on a regular basis. It may be given after every physical training session to help to identify and relieve micro trauma, ensuring that the body is fully recovered before the next training session takes place. The training massage generally focuses on the most affected areas of the body so the addition of regular full body massage can also help to contribute to the well-being of the athlete. The massage treatment will help to clear the mind as well as the body, helping to instil a positive mental attitude.

Task

Sports and remedial massage is a specialised area of manual treatment requiring a great deal of knowledge and expertise. Research some sporting activities in terms of what is required both physically and mentally of the athlete and the common injuries that occur with each sport. This information will help you to determine if this is a possible career pathway for you to follow.

Activity

Get in touch with a local sports club and offer your services as a masseur/masseuse. This will provide you with the means to gain practical experience in the application of Swedish massage of fit clients as well as gain an insight into the common injuries and problems surrounding that particular sporting activity.

Treatment tracker

SPORTS AND REMEDIAL MASSAGE

Tools

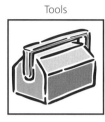

Sports and remedial massage is unlike traditional Swedish massage in that its specific purpose is to accompany a variety of sporting activities.

- The treatment is carried out using the fingers/thumbs, the heel/palm of the hands, the fist, the forearm and/or the elbow.
- The massage usually takes place with the client lying on a couch although between-event massage may take place wherever convenient.
- Mechanical massage machines are sometimes used to complement the post-event treatment.
- Heat treatments are often included as part of the post-event treatment.

Indications for treatment

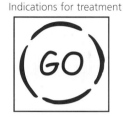

Sports and remedial massage differs from traditional Swedish massage in that the clients are predominantly fit and strong and generally have a greater sense of awareness of their own body. Sports and remedial massage may be used:

- Pre-event as part of the warming up and preparatory process involved with competitive and/or non competitive sports.
- Post-event as part of the cooling down and restorative process.
- Between events to help tired, overworked muscles to prevent excessive damage and to prepare for the next event.
- As part of a corrective programme for the treatment of injuries.
- As part of a preventative programme for ongoing training.

Contraindications

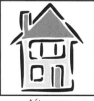

Contraindications to any form of massage are basically the same and require an element of common sense in deciding if the contraindication prevents or restricts the treatment. If in any doubt medical advice should always be sought. In addition:

- Pre-event sports massage should not be performed on a client unused to massage as it may disrupt their performance.
- Post-event massage should not be performed on any injuries for at least two days.
- Serious or suspicious injuries should not be treated without medical diagnosis and guidance.

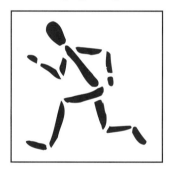

Sports and remedial massage tends to be more of an on-site treatment which may involve anything from a purpose-built treatment room to treating a client in a field. Appropriate care should be taken in the preparation of the treatment area, masseur/masseuse and client regardless of the venue.

- The working area, area to be treated and the hands of the masseurs/masseuses should be cleansed prior to any treatment taking place.
- Palpation techniques are used to locate problem areas.
- Pre-event massage tends to be brisk and fast and short in duration.
- Post-event massage always starts with light pressure until muscles are totally relaxed.

Contra actions to any form of sporting activity may include:

- Pain from tired, overworked and damaged muscles.
- Tension in the muscle fibres making them stiff and inflexible.
- Swelling and inflammation where injury has occurred.
- Weakness, breathlessness and fatigue.

Contra actions to sports massage may include:

- Increased sweating and need to urinate as toxins are released.
- Increased thirst and hunger as the body needs to hydrate and replenish nutrients.
- Reduction in blood pressure and heart rate.
- Exhaustion as the body needs to relax and rest.

Sports and remedial massage forms a useful part of the training of an athlete helping in the preparation, restoration and maintenance of the body before, during and after sporting activity. As a result care and attention should be paid to all aspects of the athletes' lifestyle to ensure that they are able to perform to optimum levels including:

- Diet, ensuring a balanced intake of nutrients and supplements as appropriate.
- Fluid intake to ensure fluid level is maintained before, during and after sporting activity.
- Frequency of massage treatment to ensure strengths are maintained and weaknesses are treated correctly.
- Rest and relaxation to maintain homeostasis.

Preparation

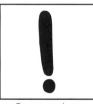

Contra actions

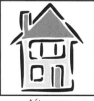

Aftercare

Knowledge review

1   Who developed the Swedish Movement Cure?

2   When is sports massage commonly used?

3   Name three Swedish massage techniques used in sports massage.

4   Which type of sports massage technique incorporates a manual pumping action?

5   Where is excess lymph drained towards and why?

6   Which sports massage technique incorporates the use of increasing pressure applied to a specific point?

7   What technique is used to identify areas in need of sports massage?

8   When using deep breathing to aid sports massage, should pressure be applied with inhalation or exhalation?

9   What does MET stand for?

10   What does stretching help to release in the muscles?

11   What does soft tissue release do to the muscle fibres?

12   What does SCS stand for?

13   What type of tissue binds the muscle fibres together to form a complete muscle?

14   Which type of sports massage is used as part of a corrective programme?

15   Which type of sports massage is used as part of a preventative programme?

16   How many individual sports are involved in a pentathlon?

17   How soon after the event should post massage be performed?

18   What do the initials RICE stand for?

19   Who makes a diagnosis of a sports injury?

20   How soon after a minor injury may treatment massage take place?

Indian head massage

Traditionally practiced by the people of India and passed from parents to children through the generations, Indian head massage involves the manual application of massage movements to the head to relieve the physical, psychological and spiritual effects of stress bringing about a sense of inner peace and tranquillity. It takes its origins from Ayurveda, the ancient medical text that prescribed the use of massage (amongst other things) as a means to encourage, strengthen and maintain the body's well-being and stimulate its own healing powers and mechanisms.

Traditionally, Indian head massage was used as part of a grooming ritual for both men and women.

- Barbers incorporated a stimulating head massage known as 'champi' as part of the grooming treatment for men.

Fascinating Fact

The word shampoo has strong associations with the word *champi*, both involving a form of head massage for grooming purposes.

- Mothers used head massage to stimulate strong and healthy hair growth in their children.

The skills associated with head massage were commonly passed through the generations by barbers to their sons and by mothers to their daughters, with each family and generation adopting their own unique way of performing the massage.

Over recent years the introduction of Indian head massage in the Western world has brought about a great deal of interest in this ancient art enabling masseurs/masseuses to add massage of the head to a treatment that commonly neglected to include this area. What has emerged as a result of this integration is a treatment that may be carried out:

- With or without clothing.
- In a seated or laying down position.
- With or without a massage medium.
- By masseurs/masseuses, beauty and holistic therapists and hairdressers alike.

Massage skills are being adapted to encourage informal almost impromptu treatments as well as more formal, structured treatments. This move has brought about the introduction of more accessible massage treatments which can be carried out with great effectiveness in a variety of situations e.g. in the workplace, on the beach, in flight etc. In addition to this, the introduction of massage to the ears, face, shoulders, neck, upper back and arms has produced a stand alone treatment that is finding its way onto the treatment lists of every salon, spa, clinic and health farm of the world. In whatever form it is applied, Indian head massage provides an extension of the therapeutic value of body massage, helping to eliminate the effects of stress and encourage greater levels of well-being.

What has also evolved from the Ayurvedic paradigm is the integration of *energy balancing*, a technique involving the interaction of energy from within a person and that which flows around the body and forms a part of the universe as a whole. Eastern beliefs generally describe this energy as being the *life force* which flows freely in good health but is blocked in ill health.

Individual Eastern belief systems all tend to agree on the fact that there exist channels within the body through which energy flows. The Ayurvedic paradigm teaches us that there also exist various *energy centres* which they refer to as *chakras*.

There are seven main chakras situated along the spine and skull through which energy (prana) enters and exits. In turn, each body system is associated with an individual chakra. A free flow of prana through the chakras is seen in good health. Poor health, however, results from stagnant prana and blocked chakras. Indian head massage aims to unblock the chakras to allow free flow of energy in a quest to restore health. This is known as 'energy balancing'.

Remember

The Chinese refer to this energy as 'chi' the Japanese as 'ki' and the Indians as 'prana'.

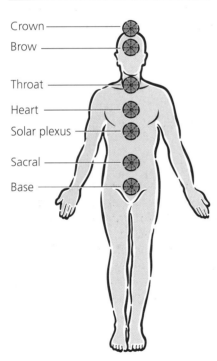

Chakras

Angel advice

The body is seen as an inverted tree. The brain is the root and the spine is the trunk. The spine supports the body in much the same way as the trunk of a tree channels support.

Where do I go from here?

The route to Indian head massage is not necessarily from a starting point of Swedish massage. However, this is possibly one of the most sensible routes as a thorough knowledge of the body as a whole enables a person to treat the part more effectively.

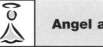

Tip

It can be common for people with no knowledge of holistic treatments and/or practitioners of a wide range of complementary treatments to study Indian head massage prior to, instead of, or at the same time as Swedish massage.

Taking Swedish massage as a natural starting point and advancing those skills with the introduction of the principles and techniques associated with the Eastern culture of India's Ayurvedic beliefs has an advantage in advancing one's physical, psychological and spiritual skills.

Angel advice

Some of these skills and subsequent effects associated with *energy balancing* are often alien to the Western world and take time for a person to 'get their head around'! Experiencing the effects of giving and receiving Swedish massage enables a person to become more open-minded in terms of alternative and complementary beliefs.

How do I advance my massage skills?

Many salons/holistic centres etc. offer day and/or weekend courses to qualified masseurs/masseuses conducted by specialists (often of Indian origin) providing a first hand insight into the Ayurvedic beliefs and traditions. Alternatively, a more formal training is offered by most colleges leading to recognised qualifications in Indian head massage incorporating detailed study of the relevant anatomy and physiology, consultation procedures and application of massage to the upper back and arms, neck and shoulders, head, face and ears.

Angel advice

It is useful to conduct further research into Ayurvedic practices before embarking on a course to ensure that you are comfortable with and share the associated beliefs. There are many books available at high street book stores and libraries and the Internet provides access to a wealth of information.

The skills associated with Indian head massage may be generally classified as being both practical (physical) and theoretical (psychological), incorporating the balanced use of body and mind. However, spirituality is often introduced as a means of treating the whole person i.e. body, mind and spirit. A masseur/masseuse may choose to adapt the use of these skills to meet the needs of their own spiritual beliefs and those of their clients.

Theoretical skills

Detailed knowledge of the anatomy and physiology of the parts of the body associated with Indian head massage is vital. A working knowledge of the other parts and systems of the body is desirable and enables the practitioner to link stress-related symptoms more effectively and provide holistic aftercare advice.

It is also important to follow developments and advances in medical science as research is constantly being carried out in areas such as neurology, endocrinology and genetics etc. which could have a bearing on the treatment of certain physical and psychological disorders.

Theoretical communication skills, e.g. treatment literature, needs to be clear and concise when explaining the origins, effects and benefits of Indian head massage in terms of the Ayurvedic beliefs so as not to confuse or even alarm prospective clients who are unaware of such practices.

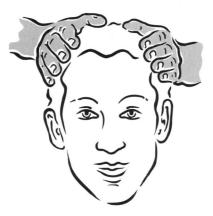

Holding

Practical skills

Practical massage skills associated with Indian head massage include:

Holding movements at the start, during and at the close of the treatment to establish/re-establish a physical connection between the client and masseur/masseuse e.g.

- Holding hands on the crown of the head to commence the treatment.
- Holding hands on the shoulders to enforce correct posture.
- Holding hands on the shoulders or feet to end the treatment.

Effleurage movements to link the treatment of the various parts together to ensure a smooth even rhythm is maintained e.g.

- Directional stroking to the upper back.
- Stroking through the hair and over the head.

Petrissage massage including kneading and picking up adapted to suit the needs of the area to be treated and the skin/muscle condition e.g.

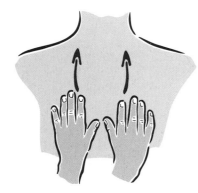

Effleurage

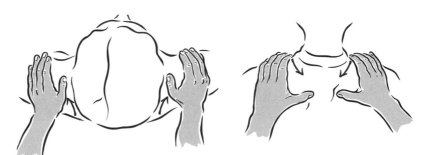

Petrissage – thumb pushes and finger pulls

- Circular kneading to the upper back.
- Picking up to the shoulders and neck.
- Picking up with the thumbs at the shoulders and sides of the neck; also referred to as *thumb pushes*.
- Picking up with the fingers at the shoulders and sides of the neck; also referred to as *finger pulls*.

Petrissage movements are often referred to as '*squeezing*' in terms of Indian head massage.

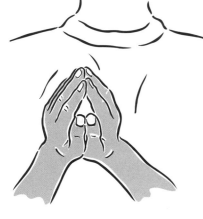

Frictions

Frictions are used deeply to release muscle from bone and more superficially to release tension in the layers of the skin e.g.

- Deep transverse frictions to the upper back.
- Deep circular friction to the head and face.
- Superficial frictions to the base of the head.

Frictions are often referred to as '*rubbing*' in terms of Indian head massage.

Tapotement/percussion movements may be used to stimulate and invigorate e.g.

- Hacking to the upper back, shoulders and head.
- Butterfly and plucking to the head.

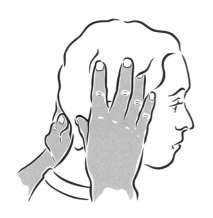

Tapotement (champi)

Traditional Indian head massage incorporate 'champi' which is a form of hacking performed with the hands together. The tips of the fingers and thumbs touch forming a cage like structure with the hands. Hacking is then performed with both hands together.

 Fascinating Fact

The gentle tapping movements performed with the fingertips associated with butterfly are traditionally known as *tabla playing*. Tabla is a popular percussion instrument of North Indian classical music incorporating a pair of drums that are rhythmically tapped with the fingers.

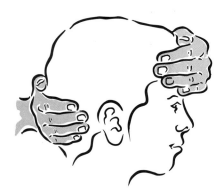

Head rocking

Joint manipulation movements are used to release tension in the joints and encourage greater ease of movement e.g.

- Gentle stretching or pulling of the ears.
- Supported head rocking is used to ease the synovial joints of the neck between the atlas and axis bones.

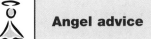

Angel advice

Supported head rocking is interspersed with deep breathing techniques to enhance the movement by encouraging greater supplies of oxygen to the area and a greater release of carbon dioxide. This in turn aids relaxation and associated muscle tension.

Acupressure is used on key points or pressure points known as *marmas*. These are similar to the acupoints and are described as being 'junctions' in energy channels. There are 107 marmas, 14 of which are on the back and 37 in the neck and head.

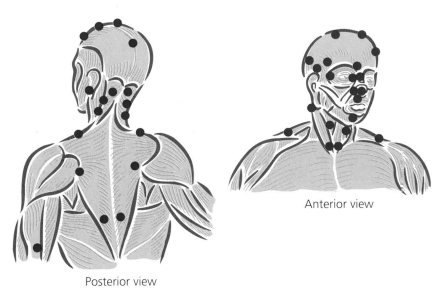

Anterior view

Posterior view

Marmas

The application of these practical massage skills may be performed with or without the use of a massage medium.

If a massage medium is used care should be given to the choice and subsequent use. Oils, creams/emulsion, gels and powder may be chosen in the much the same way as they would be for body massage. However, the use of specific oils is often recommended for the application of Indian head massage, especially when the emphasis is on the treatment of the scalp and/or hair. Suitable oils include vegetable oils that may be used for their specific therapeutic value including:

- Almond oil – popular with both Eastern and Western massage treatments for its nourishing properties and light texture.
- Coconut oil – a popular choice of oil for head massage in India because of its aroma together with its moisturising and softening properties.
- Grapeseed oil – a popular all purpose oil that may be used on all types of skin and hair.
- Mustard oil – a popular choice of oil for head massage in India especially in the treatment of men when a stimulating, warming effect is required.
- Olive oil – a popular Western choice of massage medium due to its purity. It is a heavy oil suitable for dry hair and skin.
- Sesame oil – a popular choice of oil for head massage in India because of its high mineral content, making it very nourishing and protecting for the hair and skin.

Other popular oils include jasmine, evening primrose, avocado, apricot kernel, peach kernel, calendula, hazelnut, wheatgerm, jojoba, macadamia, St John's Wort, soya and sunflower.

Tip

Care should be taken to ensure that a client is not allergic to the choice of oil e.g. nut oils.

Spiritual skills

The combination of the choice and application of massage oils, the choice and adaptation of massage movements together with energy balancing may be referred to as **Indian champissage**.

Champissage is therefore more than just head massage and as such requires specific skills including:

- A ritual application of massage oil.
- Massage skills that are adapted to meet the needs of the client.
- Balancing of subtle energy in the energy channels and energy centres.

Ritual application of massage oils involves three separate points of application including:

1   The first point is located within the hairline. Count eight finger widths from the centre of the eyebrows back towards the hair. Oil is poured onto this point so that it can be distributed down both sides of the head with circular movements using the fingers.

2   The second point is on the midline of the head at the natural crown where the hair grows in a circular pattern. Oil is poured

onto this point so that it can be evenly distributed down both sides of the head with the fingers.

3   The third point is located at the base of the skull in the occiput. Oil is poured onto this point with the client's head at an incline. The oil is evenly distributed along each side of the head towards the ears.

Massage skills incorporate a mix of all types of massage movements with varying pressure, speed and application to suit the specific needs of each individual client.

Energy balancing is an intuitive technique whereby the hands are used to create a sense of harmony between body, mind and spirit.

It is performed by:

- Placing the hands directly onto the area being treated allowing them to relax and as a result slowly start to hover above the area feeling a warmth, a tingling and/or even a slight vibration as the hands pick up on the subtle energy within and surrounding a person.
- Gradually moving the hands from a distance towards the area to be treated until a slight resistance is felt – this constitutes the energy surrounding a person.

Energy balancing may be performed for two specific purposes:

1   To balance the energy in the energy channels.
2   To balance the energy centres – chakras.

Balancing the energy channels occurs towards the end of the treatment once the massage techniques have been performed and the associated effects been achieved. The results of the massage may be likened to the fact that the energy has been unblocked and is flowing more freely through the channels. As such, it needs to be balanced to even the flow and encourage homeostasis. The masseur/masseuse stands behind the client and gently places their cupped hands in four separate positions:

1   Over the lower face
2   Over the eyes
3   Over the forehead
4   On the crown.

The hands are held in each position for a few seconds in which time the client may expect to experience a sense of clearing and calm as the circulating energy becomes more even in flow.

Balancing the energy centres occurs at the close of the treatment once the channels have been balanced.

Champissage concentrates on the three higher chakras including:

- The throat or *vishuddha* chakra – located in the throat and associated with communication and the colour blue.

- The brow or *ajna* chakra – located in the middle of the forehead and associated with intuition and the colour indigo.

- The crown or *sahasrara* chakra – located on the crown of the head and associated with higher thinking and the colours violet and white.

One hand supports the base of the head whilst the other hand is placed on the surface or slightly above the surface of the corresponding chakra at the throat, forehead and crown. The hands are held for a few seconds in which time the client may expect to experience a peaceful, calming sensation and also possibly be able to 'see' the associated colours in their mind's eye.

 Angel advice

As the hands are released from the balancing positions, a gentle downward shaking will transfer any negative energy to the earth where it may be freed and neutralised, ensuring that its effects are not transferred from the client to the practitioner or vice versa.

 Task

Research the seven main chakras finding out the associated functions of the body, colour and effects of holistic treatment on each. This fact-finding task will serve to inspire you to undertake further training or divert you from this style of massage.

Activity

Try to visit a local mind, body and spirit exhibition (details can be found on the Internet) where you will get the opportunity to talk to a range of people about the Ayurvedic art of massage as well as try variations of the treatment for yourself.

Treatment tracker

INDIAN HEAD MASSAGE

Tools

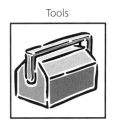

Indian head massage is a manual treatment incorporating the use of the whole of the palmar surface of the fingers/thumbs and hands as well as the forearms.

- Clients may be seated in a comfortable upright chair with arm and back rests. The masseur/masseuse works predominantly from the side and back of the client and may be seated when massaging the back and shoulders and standing when massaging the arms, neck, head, face and ears.
- Alternatively a client may be seated in a chair leaning their upper body forward onto a couch and supported with a pillow. The masseur/masseuse is positioned behind the client for treatment of the back. The client resumes a seated position for the rest of the treatment.
- Another alternative incorporates the client sitting forward on a flat couch with legs outstretched for treatment to the back and then adopts a supine laying down position for treatment of the arms, neck, head, face and ears.

Whatever the position, the emphasis should be on client comfort and the maintenance of correct posture for the masseur/masseuse.

Although Indian head massage is an ideal treatment to perform in an informal setting, it is always necessary to conduct a consultation to establish suitability.

In addition care should be taken to ensure:

- Upper clothing is removed if necessary and the client provided with a towel or robe to maintain modesty.
- Client is positioned comfortably.
- It is advisable to ensure arms and legs are kept uncrossed.
- Jewellery that may hinder the treatment may be removed e.g. necklace, ear rings etc.
- Hair should be brushed to remove excess hair products that may hinder the treatment e.g. thick gel, hairsprays etc.
- Clients may be encouraged to close their eyes during the treatment (receiving a treatment in a seated position may at first appear less relaxing to the client and so they are often reluctant to close their eyes without encouragement).

Preparation

Indications for treatment

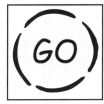

Traditionally Indian head massage was used for treatment of the scalp by a barber as part of male grooming and/or the treatment of the hair by mothers and daughters. Nowadays, Indian head massage is used to aid stress-related conditions including:

- Tension – helping to reduce the symptoms associated with muscular and emotional strain.
- Hair loss – stimulating blood flow to the follicles helping to restore temporary hair loss associated with hormonal disturbances and stress.
- Skin problems – helping to balance endocrine and exocrine glandular functions.
- Anxiety and phobias – helping to restore a sense of perspective.
- Lethargy and loss of motivation – stimulating the body and mind.
- Loss of concentration – helping to clear the mind and restore order.
- Low self-esteem – promoting well being and awareness.

Indian head massage is seen as being an holistic treatment in that treatment to the part has the potential to produce a positive effect on the whole of the body.

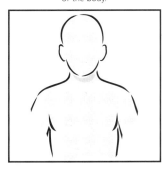

As with any form of massage treatment a person may expect to experience a reaction that may be viewed as being adverse i.e. their condition appears to worsen before it gets better. This is usually associated with the body's need to release and/or replenish e.g.

- Weeping – release of emotions.
- Sweating – release of toxins.
- Increased need to pass urine – release of excess water and waste.
- Increased need to defecate – release of waste.
- Increased hunger and thirst – replenishment of nutrients.
- Exhaustion – denoting the body's need to sleep in order to aid cellular function.

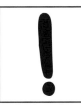

Contra actions

Contraindications

The contraindications that apply to Swedish massage also apply to Indian head massage.

Extra care should be taken with regard to problems associated with the upper body and any undiagnosed pain and/or swellings in the area should be referred to the medical profession for diagnosis and advice.

Although Indian head massage may be carried out without the use of a massage medium, the use of specific oils may be recommended for the treatment of the hair. Such oils are vegetable based and may include nut oils. As many people experience nut allergies this needs to be discussed during the consultation.

Oils to be avoided if a nut allergy exists include:

- Almond oil
- Coconut oil
- Hazelnut oil
- Macadamia nut oil

If in any doubt always choose an alternative oil. Other oils suitable for use in Indian head massage include: apricot kernel, avocado, grapeseed, jasmine, jojoba, mustard, olive, peach kernel, sesame, soya, St. John's Wort, sunflower, wheatgerm etc.

As with any form of massage, aftercare advice provides vital information to complement the treatment and encourage a sense of responsibility in the client's personal quest for improved well-being.

Care should be taken to:

- Avoid anything in excess post-treatment e.g. activity, alcohol, caffeine, rich foods etc.
- Ensure the signs that demonstrate the body's needs are adhered to e.g. hunger, need to visit the loo, thirst, need for sleep etc.

Self-treatment and further treatment advice ensures that a person continues to take responsibility for their well-being.

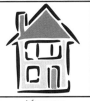

Aftercare

Knowledge review

1 Where does Indian head massage take its origins from?

2 What was the name given to the traditional head massage performed by barbers?

3 For what reasons did mothers apply head massage to their children?

4 List the areas of the body that are commonly treated as part of an Indian head massage treatment.

5 What may be described as being the life force as part of Eastern beliefs?

6 What is energy referred to as in China, Japan and India?

7 What are energy centres called?

8 How many chakras are directly associated with the Indian head massage treatment?

9 What is it that makes up a whole person?

10 Which movements start an Indian head massage treatment?

11 Which movements are used to link the treatment to ensure even rhythm and flow?

12 Which type of massage are finger pulls and thumb pushes?

13 Which type of massage movements are also referred to as 'squeezing'?

14 Which type of massage movements are also referred to as 'rubbing'?

15 Which type of massage movement is champi similar to?

16 What may be interspersed with head rocking to enhance the effects of the movements?

17 Give three popular choices of massage oils used for Indian head massage.

18 What is the term given to describe the application of massage oils, adaptation of massage and energy balancing?

19 How many points are traditionally used for the application of massage oil to the head?

20 Which chakras are treated during an Indian head massage treatment?

Aromatherapy massage

A combination of ancient and modern massage techniques combined with essential oils from plants, fruits, flowers, bark, roots or resin to bring about physiological and psychological well-being. Essential oils are added to a base oil to create a unique blend suited to each person's individual needs. Essential oils have long been used for their fragrant and healing properties for cosmetic, religious and therapeutic purposes e.g. perfume, beauty products, incense, medicines etc. They have been used both during life and after life – the Egyptians used essential oils for beautification as well as for embalming and mummification. The aromatherapy of today takes its origins from the art associated with the ancient experimental and experiential use of essential oils and the science associated with modern times.

The early twentieth century brought about scientific research into the effects and benefits of essential oils more by accident than by design. It is reputed that a French chemist and perfumer Rene Maurice Gattefosse suffered burns to his hands as a result of a laboratory explosion. He subsequently used lavender oil on his wounds which had developed gas gangrene (a serious form of infection). The lavender oil speeded up the healing process with great effect. This led him to investigate the chemical properties of essential oils in terms of healing. He shared his knowledge with a friend and colleague Dr Jean Valnet who during the Second World War used essential oils for the treatment of wounded soldiers. He utilised their powerful effects in combating and counteracting infections thus saving many lives that would otherwise have been lost. Students of Dr Valnet went on to investigate further the antiviral, antibacterial, antifungal and antiseptic properties of essential oils.

The integration of essential oils and massage for the use in beauty therapy was pioneered by an Austrian biochemist Marguerite Maury in the mid 1990s. She combined beauty therapy techniques with essential oils, introducing aromatherapy as a massage treatment. A student of both Madame Maury and Dr Valnet called Micheline Arcier was also a key player in the development of aromatherapy as an holistic treatment. She contributed to the treatment and training of the aromatherapy that we recognise today.

Experimentation over many thousands of years has led to the passing down of remedies and potions throughout the centuries and throughout the world. Recent clinical research has confirmed and subsequently theorised the effects and benefits for use in modern day aromatherapy.

Aromatherapy works in three ways:

1   Essential oils are absorbed into the skin. Because of their molecular structure, they are able to pass through the layers of the skin where they are picked up by the blood circulation and transported via the blood to all organs and body systems.

2   Essential oils are also inhaled through the nose, pass into the blood circulation via the alveoli in the lungs and are transported around the body.

3   Essential oils are picked up by the sensory functions of the nose (olfaction). This in turn produces a message in the form of an electrical impulse which passes to the brain via nerves. The brain interprets the message and recognition of the aroma takes place.

Fascinating Fact

The part of the brain associated with recognition of smell is called the limbic centre and this is also associated with memory and emotions. Therefore certain smells are able to stir up associated memories and emotions in an individual. It is believed that the human nose is able to distinguish between 10,000 different smells!

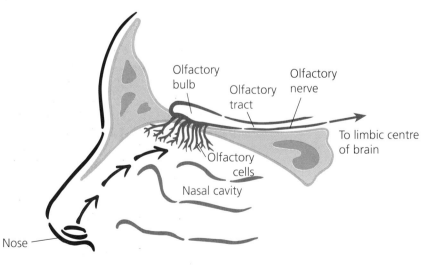

The nose

An essential oil has three effects on the body:

1　**Physiological** – essential oils are able to interact with the way the body functions thus changing its reactions e.g. calming, stimulating etc.
2　**Psychological** – the sense of smell is strongly linked with emotions and as such, essential oils can bring about a change in emotions through the brain's interpretation of their aroma.
3　**Pharmacological** – essential oils are chemical substances and as such interact and subsequently have an effect on the chemical make-up of the human body.

Essential oils are commonly used in perfumes, drugs and foods for their fragrance, colour and unique properties. However, it is the use of essential oils together with massage that forms an aromatherapy treatment.

Where do I go from here?

One of the most popular routes to follow in terms of manual massage treatment is from traditional Swedish to aromatherapy massage. Aromatherapy provides the means of enhancing and advancing the basic Swedish massage skills as well as introducing a unique range of massage mediums in the form of essential oils and base oils that require skill and sensitivity in their choice, blending and application.

How do I advance my massage skills?

Once a practitioner has acquired the basic skills associated with Swedish massage a natural progression is often towards the use of essential oils and aromatherapy. It is not enough to combine basic massage with the use of essential oils or indeed try to blend the oils without the necessary training. The art and science of aromatherapy is complex and requires careful study and guided experiential learning before a practitioner can call themselves an aromatherapist in the true sense of the word. Aromatherapy may be studied at varying levels, incorporating the choice of working with pre-blended oils and/or working with essential and base oils to create a blend that is individual to each client and their specific needs.

Aromatherapy may be divided into two distinct areas of study that are integrated to form a complete treatment:

- Essential oils
- Massage

Essential oils

Essential oils are concentrated liquids (not always oils) that are produced in specialist cells of certain plants. These specialist cells are found in various parts of the plants including:

- Petals e.g. Rose
- Flowering tops e.g. Lavender
- Whole flowers e.g. Jasmine
- Leaves e.g. Eucalyptus
- Twigs e.g. Tea Tree
- Grasses e.g. Palmarosa
- Seeds e.g. Fennel (sweet)
- Berries e.g. Juniper berry
- Fruit peel/rind e.g. Lemon
- Wood and bark e.g. Sandalwood
- Roots e.g. Vetiver
- Resins and gums e.g. Frankincense.

Essential oils are extracted from the plant by a variety of means including:

- Enfleurage – an ancient method of extraction involving several layers of glass sheets covered in fat held together by a wooden frame. Plant material is placed onto the glass sheets whereby the fat absorbs the essential oils. This process is repeated until the fat becomes saturated with the essential oil. Alcohol is used to separate the essential oil from the fat. Flowers that retain their fragrance for some time after picking may be treated in this way e.g. jasmine.
- Steam distillation – the plant material is placed into a still with water. The water is boiled and the accompanying heat releases the essential oil from the plant material. As the steam rises from the boiling water it carries the molecules of essential oil which enter a pipe. The pipe is cooled so that the steam returns to its liquid form of essential oil and water. The essential oil separates and is siphoned off. This is the most common method of extraction used.
- Dry steam distillation – the plant material is placed on a grate within a still. Water below the grate is heated and the resulting steam passes up and over the plant material releasing the essential oils which are then carried by the steam, cooled and siphoned off.
- Hydrodiffusion – steam is applied from above rather than from below. The steam percolates through the plant material and the essential oils are extracted in the same way as for steam/dry steam distillation.
- Expression – the plant material is pressed or crushed to extract the essential oils. This method is commonly used to extract the essential oils from the peel/zest of citrus fruits e.g. lemons, oranges etc.

- Maceration – plant material is placed in oil or fat and then heated to 60–70° Centigrade. The essential oils are released and become absorbed into the oil/fat. The essential oil is then separated.

- Solvent extraction – chemicals are used as solvents. They are combined with the plant material and heated. The essential oil is released from the plant material and the chemical solvent evaporates. The resulting semi-solid mass is treated with alcohol to produce a concentrated form of essential oil known as an *absolute*. This is the most modern method of extraction.

Each essential oil has a unique fragrance which identifies it and reflects its chemical composition. The fragrance of individual crops of plants will differ depending on the conditions of growth, methods of extraction, storage and care.

Essential oils are *volatile* which means that they evaporate in the air. Essential oils evaporate at different rates depending on their chemical structure and can be categorised as different *notes* i.e. top, middle or base notes:

- Top notes are oils that are most volatile and evaporate quickly. They have a sharp aroma are very stimulating and have a short-term effect on the body (up to 24 hours) e.g. lemon, orange, tea tree, and eucalyptus etc.

- Middle notes are oils that are moderately volatile evaporating at an average rate. Their effects last up to two to three days in the body e.g. lavender, fennel, geranium, camomile and rosemary etc.

- Base notes are oils that are the slowest to evaporate and have the most lasting effect on the body. They tend to have more soothing and calming effects that can last up to seven days e.g. rose, frankincense, jasmine, sandalwood and ylang ylang etc.

Essential oils are never used neat on the body for massage; instead they are diluted into vegetable fats to form a suitable massage medium. Individual or blends of vegetable fats form a **base oil** (sometimes referred to as a carrier oil). Base oils are known as 'fixed oils' because they do not evaporate.

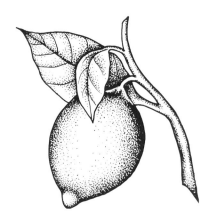

Lemon

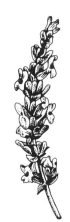

Lavender

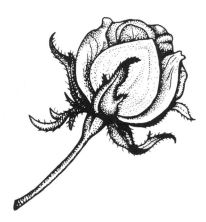

Rose

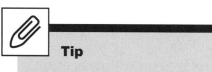

Tip

Essential oils evaporate more quickly in the heat.

Angel advice

Essential oils should *not* be diluted in animal fats, fish oils, petroleum or mineral oils or any synthetic or chemically treated vegetable oils. Baby oil is a petroleum oil and should not be used as a base for essential oils.

Base oils enhance the effects of the essential oil as well as provide therapeutic effects of their own e.g.

- Grapeseed oil – provides good slip and is suitable for all skin types.
- Sweet almond oil – light in texture, easily absorbed into the skin providing a nourishing and soothing effect.
- Hazelnut oil – moisturising, revitalising, soothing and softening to the skin.

Remember

A blend of oils that smells unpleasant to the client will not produce the desired outcome regardless of its properties.

The dilution of essential oils into a base oil is a highly skilled art and requires detailed knowledge of the essential oils and base oils as well as knowledge of the client and their physiological and psychological needs. More than one essential oil and base oil may be used to create a blend depending on the treatment plan. Essential and base oils work together and the ideal blend is one that contains therapeutic properties that are complementary to each other, suitable for the client's needs with an aroma that is pleasant for the client.

Task

Choose six essential oils i.e. two top, middle and base notes that you like the sound of and/or already know that you like the aroma of and two base oils. Find out which part of the plant they come from, the method of extraction, country of origin and general effects and benefits. Find out if they have any specific contraindications and which other oils they blend well with. Use this research to help you determine if aromatherapy is a possible career route for you.

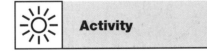

Activity

Book an aromatherapy treatment and pay particular attention to the choice and blend of oils and the effects they have on you.

Aromatherapy massage

Aromatherapy massage – massage that incorporates the use of blended essential/base oils – may be applied to all areas of the body and incorporates the use of the movements associated with traditional Swedish massage together with advanced massage techniques.

Swedish massage movements include:

- Effleurage to start, link and complete the treatment.

- Petrissage movements to stimulate circulation and encourage deep relaxation.
- Frictions to stimulate, relax and ease the tension in the muscles.
- Tapotement/percussion to invigorate and energise.
- Vibrations to release tension.

Advanced massage techniques include:

- Relaxation – holding and breathing techniques.
- Lymphatic drainage – pumping, pushing, scooping and draining towards appropriate lymph nodes for filtering of waste.
- Neuromuscular techniques – for the relief of specific areas of pain and tension.
- Acupressure – pressures applied to key points (acupoints) to free stagnant energy and unblock energy channels.
- Stretching – gentle stretching techniques may be used to alleviate tension, break down adhesions and reverse the reflex action associated with tight muscles.
- Balancing – the use of holding, visualisations, affirmations and breath awareness may be combined and adapted to enhance the therapeutic effects of the essential oils.

Aromatherapy massage is not prescriptive in that it does not draw from one method. Instead, practitioners are encouraged to adopt different techniques and learn to adapt them to meet the needs of the client and to enhance the properties of the chosen essential oils.

Task

Conduct your own research into the specific differences between pressure techniques associated with acupressure e.g. shiatsu and neuromuscular techniques. Many colleges offer day courses in such techniques to qualified masseurs/masseuses. This gives the opportunity to advance your massage skills as well as help to decide a possible career pathway.

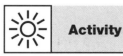

Activity

Book an aromatherapy treatment with a few different practitioners. Try to determine their style and influence of massage.

Treatment tracker

AROMATHERAPY MASSAGE

Tools

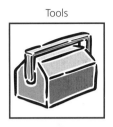

Aromatherapy is a manual treatment incorporating the use of massage with essential base oils.

For aromatherapy massage treatment it is useful to have a good choice of essential oils and base oils in order to create a variety of blends to suit the individual needs of the clients.

In addition the following are needed:

- Absorbent paper strips for testing the aroma of individual oils and blends.
- Glass dishes for blending essential and base oil together.
- Glass measures for blending base oils.
- Glass droppers for accurate blending of essential oils.
- Glass rod for stirring.
- Amber glass bottles for storing blends.

Indications for treatment

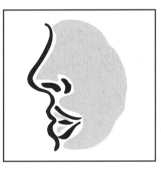

Aromatherapy is an holistic treatment in that the use of the oils and accompanying massage has the potential to affect the body as a whole.

Essential oils may be chosen to aid specific problems, for example stress, with the emphasis on:

- Top notes for stimulating and uplifting effects.
- Middle notes for therapeutic effects on specific body systems and organs.
- Base notes for calming and soothing effects associated with relaxation and mental and physical regeneration.

Contraindications

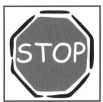

The contraindications that apply to Swedish massage also apply to aromatherapy massage.

In addition extra care should be taken with regard to the following:

- Atopic clients i.e. anyone who suffers from hay fever, eczema, asthma, allergies to dust, animal hair etc. are likely to have a reaction to essential oils so a sensitivity test should be conducted 24 hours before the treatment.
- Allergies such as those associated with nuts, wheat etc. should be noted and appropriate oils chosen that in no way put a client at risk.
- Skin prone to large/dark moles as citrus oils may increase the possibility of malignancy.
- Toxic oils should not be used or recommended in any circumstances e.g. aniseed, camphor, wormwood, mustard, sage etc.

Aromatherapy massage is usually performed with the client lying on a couch as for Swedish massage.

- A full consultation should be conducted and a treatment plan agreed.
- A sensitivity test should be conducted up to 24 hours prior to treatment if an allergic reaction is anticipated.
- The blend of oils chosen with the client allowing them to smell the individual and blend of oils.
- Skin should be cleansed to avoid cross-sensitisation with other perfumed products that may be on the skin.
- Product exfoliation or manual friction rubs may be used to remove dead surface skin cells in preparation for the treatment.

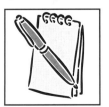

Preparation

Overuse and/or overly concentrated blends may have the following effects:

- Headaches/migraines
- Nausea
- Nightmares
- Diarrhoea
- Exhaustion
- Hyperactivity
- Light or 'fuzzy' headedness.

Contra actions

The general aftercare associated with Swedish massage is also associated with aromatherapy massage.

In addition attention should be paid to the following:

- Refrain from bathing or showering for 12–24 hours to get the maximum benefit of the oils.
- Avoid heat treatments e.g. sauna, steam and spa for at least 24 hours.
- Avoid use of the sunbed and/or sunbathing for at least 24 hours.
- Avoid waxing over an area that has been treated with essential oils.

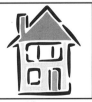

Aftercare

Knowledge review

1   What are used in combination with massage to form an aromatherapy treatment?

2   Which oil was reputed to have been used to aid the healing of the burns of the French chemist and perfumer Rene Maurice Gattefosse?

3   Who pioneered the use of essential oils and massage for use in beauty therapy?

4   How are essential oils absorbed into the body?

5   Which part of the nervous system is responsible for interpreting the fragrance of an essential oil?

6   Give three areas of a plant from which essential oils may be extracted.

7   Which method of extraction incorporates the pressing or crushing of fruit peel?

8   Which four factors may affect the fragrance of an essential oil?

9   What are the three types of 'notes' associated with essential oils?

10   Which type of essential oil evaporates quickly?

11   What are essential oils diluted into?

12   What is a base oil?

13   Why are base oils known as 'fixed oils'?

14   Give an example of a base oil.

15   When is effleurage used in an aromatherapy massage?

16   What do vibration movements help to release in the muscles?

17   Which advanced massage skill helps to relieve pain?

18   Where is lymph drained towards during lymphatic drainage massage?

19   What do acupressure movements aim to do?

20   What is the term given to a positive visual image that may be used to focus on during a massage treatment.

Reflexology massage

Reflexology incorporates the application of finger/thumb pressure techniques to points on the feet, hands or ears to stimulate the body's own healing mechanisms. These parts are viewed as microcosms or miniature representations of a larger system – the whole body – based on the belief that by stimulating the part, one can stimulate the whole. The history of reflexology has many parallels with that of massage and has over the years been subject to ancient Eastern and more recent Western influences. The reflexology studied today takes its origins from both cultures; the practical emphasis is based on medical research and science and the intuitive emphasis is taken from the psychological and spiritual aspects very much associated with art and creativity.

When physicians in the Western world were experimenting with massage techniques to aid medical problems, there were also those who were experimenting with an alternative form of treatment which was originally known as zone therapy before becoming compression therapy and eventually reflexology.

We have evidence similar to that depicting the origins of massage that reflexology has been practiced in some form throughout history. However, it was not until the early 1900s that an American ear, nose and throat specialist, Dr William Fitzgerald, experimented with the use of pressure to block pain. He discovered that by applying pressure to a part of the body e.g. the fingers, pain could be effectively blocked and tracked through zones in the body. He developed the concept that the body has ten longitudinal zones that correspond with the fingers and toes and run along the body.

This discovery tied in with the Eastern belief associated with meridians and energy flow and with the more recent Western discovery in the late nineteenth and early twentieth century by neurologists of dermatomes.

Meridians are channels running through the body resulting in separate pathways through which energy flows in a twenty-four hour cycle that divides night from day. Dermatomes are segmented regions of the body, each of which are supplied with a spinal or cranial nerve linking the body with the brain and vice versa.

The medical profession continued to experiment with the concept of zone therapy which was further developed by Dr Edwin Bowers and Dr Joseph Shelby. Both these physicians worked closely with Dr Fitzgerald in developing and confirming the zone theory. But it was a colleague of Dr Shelby who moved the concept on to the treatment we recognise as being the reflexology of today. Eunice Ingham, a physiotherapist, worked on many of Dr Shelby's patients in the 1930s and discovered that if she used alternating pressure instead of just compression she could bring about a healing effect within the zones. She went on to map out the organs of the body on the feet and devoted her life to confirming the theory that the

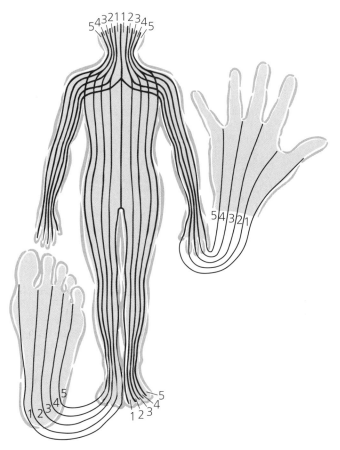

The longitudinal zones of the body

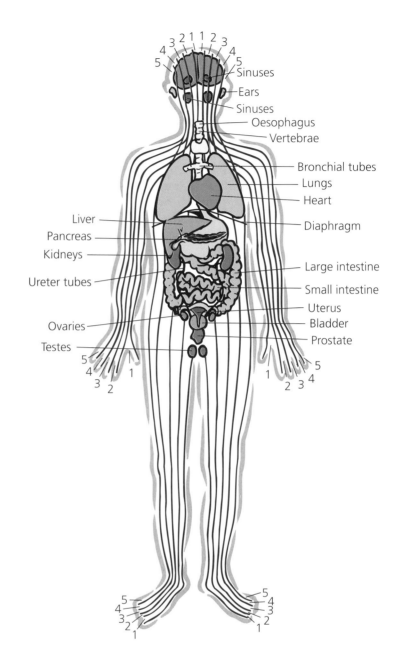

The following labels appear on the body map:

Sinuses
Ears
Sinuses
Oesophagus
Vertebrae
Bronchial tubes
Lungs
Heart
Liver
Diaphragm
Pancreas
Kidneys
Ureter tubes
Large intestine
Small intestine
Uterus
Bladder
Ovaries
Prostate
Testes

The body map

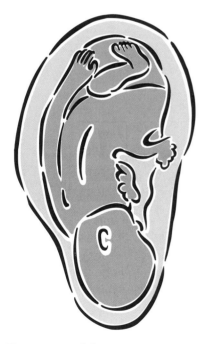

The inverted foetus

organs could be treated effectively by working on corresponding reflex points on the feet. This theory could also be adapted for the hands although it was felt that the feet were more receptive to treatment and easier to work with.

At around the same time a French physician, Dr Paul Nogier, identified through his work and research the correlation between points on the ear and various parts of the body based on the concept of the inverted foetus.

These theories form the basis of the reflexology practiced today.

Where do I go from here?

Reflexology is a very popular progression route from Swedish massage as it incorporates the use of the basic massage techniques with a set of specific techniques to focus on the treatment of a part of the body with the overall aim of aiding the whole of the body. The study of reflexology requires:

- Knowledge and understanding of the treatment.
- Massage skills for the application of the treatment.
- Intuitive skills for the interpretation of the treatment.

Reflexology offers a challenging and rewarding progression route for a masseur/masseuse to follow in order to extend their provision of services in the treatment of stress-related disorders.

How do I advance my massage skills?

Reflexology is a complex area of study that requires formal learning together with experiential learning to be able to develop the associated science and art into a commercial treatment. As such it may be studied at a basic level which generally involves the treatment of the feet only and at an advanced level which incorporates treatment of the feet, hands and ears.

The skills required for reflexology may be divided into three main categories:

- Theoretical skills – a detailed study of anatomy and physiology.
- Practical skills – study of specific practical massage techniques.
- Psychological skills – associated with the mind.

Theoretical skills

One of the most important tools for a practitioner of reflexology is having a working knowledge of the anatomy and physiology of the whole body, because the theory relating to the structure and function of the parts forms the basis of the treatment. Detailed knowledge of the body systems is vital and should include the systemic systems that pertain to or affect the body as a whole and are treated generally; as well as the individual systems that are treated specifically.

Systemic systems include:

- Nervous system – the central, peripheral and autonomic nervous systems.

- Circulatory systems – the heart, blood and blood vessels.
- Integumentary system – the skin, hair and nails.
- Immune system – the special cells, tissue, glands and organs associated with fighting disease.

The individual systems include:

- Skeletal/muscular systems – bones, joints and muscles.
- Respiratory system – bones, muscles, organs and glands associated with the intake of oxygen and the output of carbon dioxide.
- Digestive system – the ingestion, digestion, absorption of nutrients and the excretion of waste.
- Genito-urinary system – reproduction and the excretion of excess water and waste.
- Endocrine system – the production, circulation and function of hormones.
- Lymphatic system – lymph, lymphatic vessels, nodes and ducts.

In addition to having an understanding of the structure and function of the human body, a working knowledge of the common diseases and disorders that affect the systems is useful.

Tip

It is useful to have a **Nurse's dictionary** and a **Dictionary of Drugs and Medication** available to look up medical conditions and associated drugs that you are not aware of.

Practical skills

Reflexology is based on the combination of Swedish massage techniques to start and end the treatment together with additional compression or pressure techniques to treat the zones and reflex points.

Swedish massage techniques include:

- **Holding** – used as a form of 'greeting' at the start and close of the treatment.
- **Effleurage** – non-directional and directional movements used to encourage relaxation at the start and close of the treatment and to link other massage movements as necessary.

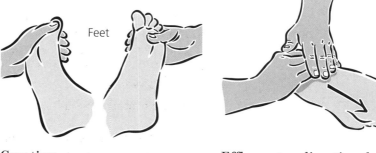

Feet

Greeting   Effleurage – directional

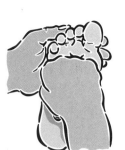

Petrissage

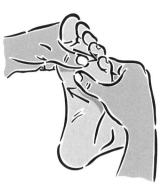

Frictions

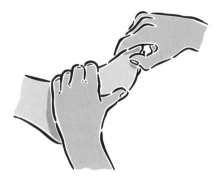

Tapotement

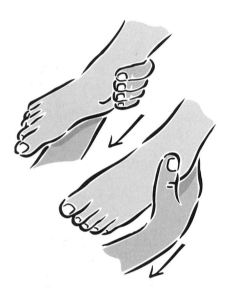

Joint manipulation – stretch

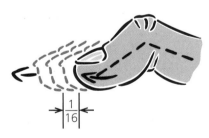

Thumb walking

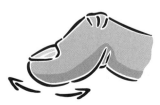

Thumb slide

- **Petrissage** – kneading and knuckling are commonly used to encourage further relaxation and stimulate the systemic systems i.e. circulation, nerve supply etc.
- **Friction** – circular and/or transverse friction may be used to provide localised stimulation and release of tension.
- **Tapotement/percussion** – gentle hacking, cupping and pounding may be used together with butterfly, flicking and plucking to stimulate and energise.
- **Joint manipulation** – rotation, stretching and twisting may be used to encourage greater ease of movement in the joints.

Compression or pressure techniques are exclusive to the treatment and are used to:

- Locate the reflex points.
- Determine the level of stress associated with each reflex point.
- Treat the reflex points.

Compression or pressure movements include:

- **Thumb/finger walking** – with thumb/finger bent at the first joint small movements that mimic a caterpillar walking are made feeling the underlying tissue as the 'walk' progresses.
- **Thumb/finger slide** – same position as for 'walking'. The thumb/finger gently slides back and forth over an area to soothe a stressed reflex point.
- **Pivot-on-a-point** – extra pressure is applied by focusing on a specific reflex point and applying pressure in a circular motion.
- **Hook-in-back-up** – deeper and more specific pressure may be applied to locate a deep-seated reflex point. The thumb is flexed and hooked into a point before being pulled back.
- **Rocking** – the thumb/finger is used on the spot and gently rocked from side to side gaining greater access into the reflex point.

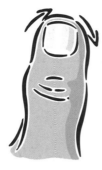

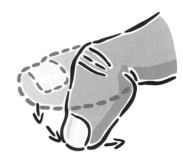

Pivot-on-a-point   Hook-in-and-back-up

- **Thumb/finger press** – an on the spot press and release using the thumb/finger to gently focus on a specific reflex point.

A reflexology treatment commences with the application of Swedish massage techniques to relax the client before performing compression or pressure movements to the specific reflex points. Any irregularities in the feel of each reflex point are noted and discussed with the client to determine a possible cause and appropriate aftercare is provided along with further treatment advice.

Psychological skills

Psychological skills are those that are associated with the mind – some we can quantify, others are not so easily described.

The left side of the brain is responsible for the quantifiable skills associated with logical thought and the right side of the brain is responsible for more intuitive thought:

- The left side of our brain will make us believe that someone is fine just because they say they are.
- The right side of our brain will enable us to read beyond their words as we intuitively pick up on the fact that all is not well despite the fact that a person says that they are fine.

Reflexology, like massage, is a two-way process involving the client and the practitioner and as such requires a balance of psychological skills between the left and right brain activity in order to provide the best possible treatment.

Psychological skills include:

Communication skills

- Verbal – including the tone, volume, pitch and speed as well as articulation and emphasis.
- Non-verbal – including facial expressions, eye contact, eye movements, posture, gestures, appearance and proximity.

- Tactile – including permission and pressure.
- Non face-to-face – including written and extra sensory communication.

Counselling skills

- Active listening – using sensory skills associated with our ears to hear the sounds and the interpretation skills associated with our brains to listen to the meaning.
- Empathy – try to get a view of what a person is feeling from their perspective rather than our own.
- Openness – whilst we do not have to agree with everyone's values and opinions, we need to be open to the fact that these may differ from person to person and approach each new client and situation with an open heart and mind.
- Acceptance – demonstrating an attitude that is non-judgemental, supportive, positive and confidential.

These skills are not exclusive to reflexology, nor do they make a person a counsellor. They are advanced psychological skills that develop with experience and insight and may be used to enhance any form of treatment.

Reflexology at its best forms an extension of the practitioner's theoretical, practical and psychological skills and as such is best studied after the completion of a massage course. This makes the transition from treating the whole to treating a part that reflects the whole all the more easy and natural.

Activity

Book an appointment for a reflexology treatment and take note of the integration of Swedish massage movements with the use of specific reflexology techniques. Examine how the treatment to a part differs from the treatment of the whole body and monitor your reactions prior, during and post-treatment.

Task

Many clients who come to you for massage treatments will inevitably enquire about reflexology. Devise an information sheet for clients showing them that you have the knowledge. This will also help you to determine whether or not reflexology is a career progression for you. If you choose not to offer a particular treatment to your clients it is wise to offer them a suitable alternative and/or refer them to someone who you know is reputable.

Treatment tracker

REFLEXOLOGY MASSAGE

Tools

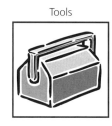

- The treatment is carried out using the thumbs, fingers and whole hand.
- The client may be positioned on a couch or chair.
- Products are not needed for the treatment although creams/emulsions may be used for the relaxation movements at the start and close of the treatment.

Indications for treatment

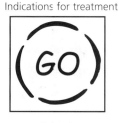

- Relaxation.
- Stress relief.
- Pain relief e.g. during childbirth.
- Addictions e.g. drugs or alcohol.
- Treatment of the terminally ill to improve quality of life.
- Mental health e.g. as a means of communication.

Contraindications

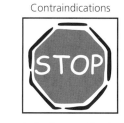

Few contraindications to reflexology exist but care should be taken with:

- Infectious disorders that may result in cross-infection e.g. verruca on the feet, warts on the hands etc.
- Conditions requiring surgery and/or recent surgery.
- Circulatory disorders e.g. varicose veins, thrombosis and heart conditions.
- Early stages of pregnancy.
- Undiagnosed swellings and/or lumps.
- Some medication – seek medical advice.
- An excessively full or empty stomach.
- Under the influence of alcohol.

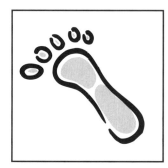

Reflexology may be carried out with the client sitting or lying on a couch or chair with the part to be worked on exposed i.e. feet, hands or ears.

- Conduct a full consultation.
- Agree a treatment plan with the client.
- Position the client on a couch or chair paying attention to safety and comfort.
- Positioning of practitioner for ease of access to the part as well as safety and comfort.
- Cleansing of the part with antiseptic wipes or spray.
- Application of Swedish massage movements to the part for relaxation.
- Application of compression/pressure movements to the reflex points.
- Swedish massage to complete the treatment.
- Feedback and aftercare advice.

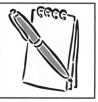

Preparation

- Increased feelings of hunger and/or thirst.
- Increased feeling of tiredness and exhaustion.
- Release of emotions e.g. weeping.
- Release of toxins e.g. sweating, need to urinate and/or defecate.
- A general worsening of a condition before it gets better.

These contra actions are sometimes referred to as being part of the **healing crisis** or disturbance of the state of balance which signifies a turning point.

Contra actions

- Respond to the releasing requirements of the body e.g. urination, defecation.
- Allow the body time to rest by avoiding excesses.
- Respond to the replenishing needs of the body i.e. drink water and eat a light meal
- Avoid caffeine, alcohol and rich spicy foods that are difficult to digest.
- Monitor the body over a 24–48 hour period and respond to its needs.

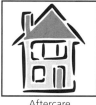

Aftercare

Knowledge review

1   Which parts of the body may be treated with reflexology?

2   How many longitudinal zones did Dr Fitzgerald develop?

3   What flows through meridians according to Eastern belief?

4   What are the segmented regions of the body that are supplied with a cranial or spinal nerve called?

5   Who developed reflexology as we know it today?

6   When are traditional Swedish massage movements used in reflexology?

7   Which part of the hand is used for 'walking' pressure techniques?

8   What is the benefit of the thumb/finger slide?

9   What technique is used to apply circular pressure to a specific reflex point?

10   What types of reflex points require the hook-in-back-up technique?

11   Which side of the brain is associated with logical thought?

12   Give three examples of how verbal communication may differ.

13   Give three examples of non-verbal communication.

14   What is empathy?

15   Why are verrucas and warts classified as being contraindicated to reflexology treatment?

16   What type of emotional release may someone experience post-reflexology?

17   What action does reflexology have on the general circulation of the body?

18   Is reflexology indicated for stress relief?

19   What type of foods should be avoided post-reflexology treatment?

20   Give an example of when reflexology may be used to help in the relief of pain.

Glossary

ACTH adrenocorticotrophic hormone

acupoint pressure points used in acupressure

acupressure ancient Chinese method of healing

acupuncture the Chinese practice of piercing specific areas of the body with fine needles for therapeutic purposes

acute used to describe a condition that is sudden, severe and short in duration

adenoids lymphatic tissue in the throat

adrenal glands endocrine glands situated above the kidneys

adrenalin hormone produced by the adrenal glands in response to stress

affirmation positive words to 'voice' intent

aldosterone hormone produced in the adrenal glands controlling the levels of salts in the blood

allopathy a system of therapy based on the production of a condition incompatible with the condition being treated

alveoli tiny air sacs in the lungs where the interchange of gases takes place

anal canal final section of the large intestine

anatomy structure

androgens male hormones

andropause male menopause

anterior front

antibody defence against an antigen

antidiuretic hormone hormone produced in the pituitary gland to control water levels in the body

antigen harmful substance

antioxidants nutrients that counteract free radical attack e.g. vitamins A, C and E

anus final part of the large intestine

apical breathing shallow breathing

appendix lymphatic tissue in the digestive system

arteries blood vessels leading away from the heart

auditory canal internal portion of the ear

aural by ear

auricle earflap or pinna

autonomic nervous system sympathetic and parasympathetic nervous systems responsible for automatic functions

axon nerve fibres which carry impulses away from the cell body

balancing to bring about a state of equilibrium

beating a form of percussion massage

bile secretion of the liver which is stored in the gall bladder

bladder organ that stores urine

blood pressure pumping action of the heart

body systems groups of associated organs and glands that have a common function

bone marrow red bone marrow is found in cancellous bone and is responsible for the formation of new blood cells. Yellow bone marrow is made up of fat cells and is stored in the length of some compact bone

bronchi air passageways leading into the lungs

bronchioles small air passageways in the lungs

caecum start of the large intestine

calcitonin hormone produced in the thyroid gland

cancellous bone spongy bone tissue

capillaries single cell structures at the end of blood and lymph vessels

carbohydrates energy-producing foods

carbon dioxide gas produced in the cells as a result of using oxygen

cardiac muscular tissue muscle tissue exclusive to the heart

cardiac sphincter ring of muscle between the oesophagus and the stomach

carpals bones of the wrist

cartilage connective tissue providing additional support for the skeletal system

cartilaginous joints slightly moveable joints

case history details gained during a consultation relating to personal, medical, physical, emotional and lifestyle factors

catabolism chemical reaction within a cell that causes the break down of nutrients into the smallest possible form for energy production

cell microscopic part of an organ

central nervous system the brain and spinal cord

cerebral hemispheres left and right halves of the brain

cerebrum the forebrain

cerumen earwax

cervical vertebrae the seven bones of the spine forming the neck

chakras energy centres

chi traditional Chinese term for energy

chronic term used to describe a condition which is long in duration

chyme broken-down food in the stomach

cilia tiny hairs attached to a cell

circulatory systems transport systems for blood and lymph

clavicle collar bone

coccyx the four fused bones of the spine forming the tail bone

code of ethics a specific set of rules laid down by a regulatory body

collagen protein found in connective tissue e.g. skin, bones

colon large intestine

communication a means to convey a message

compact bone hard bone tissue

conception vessel controlling vessel of yin meridians

connective tissue groups of cells forming a protective and supportive tissue

consultation establishing whether or not a client is suitable for treatment. A consultation forms a continuous and progressive part of the massage treatment

contra action an adverse reaction to a treatment, 'a disturbance of state'

contraindication a condition which could be made worse by treatment or be a possible cause of cross infection

cortisol mineralocorticoid produced in the adrenal glands

COSHH Control of Substances Hazardous to Health Regulations 1999

counselling a way of conveying a message in a helpful manner

cranial nerves twelve pairs of nerves leading from the brain to all parts of the face

cranium the head

cupping a form of percussion massage

dehydration lack of moisture

dendrite nerve fibre which pass impulses to the cell body

deoxygenated lacking in oxygen

dermatomes segmented regions of the body each of which are supplied with a nerve

dermis layer of connective tissue below the epidermis of the skin

diaphragm muscle separating the abdomen and the thorax

diaphragmatic breathing deep breathing

digestive system responsible for the intake of nutrients and the release of waste

distal the point furthest away from an attachment

diuretic a substance that increases urine production

DNA deoxyribonucleic acid

dorsal back or posterior surface

ducts tubes

duodenum first part of the small intestine

effleurage soothing, surface massage movements

embryo early stages of a fertilised ovum

empathy understanding another person's feelings

endocrine system responsible for controlling the body through chemical messengers in the form of hormones secreted by endocrine glands

epidermis top layer of skin

epithelial tissue groups of cells forming layers of protective tissue

eustachian tube connecting the middle ear with the nasopharynx

excretion the process of eliminating waste from the body

exhalation breathing out

exocrine glands glands lined with epithelial tissue that secrete substance through a duct to another part of the body

faeces waste product of the digestive system

fallopian tubes passageway leading from the ovaries to the uterus

fats foods that provide the body with a source of energy

fertilisation the impregnation of an ovum by a sperm

fibre food which is indigestible and is needed to aid elimination of waste from the digestive system

fibrous joints fixed joints without movement

foetus developing baby

follicle stimulating hormone hormone produced in the pituitary gland which has an effect on the gonads

free radicals the toxic by-product of energy metabolism

friction a form of petrissage massage

FSH follicle stimulating hormone

gall bladder accessory organ of the digestive system. Stores bile to aid digestion

GAS general adaptive syndrome

genitalia reproductive organs

genito-urinary system the male and female genitalia responsible for reproduction and the urinary organs responsible for helping to maintain the body's fluid balance

gland a structure lined with epithelial tissue which secretes a substance

glucagon hormone produced in the pancreas; it helps control blood sugar levels

glucocorticoids hormones produced by the outer cortex of the adrenal glands

gonadocorticoids hormones produced by the outer cortex of the adrenal glands

gonads reproductive organs

governing vessel controlling vessel of yang meridians

growth hormone hormone produced in the pituitary gland

hacking a form of percussion massage

haemoglobin substance that allows the blood cells to carry oxygen and carbon dioxide

HASAWA Health and Safety at Work Act 1974

healing to make or become well

healing crisis extreme reaction, a 'turning point' or 'danger point' characterised by the body's need to 'get worse before getting better'

helix upper section of the ear flap

hepatic flexure bend in the large intestine

holding used at the start and finish of a massage treatment

holistic considering the complete person; the whole self; body, mind and spirit

homeopathy remedies that produce similar symptoms as the disease to be cured

homeostasis physiological stability

hook-in-back-up a pressure technique used in reflexology

hormones chemical messengers produced by endocrine glands

human energy field (HEF) energy surrounding living things

human organism body systems function together to form a living human being

hypersecretion over-secretion

hyposecretion under-secretion

hypodermis layer of fatty tissue lying directly below the dermis of the skin

IBS irritable bowel syndrome

ileocaecal sphincter ring of muscle at the end of the ileum

ileum final part of the large intestine

immune system responsible for protecting the body against disease

infectious a condition that can be passed from person to person

inflammation a localised protective response

inhalation breathing in

insulin hormone produced in the pancreas which helps to regulate blood sugar levels

integumentary system consisting of the skin, hair and nails

Islets of Langerhans endocrine section of the pancreas

jargon technical terms relating to treatment. Questions directed at the client should be jargon-free

jejunum middle section of the small intestine

joint the point at which two or more bones meet

joint manipulation a type of massage

ki traditional Japanese term for energy

kidneys two bean-shaped organs that produce urine

kneading a form of petrissage massage

knuckling a form of petrissage massage

lacteals lymphatic capillaries in the small intestine

larynx upper throat

lateral away from the midline

lateral longitudinal arch arch running along the outside edges of the feet

left brain left cerebral hemisphere of the brain associated with analytical functions and logical thinking. Controls the right side of the body

legislation a general set of rules laid down by a government department

leucocytes white blood cells

LH luteinising hormone

lifestyle details relating to work, leisure, diet and exercise. Information gained during a consultation

ligaments attach bone to bone at a joint

liver largest organ of the body

longitudinal lengthways

lumbar vertebrae the five bones of the spine forming the lower back

lungs organs of respiration

luteinising hormone hormone produced in the pituitary gland affecting the gonads

lymph straw-coloured fluid

lymphatic tissue connective tissue which forms lymph nodes

lymphocytes white blood cells that produce an antibody against an antigen

master gland pituitary gland

massage the process of touching, feeling and/or kneading a part of the body

masseur a male practitioner of massage

masseuse a female practitioner of massage

medial towards the midline

medial longitudinal arch arch running along the inside edges of the feet

meiosis a process of cell reproduction to create a new organism

melanin the natural colour pigment

melanocyte stimulating hormone hormone produced by the pituitary gland affecting the production of melanin in the skin

menopause the cessation of the female menstrual cycle

menstruation the release of an unfertilised ovum from the uterus

meridians energy channels

metabolism a chemical process within the cells

metacarpals bones of the hand

metatarsals bones of the feet

midline the centre line of the body

mineralocorticoids hormones produced in the adrenal glands

minerals food that provides the body with the nutrients needed to perform its functions

mitosis simple cell division

motor nerves receive messages from the central nervous system

mucus fluid formed by goblet cells

muscular system muscles of the body responsible for voluntary and involuntary movement

muscular tissue cardiac, visceral and skeletal tissue responsible for movement

neuron nerve cell

nervous system central, peripheral and autonomic nervous systems responsible for controlling the body with electrical impulses

nervous tissue groups of neurons and neuroglia forming the nervous system

non-verbal communication the use of the body to convey a message

noradrenalin hormone/neurotransmitter produced in the adrenal glands in response to stress

oedema swelling caused by excess fluid in the tissues

oestrogen female hormone produced in the ovaries

olfactory sense of smell

open questions questions that require more than a one word answer

oral spoken

organ a structure that is made up of two or more tissue types and has specific form and function

organism the sum of cells, tissues, organs and body systems

ova eggs

ovum single egg

oxygen vital gas breathed into the body from the air

oxygenated rich in oxygen

oxytocin hormone produced in the pituitary gland affecting the reproductive organs

palpation the examination of a part by touch or pressure of the hand

pancreas accessory organ of digestion. Also has endocrine functions

parathormone hormone produced in the parathyroid glands affecting mineral levels in the blood

parathyroid glands endocrine glands located in the neck along with the thyroid glands

pelvic girdle part of the appendicular skeletal system forming the hip joint with the legs

perceptive obtain knowledge through use of the senses

percussion a brisk, stimulating form of massage

peripheral nervous system 12 pairs of cranial nerves and 31 pairs of spinal nerves

peristalsis involuntary muscular action

petrissage deep massage movements

Peyer's patches lymphatic tissue in the small intestine

phalanges bones of the fingers and toes

pharynx back of the throat

picking up a form of petrissage massage

pineal gland endocrine gland situated in the brain

pinna ear flap or auricle

pituitary gland endocrine gland situated in the brain

pivot-on-a-point a pressure technique used in reflexology

plasma fluid part of blood

plexus network of nerves

pounding a form of percussion massage

practitioner a person who performs a skill

prana traditional Indian term for energy

progesterone female hormone produced in the ovaries

prolactin hormone produced in the pituitary gland affecting the gonads

prostate gland produces the fluid part of semen in males as part of the genito-urinary system

proteins food that provides the body with the nutrients for growth and repair

proximal closest point of an attachment

PRS Performing Rights Society

puberty the time when secondary sexual development starts to take place

pulse contraction and relaxation of the heart

pyloric sphincter ring of muscle between the stomach and the duodenum

rectum latter part of the large intestine

reflexes points on the feet, hands and/or ears that reflect organs of the body

respiratory system system responsible for breathing involving the intake of oxygen and release of carbon dioxide

RIDDOR Reporting of Injuries, Diseases and Dangerous Occurrences Regulations 1995

right brain right cerebral hemisphere of the brain associated with systemic functions and creative thinking. Controls the left side of the body

rolling a form of petrissage massage

rotation a form of joint manipulation

RSI repetitive strain injury

safe stress high demands, low constraints, with high levels of support

sebum the skin's natural oil produced by the sebaceous glands in the skin

secretion a cellular process for releasing a substance

semen secretion from the testes, seminal vesicles and prostate gland containing sperm

seminal vesicles small sac-like structures responsible for secreting the fluid part of semen

sensory nerves carry impulses from the sensory organs to the central nervous system

sex corticoids hormones produced in the adrenal glands

shiatsu the Japanese practice of massage without needles

sinuses air spaces in the facial bones containing mucous lining

skeletal system bones and joints of the body

skull bones of the cranium and face

solar plexus network of nerves situated in the abdomen below the diaphragm

spinal nerves 31 pairs of nerves running from the spine to all parts of the body

spleen lymphatic tissue situated in the upper left side of the abdomen

splenic flexure bend in the large intestine

stress high demands, high constraints, with low levels of support

sweat watery substance produced by the sudoriferous glands in the skin

synovial joints freely moveable joints

systemic affecting the body as a whole

tactile sense of touch

tapotement a stimulating form of massage movement

tarsal bones bones of the ankle

tears watery substance produced by the lacrimal glands

tendons attach muscle to bone

testosterone male hormone produced in the testes

thorax the chest

thymosins hormones produced by the thymus gland

thymus gland endocrine gland situated behind the sternum

thyroid gland endocrine gland situated in the neck

thyroid stimulating hormone hormone produced in the pituitary gland affecting the thyroid gland

thyroxine hormone produced in the thyroid gland helping to regulate metabolism

tissue groups of cells with the same function

trachea windpipe

transverse running across

transverse arch arch running across the balls of the feet

triidothyronine hormone produced by the thyroid gland

tsubo specific points of the body where pressure is applied as part of a shiatsu treatment

universal energy field (UEF) energy flowing within the world around us

ureters tubes leading from the kidneys to the bladder

urethra tube leading out of the body from the bladder

urine water and waste produced in the kidneys

uterus womb

vagina passageway leading from the uterus to the outside of the female body

veins blood vessels that transport blood to the heart

verbal communication the use of the voice to convey a message

vertebrae bones of the spine

vibration a form of massage incorporating static/moving vibrations and shaking

visualisation the use of positive images and/or colour to bring about physiological changes in the body

vitamins food that provides the body with nutrients to maintain its vital functions

yang energy representing positive active polarity

yin energy representing negative inactive polarity

wringing a form of petrissage massage

zones longitudinal or transverse sections through which energy flows

zygote a complete cell that has been formed by the fusing together of a female egg and a male sperm

Index